Organ Transplants

Procurement, Procedures and Allocation Policies

snova
New York

Surgery - Procedures, Complications, and Results Series

Surgery for Crohn's Disease. Second Edition
Stephen M. Kavic, MD, FACS,
Rebecca Brown, MD, FACS, FSCRS
and Kerri Lopez, MD (Editors)
ISBN: 979-8-89530-676-5
eBook ISBN: 979-8-89530-739-7

Breast Aesthetic and Reconstructive Plastic Surgery
Ciro Comparetto and Franco Borruto
ISBN: 979-8-89530-212-5
eBook ISBN: 979-8-89530-257-6

A Closer Look at the Recurrent Laryngeal Nerve
Dr. Sachender Pal Singh
and Dr. Samiksha Singh (Editors)
ISBN: 979-8-89113-907-7
eBook ISBN: 979-8-89113-973-2

Ovarian Cancer: The "Gynaecological Challenge" from Diagnostic Work-Up to Cytoreduction and Chemotherapy. Volume 2
Christos Iavazzo, Alexandros Fotiou, MD
and John Spiliotis, PhD (Editors)
ISBN: 979-8-88697-644-1
eBook ISBN: 979-8-89113-370-9

Digital Implant Planning and Guided Implant Surgery
Niveditha S. Prasad, MDS,
Sheejith Madapathi, MDS,
Sarath Raj, DMRD, DNB
and Nivea T. Francis, MDS
ISBN: 979-8-89113-324-2
eBook ISBN: 979-8-89113-375-4

Ovarian Cancer: The "Gynaecological Challenge" from Diagnostic Work-Up to Cytoreduction and Chemotherapy. Volume 1
Christos Iavazzo, Alexandros Fotiou, MD
and John Spiliotis, PhD (Editors)
ISBN: 979-8-88697-633-5
eBook ISBN: 979-8-89113-034-0

Diabetic Foot – A Vascular Surgeon's Perspective
Martina Zavacká, PhD (Editor)
ISBN: 979-8-89113-019-7
eBook ISBN: 979-8-89113-065-4

Nosocomial Infection in Abdominal Surgery
Andrés García Marín, MD, PhD
and Jaime Ruiz-Tovar, MD, PhD (Editors)
ISBN: 978-1-68507-603-0
eBook ISBN: 978-1-68507-666-5

More information about this series can be found at
https://novapublishers.com/product-category/series/surgery-procedures-complications-and-results/

Nathalie B. Larson
Editor

Organ Transplants

Procurement, Procedures and Allocation Policies

snova
New York

Library of Congress Cataloging-in-Publication Data

ISBN: 979-8-89530-729-8 (Hardcover)
ISBN: 979-8-89530-824-0 (eBook)

Published by Nova Science Publishers, Inc. † New York

Contents

Preface

In 1984, legislation created the first computerized system for matching sick patients with the organs they need. It was called the Organ Procurement and Transplantation Network. The group that oversees and coordinates the network is the United Network for Organ Sharing (UNOS), which has nearly 400 members, including 252 transplant centers and 57 regional organizations known as organ procurement organizations (OPOs). Each OPO has a defined geographic service area. Serious errors in the procurement and transplantation system are shockingly common. Between 2010 and 2020, more than 1,100 complaints were filed by patients and families, staff and transplant centers. These errors have cost lives; approximately 6,000 Americans die each year while waiting for an organ transplant.

Chapter 1

A System in Need of Repair: Addressing Organizational Failures of the U.S.'s Organ Procurement and Transplantation Network*

Committee on Finance

Wednesday, August 3, 2022
U.S. Senate, Committee on Finance,
Washington, DC.

The hearing was convened, pursuant to notice, at 2:30 p.m., in Room SD–215, Dirksen Senate Office Building, Hon. Ron Wyden (chairman of the committee) presiding.

Present: Senators Cardin, Brown, Casey, Cortez Masto, Warren, Grassley, Thune, Portman, Cassidy, Young, and Barrasso.

Also present: Democratic staff: Melissa Dickerson, Investigator; Daniel Goshorn, Chief Investigative Counsel; Joshua Sheinkman, Staff Director; and Ryder Tobin, Investigative Counsel. Republican staff: John O'Hara, Republican Trade Policy Director and Counsel; and Caitlin Soto, Senate Committee on the Judiciary Oversight Counsel for Senator Grassley.

Opening Statement of Hon. Ron Wyden, A U.S. Senator from Oregon, Chairman, Committee on Finance

The CHAIRMAN. The Finance Committee will come to order.

The last place anybody wants to hear about gross mismanagement and incompetence is in the business of saving lives. That's precisely and unfortunately what the Finance Committee meets to discuss today. This morning's hearing is an update on an investigation Senator Grassley and I, along with Senator Cardin and Senator Young, have been conducting for more than 21⁄2 years. It examines the network of dozens of organizations that manage organ transplants, and particularly the group that oversees and coordinates them, the United Network for Organ Sharing, or UNOS.

---

* This is an edited, reformatted and augmented version of Hearing Before the Committee on Finance United States Senate, Publication No. S. HRG., 117–878., dated August 3, 2022.

In: Organ Transplants: Procurement, Procedures and Allocation Policies
Editor: Nathalie B. Larson
ISBN: 979-8-89530-729-8

We have reviewed 100,000 UNOS documents totaling more than a half-million pages. Before I get to specific findings, I want to frame what we have learned as simply as possible.

Far too many Americans are dying needlessly because UNOS and many of the transplant organizations it oversees are failing and seem uninterested in improving. These issues involve an alphabet soup of acronyms and organizations, so I will start out with a bit of background. A 1984 law created the first computerized system to match sick patients with the organs they need. It was named the Organ Procurement and Transplantation Network.

Someone needed to manage that system for the whole country, so the government sought to contract an organization to run it. UNOS was the only bidder for that first contract in 1986. The contract has come up for bid seven other times. UNOS has won all seven.

Today, the network UNOS oversees is made up of nearly 400 members, including 252 transplant centers and 57 regional organizations known as organ procurement organizations, or OPOs. Each OPO has a defined geographic service network. A family sitting in a hospital room thinking about donating a loved one's organ does not have a choice of OPOs.

Those are the important terms to remember here. When a kidney donated in Corvallis needs to get to a patient in Portland, that is where an OPO comes in. UNOS oversees the OPOs. As our investigation shows, UNOS does this job quite poorly.

Serious errors in the procurement and transplant system are shockingly common. Between 2010 and 2020, more than 1,100 complaints were filed by patients and families, staff, transplant centers, and others. The nature of these complaints runs the gamut. For example, in a number of cases OPOs had failed to complete critical, mandatory tests for matters like blood types, diseases, and infection.

Our investigation found one patient died after being transplanted with lungs that a South Carolina OPO marked with the wrong blood type. Similar blood-type errors happened elsewhere, and patients developed serious illness. Some had to have organs removed after transplant. Another patient was told he would likely die within 3 years after an OPO in Ohio supplied him with a heart from a donor who had died of a malignant brain tumor. UNOS did not pursue any disciplinary action. In a case from Florida, another patient contracted cancer from transplanted organs, and the OPO sat on the evidence for months.

In total, our investigation found that between 2008 and 2015, 249 transplant recipients developed a disease from transplanted organs. More than a quarter of them died.

Delivering organs has been another source of life-threatening errors. We found 53 such complaints between 2010 and 2020, as well as evidence that this was just the tip of the iceberg. In some cases, couriers missed a flight. In others, the organs were abandoned at airports. Some organs were never picked up. Many of these failures resulted in organs being discarded.

It is reasonable to assume that many more errors are going unreported. Why? Because filing official complaints with UNOS appears to accomplish zero productive oversight or reform. Organ transplant professionals repeatedly told the Finance Committee that the UNOS complaint process was—and I quote here — "a black hole." Complaints went in, UNOS went quiet.

In interviews with the committee, UNOS leaders have dragged their feet, dodged tough questions, and shifted responsibility onto others. Investigations and disciplinary measures rarely amount to much more than a slap on the wrist. Only one time—just once— has UNOS recommended that an OPO lose their certification.

The bottom line is that the failures we uncovered cost lives. Thousands of organs donated each year wind up discarded, including one in four kidneys. Yet according to Federal data, roughly 6,000 Americans die every year while waiting for an organ transplant. This kind of mismanagement has a disproportionate impact on minority Americans. African Americans, for example, have a greater need for kidney transplants than other demographic groups.

The Centers for Medicare and Medicaid Services recently issued new standards for OPO performance, and more than a third of OPOs are failing to meet them. Fixing what's broken could substantially increase the supply of lifesaving organs available for transplant.

Finally, another area of the committee's investigation has examined the IT, the information technology, used by UNOS to run the transplant network. This system is outdated, mismanaged, and insecure. Using such decrepit technology to run the transplant network puts lives in danger and puts sensitive data at risk, and apparently there is no solution in sight.

In a report issued last year titled "Lives Are at Stake," the U.S. Digital Service flatly concluded that UNOS does not have the technical capability to modernize the system.

I am going to close like this: if you looked at the staff at UNOS and many of the Nation's OPOs, I would wager the vast majority are hardworking, good people doing their best to save lives. The glaring issues uncovered in our investigation stem from failures at the top—leadership failures. Our investigation is ongoing. It's clear the system needs reform badly. We are going to keep digging into issues at UNOS and the OPOs, as well as the policies that need changing at the Federal level. This is not a partisan subject. Everybody wants the system to work with as few errors as possible.

We have been conducting a bipartisan investigation on this for some time. I want to commend Senators Grassley, Cardin, and Young. The three of them have been working very closely with us. This is a thoroughly bipartisan inquiry. I want to thank Senator Cardin, who is here, Senator Grassley who is here. I also see Senator Thune here. So, we are going to have a lot of members interested in this. I see Senator Warren as well.

And I want to thank our witness panel for joining the committee today.

[The prepared statement of Chairman Wyden appears in the appendix.]

The CHAIRMAN. Senator Grassley?

Opening Statement of Hon. Chuck Grassley, a U.S. Senator from Iowa

Senator GRASSLEY. Yes, thank you, Mr. Chairman. Today we want to talk about the U.S. Organ Procurement and Transplantation Network and its government contractor overseeing this program, the United Network for Organ Sharing.

In 1984, Congress passed the National Organ Transplant Act, a bill cosponsored by the late Senator Orrin Hatch, a friend of mine and former chairman of this committee. A few years later in 1998, the Federal Government contracted with the United Network for Organ Sharing to oversee the transplantation network.

The network performs three critical functions on behalf of the Federal Government: policymaking, technology delivery, and oversight of member compliance with its policies and with its procedures. However, for more than a decade now, government watchdogs and the media have questioned the adequacy of the network's oversight. That is because of multiple reports of fraud, waste, and abuse; criminality; deadly patient safety; and failure to recover organs.

Some have even observed that the network is 15 times more likely to lose, damage, or mishandle an organ in transit than a passenger airline is to lose its luggage. I have written about all these issues and more, going way back to 2005.

Sadly, the Federal Government has only recently begun to take action. As a result, thousands of organs go to waste each year, resulting in lives lost and billions of dollars wasted. This system is even worse for people of color and rural residents, who are less likely to get on the wait list, and less likely to find a match. At least among themselves, the network's senior leadership admits these facts.

One official's response to these concerns was to suggest rural Americans were dumb and should be just moved somewhere else to obtain lifesaving treatment. And of course, that attitude is totally unacceptable.

Now a bit more about the investigation into the network. In February of 2020, this committee sent a letter to the network requesting information and data on its oversight of the transplantation organization. We found that there is a huge variability in how well organ procurement organizations, known as OPOs, are serving their communities. In fact, according to the Centers for Medicare and Medicaid Services, as many as 22 of the 57 OPOs are failing outcome and performance metrics. This variability has negative consequences for the transplantation network and causes transplant hospitals to have fewer organs for patients on the wait list. We also found that the network has a broken governance system that fails to hold its members accountable for reoccurring patient safety issues. Now as I said, once again when I started looking into this way back in 2006, the network acts like, quote, "the fox guarding the chicken house," end of quote, instead of a trustworthy and independent oversight body that holds its members accountable. As such, transportation failures, ABO blood type testing, and allocation errors are common occurrences at underperforming OPOs.

So, Mr. Chairman, it is about time, and very timely that we hold this hearing. Congress has waited too long to fix a broken system. We must insist upon accountability moving forward. Patients' lives are at stake.

Thank you.

The CHAIRMAN. Thank you very much, Senator Grassley. As I noted in my opening statement, I am very glad that we have Senator Young here as well. Senator Young, Senator Grassley, Senator Cardin, and I have been at this for some time, and this has been thoroughly bipartisan.

The committee has made a number of important findings during this bipartisan inquiry. We believe it is in the public's best interest to see these results.

Therefore, I ask unanimous consent to enter the committee's hearing memo and all supporting documents related to that memo into the record.

[The documents have been posted to the committee's website.]

The CHAIRMAN. Let me now introduce our guests. We are pleased that they are here. Mr. Shepard is the chief executive officer of United Network for Organ Sharing. His organization currently holds the government contract for the Organ Procurement and Transplantation Network. He has been in this role since 2012. Prior to joining UNOS, he served for 15 years in various positions with the Virginia State Government.

Diane Brockmeier is here. She is the president and CEO of Mid-America Transplant, an organ procurement organization located in St. Louis, MO. A nurse by training, Ms. Brockmeier started her career at Mid-America as the organ procurement coordinator in 1986. In 2016, she became the president and CEO, overseeing the organization's operations, including partnerships with more than 120 hospitals and transplant centers located throughout Missouri, north-east Arkansas, and southern Illinois.

Mr. Barry Friedman is here. He is the executive director of the AdventHealth Transplant Institute in Orlando, FL. This is a position he has held since January of 2020. He began his civilian career in organ transplantation as an ICU staff nurse in St. Louis, MO in 1985 and has over 30 years of experience in the transplant community, including roles in leadership positions at transplant centers around the country. He has also had a distinguished military career.

Calvin Henry is the Region 3 representative on the OPTN Patient Affairs Committee. In 2012 he received a double lung transplant at Houston Medical Hospital after being diagnosed with an untreatable lung disease considered to be a terminal illness. Now a successful lung transplant recipient, he runs marathons. Mr. Henry has a professional background in health information. He also volunteers as a patient mentor for his local transplant center in Georgia to connect those on the wait list with education on financial resources. Mr. Henry asked that a letter from the Patient Affairs Committee urging immediate reforms in the transplant system be entered into the record. Before he begins his statement, I ask unanimous consent to do so.

And Dr. Jayme Locke is an abdominal transplant surgeon at the University of Alabama, Birmingham, where she is a professor and the chief of the Division of Transplantation, among other positions. A graduate of Duke University, she completed her medical degree at East Carolina University and her surgical residency at Johns Hopkins.

We want to thank all our guests for their participation, and we will begin with Mr. Brian Shepard.

Statement of Brian Shepard, Chief Executive Officer, United Network for Organ Sharing (UNOS), Richmond, VA

Mr. SHEPARD. Thank you, Mr. Chairman, members of the committee. Thank you for inviting me to discuss our Nation's organ donation and transplant system, the role of the United Network for Organ Sharing, or UNOS, and our community's ongoing efforts to increase transplantation.

My name is Brian Shepard. I am the CEO of UNOS, the mission-driven nonprofit which holds the Federal contract to serve as the U.S. organ donation and transplant network. In my role, I have seen up close the power of organ donation and transplants, lifting and sustaining the families of organ donors and restoring and inspiring transplant recipients.

Through NOTA, Congress intentionally put organ allocation policy in the hands of the clinical, professional, and patient community. UNOS works with transplant hospitals, OPOs, and patients to address the most important issues in donation and transplant, and we leverage experts in the fields of technology research and science to continually improve the national system.

We convene a community of diverse professionals and patients, sometimes with very strongly held opinions, and leverage that very diverse set of opinions into a system that provides the greatest possible benefit to patients awaiting transplants. In fact, all of the committed individuals on this panel with me have served on or even led at least one OPTN committee, and two of them have even served on the board of directors. And their opinions and insights have helped shape the system that we have today.

Today I look forward to having a conversation about that system, a system that just marked its ninth consecutive record-setting year of lifesaving transplants and surpassed 41,000 transplants in the year 2021, a total never before achieved in a single year by the United States or any other country in the world.

Transplantation on that scale would have been hard to imagine in 1984 when Congress passed the National Organ Transplant Act. The law established the OPTN to maintain a national registry for organ matching, and specified that that network would be a private, nonprofit entity. And it has been an honor to serve the Nation for over 3 decades. But we also realize that UNOS is not the final word in donation and transplant. We are part of a multifaceted system of improvement and oversight that includes multiple Federal agencies, including important roles for HRSA, CMS, CDC, FDA, and NIH.

Consistent with the Institute of Medicine recommendations and best practices in health-care quality, the OPTN's authorizing regulation creates a role of peer monitoring and quality improvement that complements but is very different from the regulatory certification and oversight role granted to CMS to support their role.

UNOS's work is bounded by NOTA, the OPTN final rule, and the OPTN contract, and focuses on three main areas: developing equitable allocation policies; maintaining the national wait list and offering matches to patients through safe, secure, and modern technology; and continuing to improve performance through peer review. All of our work is closely overseen by HRSA, who serve as members on all of our 19 committees and our national board of directors.

That is the community that UNOS is so proud to be a part of, a community dedicated to the equitable distribution of organs, no matter who you are or where you live. We have made rapid and remarkable changes in the past few years alone, changes that have expanded equitable access to transplants for candidates on the list; increased priority for the sickest patients; and reduced disparities between races, ethnicities, and geographies. But there is always more to do.

There are over 100,000 Americans waiting for an organ as we speak. Even as 115 patients are successfully transplanted every day, another 17 die waiting. We cannot rest until every patient who needs a transplant is able to get one.

By building on the successes of our national system and our community's ongoing efforts, we can come together around that vision. And when we do, our work literally saves lives. UNOS stands ready to work with any Senator on potential legislation, to provide information, or to serve as a resource.

Thank you again for inviting me to discuss the status of donation and transplant, and I look forward to taking your questions.

[The prepared statement of Mr. Shepard appears in the appendix.]

The CHAIRMAN. Thank you, Mr. Shepard. Ms. Brockmeier?

Statement of Diane Brockmeier, R.N., BSN, MHA, President and CEO, Mid-America Transplant, St. Louis, MO

Ms. BROCKMEIER. Chairman Wyden and members of the committee, my name is Diane Brockmeier, and I am the president and CEO of Mid-America Transplant, the organ procurement organization serving eastern Missouri, southern Illinois, and northeastern Arkansas. Thank you for the opportunity to speak today.

At our organization, we follow the ethos of "every donor, every time." Our team is committed to giving donors and their families the care they deserve, while stewarding their gifts to patients desperately in need.

Mid-America Transplant depends on the broader national transplant system administered by UNOS to accomplish this work. We need to urgently address patient safety. Each organ lost due to system or provider failure has a consequence to the thousands of patients waiting for a transplant. Furthermore, a discarded organ fails to honor the heroic gift from a selfless donor and compounds the family's sense of loss.

UNOS lacks urgency and accountability around identifying and remediating this preventable loss of organs, and they are not required to publicly report adverse events when patients are harmed, organs are lost, or the quality of patient care is deemed unsafe.

UNOS does not require clinical training, licensure, or certification standards for OPO staff delivering critical patient care. In this environment, who is looking out for the patient? Who is being held accountable for poor patient care? No OPO has ever actually been decertified, regardless of its performance or its safety record. UNOS has failed to align its efforts to ensure patient safety at the system level, and this decision has tragic and deadly consequences. We must update the archaic technology system at UNOS. As OPOs, we are required to work with UNOS's technology—DonorNet—every day. DonorNet is outdated, difficult to use, and often slow to function when every minute counts. Manual entry subjects it to error, and OPO and transplant center staff are not empowered with the right information when time is critical. I did serve in leadership roles on the OPO committee from 2017 to 2022. Committee members and industry leaders voiced repeated requests to improve DonorNet. The consistent response was: UNOS IT did not have the bandwidth to address this work.

The limitations of the UNOS technology are delaying and denying transplants to patients who are dying on the wait list. Poor technology impacts the disturbingly high kidney discard rate in the United States, where one in four kidneys never make it to a patient for transplantation.

Critical time is lost due to the inefficiency of DonorNet, wasting time on offers that will not be accepted. Of course, an available organ should be offered to the patient in list sequence. However, far too much of the matching, particularly on older donors and organs that are difficult to place, is left to the individual OPOs and transplant centers to find each other despite, rather than facilitated by, UNOS technology.

Mid-America Transplant intentionally identifies surgeons who accept kidneys that have been repeatedly turned down many times. These are lifesaving options for those patients.

In May of 2022, one of these patients was number 18,193 on the list. Relying on DonorNet alone, that kidney would never have been placed, and the chance to save a life would have been wasted. When an OPO goes out of sequence to place an organ that would otherwise be thrown away, UNOS requires an explanation. However, when organs are recovered and discarded, UNOS remains silent.

We must remove conflicts to ensure effective governance. From 2018 to 2020, I served as a board member for the OPTN. Serving on the board of the OPTN automatically assigns membership to the UNOS board. My board experience revealed that at times UNOS's actions are not aligned with its fundamental vision of a lifesaving transplant for everyone in need.

How can you fairly represent the country's interest and a contractor's interest at the same time? Board members are often kept in the dark about critical matters and are marginalized, particularly if they express views that differ from UNOS leadership.

Preparatory small group calls are conducted prior to board meetings to explore voting intentions. And if the board member was not aligned with the opinion of UNOS leadership, follow-up calls were initiated. Fellow board members reported feeling pressured to vote in accordance with UNOS leadership.

I implore the committee, along with CMS and HRSA, to ensure that those who speak out in support of system reform are not penalized. Patients deserve a transparent, accountable system that works on their behalf.

To protect patients, I urge Congress and the administration to separate the OPTN functions into different contracts so that patients can be served by best-in-class vendors; to immediately separate the boards of the OPTN and OPTN contractors; and to ensure that patients are safeguarded through open data from both the OPTN and OPOs. Your immediate action on this matter will save lives.

[The prepared statement of Ms. Brockmeier appears in the appendix.]

The CHAIRMAN. Thank you very much, Ms. Brockmeier. Next will be Mr. Barry Friedman.

Statement of Barry S. Friedman, R.N., BSN, Executive Director, Adventhealth Transplant Institute, Orlando, FL

Mr. FRIEDMAN. Chairman Wyden, Ranking Member Crapo, Senator Grassley, and members of the committee, on behalf of AdventHealth, I am honored to provide testimony on the current state of organ transplant policy in the United States. My testimony reflects 30 years of health-care and transplant experience and my direct leadership involvement in the United Network for Organ Sharing, and the Organ Procurement Transplantation Network.

I currently serve as the executive director of the AdventHealth Transplant Institute, one of the busiest centers in the United States, having performed nearly 5,000 transplants. I take very seriously our sacred duty to the families and patients who entrust us with the gift of life to provide for organ transplants.

It is our duty to be good stewards of these organs, honoring the faith of these families and the health of our communities. Families in need of lifesaving organs have no other option but to trust the organ transplantation system that is in place. This system has failed many patients waiting for organ transplants, due to the lack of oversight and accountability. Approximately 23 percent of kidneys procured from deceased donors are not used and instead discarded, resulting in preventable deaths.

It is our responsibility to address this issue. Organ transportation is a process left to federally designated organ procurement organizations, OPOs. Currently, they develop their own relationships with carriers, rely on airlines, charter flights, ground transportation, and Federal agencies to facilitate transportation. In many cases, organs must connect from one flight to another, leaving airline personnel responsible for transfers. While anyone can track their Amazon or FedEx package, there is currently no consistent way of tracking these lifesaving organs.

The transplant community promoted the use of GPS tracking of organ shipments, and UNOS piloted an organ tracking system. This system was not dependable, therefore we opted out and now are working with a company that uses less-expensive, higher-quality trackers and can monitor shipments in real time.

Currently there is no requirement for OPOs to use tracking systems. Data availability and transparency are key to improving organ procurement, and UNOS has not proven capable of providing this function.

OPTN technology has significant interoperability challenges and lags behind other technology platforms. This contributes to a fractured flow of information between OPOs, donor hospitals, and transplant programs. I also believe there is a conflict of interest related to the management of IT functions by UNOS, as the IT tools they offer transplant centers come with additional costs, despite them being essential for the safety and management of organs.

UNOS is not effectively screening organ donors so that they can be quickly directed to transplant programs. UNOS asks centers to voluntarily opt out of certain organs via a filtering process. As a result, OPOs waste valuable time making organ offers to centers that will never accept them.

Time wasted equates to prolonged cold ischemic time and organs not placed, resulting in lost organ transplant opportunities. This creates a vicious cycle that disadvantages patients on the wait list. Due to the limited expertise that UNOS has in the placement of organs, it would be best if they were no longer responsible for the development of organ placement practices.

The UNOS policymaking process lacks transparency. Currently OPTN board members concurrently serve as the board members of UNOS, which creates a conflict of interest that contributes to this lack of transparency. UNOS committees are formed in a vacuum. There is no call for nominations, and no data shared with the transplant community to explain the rationale behind decisions that create policy change.

A perfect example of this was seen recently during the kidney allocation change in policy where a geography committee was formed. This committee that was created, created an inequitable distribution of organs. The committee was instrumental in creating this policy, which resulted in a high kidney discard rate, which also caused increased cost and challenges with transportation.

Most importantly in this equation, we are jeopardizing the trust of our most precious resource—organ donors and their families, and the recipients of those who receive these organs.

The challenges that I have detailed to you are fixable, and we need to reempower the UNOS membership and increase patient advocacy representation within the policymaking process. We can implement interoperable technology, increase transparency, adopt real-time GPS tracking of organs, improve organ offers with the placement of friendly strategies, and reduce organ discard rates.

We applaud the Senate Finance Committee for listening and learning today and thank you for providing the United States of America the opportunity to maintain the stellar clinical care for patients who require lifesaving organ transplants.

[The prepared statement of Mr. Friedman appears in the appendix.]

The CHAIRMAN. Thank you very much, Mr. Friedman.

Next, we are going to have Mr. Calvin Henry, who I believe is going to be testifying virtually. Mr. Henry, are you out there in cyberspace?

Mr. HENRY. I am.

The CHAIRMAN. Wonderful. We would like to hear from you.

Statement of Calvin Henry, Region 3 Patient Affairs Committee (PAC) Representative, Organ Procurement and Transplantation Network (OPTN), Dacula, GA

Mr. HENRY. Good afternoon, Chairman Wyden, Ranking Member Crapo, and members of the committee. My name is Calvin Henry, and I serve on the OPTN Patient Affairs Committee, the Region 3 representative for the southeastern United States and the U.S. territories of the Virgin Islands and Puerto Rico.

I am also a double-lung transplant recipient of 9½ years. I have spent much of that time as a dedicated patient advocate, in direct support of transplant candidates and recipients, organ donation, and as a strong proponent for system-wide improvements and transparency throughout the organ procurement and transplantation process.

It is a privilege to be invited here today to share my thoughts regarding the current state of this system. Let me share my experience navigating the transplant system.

Fifteen years ago, I was diagnosed with a terminal lung disease that was later identified as scleroderma and informed that my only option for survival was to receive a double-lung transplant. I was told, however, that I was unlikely to receive one, and that I should just begin making end-of-life preparations.

The next several years after that diagnosis were perilous. On three separate occasions, I nearly lost my life due to the adverse effects of the disease. I was also diagnosed with achalasia, a serious and disqualifying disorder for transplant. The rejection I received from that program launched an arduous solo effort, without the assistance of any organization, to locate another program that would take me on as a patient.

The specific circumstances of my own experiences may be unique, but the constant difficulties in accessing transplant services are all too common. I was fortunate because I had the means, including access to good insurance, that allowed me to travel to another State to receive care.

That is not always the case. I want to highlight the disparities and inequitable access to transplant services that disproportionately harm Black people and people to color who do not have the resources to access transplants in these circumstances.

This committee has previously highlighted that the organ donation system's failures are an urgent health equity issue. Across the board, the numbers for kidney failure for Hispanic Americans, Black Americans, and Native Americans are far worse than White Americans.

We also know that Black people and people of color are less likely to receive transplants. Research has also documented that often Black families receive differential treatment from OPOs. As former Surgeon General Dr. Ken Moritsugu noted: "Often, misallocation of OPO resources found that OPOs do not respond to all donation cases, or do not properly train and support their front-line staff." The impact of this, he said, unsurprisingly falls disproportionately on families of color. The donor study showed the U.S. may be recovering as few as 28,000 organs each year. According to the chief of transplant at Vanderbilt, who testified at the House Oversight hearing last year, if the system were fully functioning, there would be no waiting list for livers, hearts, or lungs within 3 years, and the kidney wait list would be dramatically reduced.

The leaders, and several of my colleagues on the OPTN Patient Affairs Committee, asked me to submit a letter, included in my full written testimony. I have joined them. Among the messages to you: antiquated technology and an apathetic culture cause patients to languish with incomplete and often incorrect information and leave people to die every day on the wait list.

OPTN PAC members have raised these points often with UNOS leadership and have seen our calls for reform ignored. We have been aghast at the absolute failure of UNOS to operate the practice and business of transplant, and to acknowledge, much less effectively serve, patients who are waiting and dying on the organ wait list.

We ask that you ensure that the Federal Government makes the fast-approaching contracting OPTN cycle competitive for the first time since the original OPTN contract was awarded in 1986, and we implore you to ensure that UNOS does not hold patients hostage in the process.

Senators, I urge you all to act to ensure that we make better use of the organs that are donated, to ensure that health equity issues with Black people and people of color are addressed, and that the glaring technology issues causing patients harm are quickly remedied.

I thank you for your time.

[The prepared statement of Mr. Henry appears in the appendix.]

The CHAIRMAN. Mr. Henry, thank you very much, sir, for your participating. And also, colleagues, I want to note that he has asked that a letter from the Patient Affairs Committee urging immediate reforms in the transplant system be entered into the record. Mr. Henry and colleagues, that has been done. [The letter appears in the appendix on p. 66.]

The CHAIRMAN. Dr. Jayme Locke is next.

Statement of Jayme E. Locke, M.D., MPH, Director, Division of Transplantation Surgery, Heersink School of Medicine, University of Alabama, Birmingham, AL

Dr. LOCKE. Chairman Wyden and members of the committee, my name is Dr. Jayme Locke, and I am the director of the Division of Transplantation Surgery at the University of Alabama at Birmingham.

At UAB we currently have 1,022 patients wait-listed for kidneys. The majority self-identified as African Americans or Blacks. Transplantation was always supposed to be about the patient, but the system we operate now has almost a complete lack of ownership and responsibility, whether it is a failing OPO or UNOS failing at the most basic responsibilities of getting recovered organs matched and safely to their intended recipients.

These are the government's own contractors. My patients, your constituents, need your help. We know that thousands of kidneys are recovered and discarded every year, and that thousands more are never recovered at all. Discards have increased since the most recent allocation change, as the new system increased complexity, and to date, UNOS has shown no ability to manage even simple logistics.

The most powerful thing to know about this is that every organ represents a life. We can never forget that. Imagine having a medication you need to live being thrown away simply because someone took too long to get it to you—your life, quite literally, in a trash can.

Organs are no different. They too have shelf lives, and they are measured in hours. Discarded organs and transportation errors may sound abstract, but let me make this negligence real for you.

In 2014, I received a kidney that arrived frozen. It was hard as a rock, like an ice cube you could put in your drink. The intended recipient was sensitized, meaning difficult to match. The only thing we could do was tell the waiting patient that due to the lack of transportation safeguards, the kidney had to be thrown in the trash—the final generous act of a donor in Maryland.

In 2017, I received a kidney that arrived in a box that appeared to have tire marks on it. The box was squished, and the container inside had been ruptured. We were lucky and were able to salvage the kidney for transplant. But why should luck even play a role? Since the frozen kidney and the box with tire marks, I have received other kidneys that had to be discarded, either due to handling issues or UNOS transportation errors. But one week this May was particularly difficult. In one week, I received four kidneys from four different OPOs, each with basic errors that led to the need to throw away those lifesaving organs; one due to a botched kidney biopsy into the kidney's collecting system, another because of a lower artery that had been cut during procurement that could have been fixed if someone involved had assessed the kidney for damage and flushed it before packing. But that did not happen. Two others arrived to me blue, meaning they had not been flushed either.

Opacity at UNOS means that we have no idea how often basic mistakes happen across the country, nor can we have any confidence that anything is being done to redress such errors so they do not keep happening.

All I know is that in one week I received four kidneys, two from Tennessee, one from Florida, and one from Georgia, that could not be used. What was particularly heart-breaking was that two of these kidneys were for sensitized African American or Black women. Women who have been pregnant, especially multiple times, are harder to match, contributing to both gender and racial disparities in access to transplant.

This is a very real example of how a constrained pool of organs and high discards disproportionately hurt women and women of color, who are more likely to have multiple pregnancies.

I know others have spoken up, and more still who want to speak up, but, Senators, please know that every person I have talked to who has spoken up about system failures has told me they have been punished in some way, through both micro- and macro-aggression.

The very highest level of leadership within UNOS is an insular club that has turned its back on patients by ignoring their own unconscious biases, and even impugning patients behind closed doors. We need reform now. I am asking for your urgent help on behalf of my patients and all the other patients waiting around the country.

Number one, immediately separate the OPTN board from any of the boards of any contractors. Number two, bring in real experts to ensure our patients are served by the best of the best in each field, separating out key functions of the OPTN, including policy, technology, and logistics. And number three, ensure that patients are safer by holding all contractors accountable through event reporting and immediate redressing of problems.

One final and critical point. I cannot tell you how disturbing it was to read of the way UNOS has allegedly held the UNOS transplant system hostage. According to The Washington Post, quote, "UNOS also has at times even threatened to walk away and continue operating without a contract, despite the fact that it would be illegal," end quote.

Doing anything to jeopardize patients, even threatening to walk away, violates a basic principle of health care. It is called "patient abandonment." You simply cannot do that, or even threaten to do that. I would lose my medical license for walking away from a patient.

If it is true that UNOS has suggested that it might walk away or not cooperate with a transition to new contractors, that would make it an organization that cannot be responsible for taking care of lives. There is very little in health care that has the immediate life-and-death stakes of organ transplantation.

Please realize that every day that passes that these failing systems are in place, it means more of our neighbors will die. My patients need the Senate to act.

Thank you.

[The prepared statement of Dr. Locke appears in the appendix.]

The CHAIRMAN. Thank you all. And these are terrible accounts that you have just given us, Dr. Locke: the idea that kidneys arrive with tire marks; the reprisals against those who speak the truth about the inefficiencies and gaps in quality with respect to these services. I mean, this is really a wake-up call, and you have delivered it powerfully, and I thank you.

I will start with this question that a number of you have referred to: the issue of the recovered organs being discarded. And obviously, the purpose of the transplant network is to match organs with patients who need them.

Unfortunately, one in seven organs recovered by an organ procurement organization is not transplanted, at a rate, as far as I can tell, that is increasing and has been since 2018. For kidneys, the most needed organ, the situation is even worse. One in four recovered kidneys are discarded before transplant, a rate that is also increasing.

Now obviously, there are instances where an organ cannot be transplanted for legitimate medical reasons, but in the course of this Finance investigation, we discovered an endless number of cases of organs being discarded because of errors at the OPOs. In several cases, organs were discarded because they were delayed or lost on their way to a transplant center. In another case, a heart was discarded because an OPO had a policy disagreement with a hospital. And yet in another case, an OPO literally threw two kidneys in the trash—in the trash—immediately after recovering them.

So, Mr. Henry, let me start with you. We have over 90,000 people waiting for a kidney transplant in this country, yet one in four kidneys recovered are not being transplanted. So my question to you, Mr. Henry—you have been a patient advocate, and spoken eloquently today—how does this high discard rate, and the practices that are being documented and that you found, how does this affect the public's willingness to donate when they hear this?

Mr. HENRY. Well first, hearing about the, in my mind, inexcusable recovery rate, it is absolutely heartbreaking. And we talk about the fact that a little over 90,000 kidney candidates are on the waiting list, and 106,000 total organ recipients. As an advocate, I am asked to go out into the community, which I willingly do, because organ donors save lives.

So I willingly and eagerly advocate for organ donation. But when you hear about this high non-use rate, people think, "We are asked to donate, and the individuals, the OPOs and UNOS, who are in charge and are supposed to be stewards of ensuring efficient recovery, do not seem to be doing the job necessary."

So again, it is absolutely heartbreaking.

The CHAIRMAN. So, Mr. Shepard, we have this tremendous sacrifice by donors and families. You heard what Mr. Henry said: all the time and money and effort, and recovered organs are not being translated into patients who need them.

Is it acceptable that 25 percent of kidneys are being discarded? Is that okay with you?

Mr. SHEPARD. No, Senator, absolutely not.

The CHAIRMAN. So, it is not acceptable?

Mr. SHEPARD. We find that number to be entirely too high and think that every missed opportunity for transplant is a tragedy.

The CHAIRMAN. So why are they too high? And what are you doing about it?

Mr. SHEPARD. There are any number of reasons that an organ would not be used. There are a few that are specific operational events at OPOs, and I think your research and your review of the MPSC files shows that. I think a much larger number are simply deemed not viable for transplant by the centers that they are being offered to.

One of the things that UNOS is doing about it, we just adopted a new metric for our evaluation of transplant centers. This year we have adopted a metric to measure transplant centers on their organ acceptance rate. So, in the past we have measured them— and we still will—on their post-transplant success rate. How long did their patients last? How long did their grafts last? But now we will also be measuring transplant hospitals on whether or not they are accepting organs at an acceptable rate.

The CHAIRMAN. Ms. Brockmeier, do you think that is the heart of the problem? I mean, Mr. Shepard says the big problem is you have a high discard rate because the transplant centers are refusing organs for medical reasons. That seems pretty farfetched to me, but I would like your thoughts.

Ms. BROCKMEIER. Certainly, Senator, there are at times occurrences when we would discover that a potential donor might have cancer or something during the interoperative procedure. So those kidneys obviously could not be allocated for transplantation. So on occasion, yes, sir, that does happen.

But the cumbersomeness of the technology by which we can identify the best homes for those kidneys certainly complicates and, I think, compounds the discard rate.

The CHAIRMAN. That is, to me, the heart of the problem, that, yes, there are medical instances where it is warranted. You said that. I have said that. I think that is the consensus sentiment. But I think the heart of the problem is that the system does not work, and it is way too cumbersome and inefficient, and we have got to turn it around.

Senator Grassley?

Senator GRASSLEY. I would like to have any one or two of you who could answer this question to do it. You heard me in my opening comments refer to the fact that the system does not seem to be fair to racial minorities or people living in rural communities. So what are your efforts underway to understand the root causes and help make the system fairer to patients on the waiting lists? Explain the factors that result in the disparity for minorities and rural populations in the process, and how can the Federal Government address the problem if we have to be involved in addressing it?

Dr. LOCKE. One of the most important things that we do not currently do is, we do not actually account for disease burden in terms of examining our waiting list. So we have no way of knowing if we are actually serving the correct people, if the correct people are actually making it to the waiting list.

Disease burden is super important because it not only identifies the individuals who are in need of transplantation, but it also speaks to supply. So areas of high rates of end-stage kidney disease burden like the southeastern United States are going to have much lower supply. And they also are predominantly—those waiting lists predominantly consist of African American or Black individuals.

So, if you want to make a truly equitable organ system, you have to essentially get more organs to those areas with higher disease burdens.

I think the other thing is that we have to have more focus on how we approach donor families and make sure that we have cultural competence as a part of our OPOs in how they approach families to ensure that we are not marginalizing minority families with regard to the organ donation process.

Senator GRASSLEY. Mr. Shepard, UNOS has responsibility to conduct oversight of membership. There is little indication that your organization is capable of doing it. So if, in fact, this committee found that less than 40 percent of all patient safety cases are referred to the Membership and Professional Standards Committee— which is responsible for monitoring member compliance with the transplantation network's policies and procedures—how does UNOS staff determine what cases are referred to this committee? Mr. SHEPARD. Thank you, Senator. UNOS staff refers cases to the MPSC—that is the peer committee—and again, our statute and regulation require us to use peer review to do the quality improvement work that we do.

Our staff is approved by the peer committee. The peer committee has given them a set of guidance rules to say, these are the types of cases that we would like to see, these are the types of cases that, when you evaluate them, do not need to be referred to the committee.

Our staff do not make those judgments independently. All of those staff decisions as to whether a case meets the MPSC rubric for referral are referred in a group of the member quality staff, including the chief medical officer of UNOS.

Senator GRASSLEY. Well, with the committee's findings in mind, should your organization reevaluate its oversight efforts so that more cases are referred to the committee? And if you disagree with that, why not?

Mr. SHEPARD. I would say one of the things that our conversation with your staff has led us to understand is that the current committee may not be as aware of some of the past decisions that past committees have made in establishing those rubrics. So we have created a new process where, at the seating of each new MPSC committee, we go over that rubric so that each committee can endorse, amend, or otherwise alter the description of what types of cases they would like to see, and not simply rely on what a past committee has decided.

Senator GRASSLEY. Mr. Friedman, in 2021 the U.S. Digital Service found that UNOS cannot properly modernize its IT system and its core systems are fragile. This is concerning, especially since the organization is the only government contractor responsible for making transplants possible.

Can you give us an example of a time when UNOS's technology caused an adverse patient safety event? And generally, do you think AdventHealth is getting the best value with regard to the services offered by UNOS?

Mr. FRIEDMAN. Senator Grassley, I agree with you that the IT system is fractured. There are situations where organs are not offered in a timely manner. The IT system that UNOS currently utilizes does not easily allow transplant centers opportunities to turn down organs or ensure that the right organ is going to the right patient.

I also believe with IT technology, as I stated, monitoring organs and organ placement—when I was in the military, I did medical airlift. My crews out of Scott Air Force Base knew where I was, worldwide, with my patient.

I could not even get a kidney that was 20 miles away from my transplant center with UNOS thinking that it was in Miami, when it was actually in Orlando, 20 miles away. Lack of IT systems, lack of technology, has caused harm potentially to patients, or delayed patient treatment, or increased the cost of care for patients.

This is deplorable and needs to be fixed.

The CHAIRMAN. Thank you, Senator Grassley. Senator Cardin?

Senator CARDIN. Thank you, Mr. Chairman. And I thank you for your leadership on this issue, and I want to thank our witnesses today.

Our committee report verifies our fears that the system today is badly broken. And our witnesses today have reinforced that view. That is a tragedy that needs to be corrected.

Unless you have transparency, unless you have accountability, there is no way that you can correct a system. And if those who want to report a problem are retaliated against, it makes the matter much, much worse.

If we have to change the law to accomplish that, then we have to change the law to do that. I am hearing about numerous mistakes in harvesting and preparations and matching and transportation. But if you do not have timely knowledge of those errors, you cannot correct those errors. And from what I can tell, most of these errors are being hidden rather than acted upon and changed.

So you know, all of us are involved in buying products that are tracked, and we are amazed at how we can see where they are at every step of the process. The technology is widely utilized.

So, Mr. Shepard, let me just ask you about the technology that you are using. According to our reports, your system has crashed on several occasions. And when your system is down, you cannot do the match, so time is lost. We are seeing all these challenges. Is there a financial problem as to why you cannot update the technology? Is there a reason why we cannot get much better performance on vital organs being tracked or matched? What is the problem here?

Mr. SHEPARD. Senator, the OPTN IT system that UNOS operates has 99.99 percent up-time. It is a highly reliable system. We are audited annually by HRSA.

Senator CARDIN. My information is you have had 17 days down since, I think, 1999. That is not correct?

Mr. SHEPARD. In 23 years, yes, sir.

Senator CARDIN. Okay. Well, every day there is a loss of life, isn't it?

Mr. SHEPARD. That is the total amount of time over the——

Senator CARDIN. I hope our national defense system is not down 17 days a year.

Mr. SHEPARD. The system has never been down for a day, to my knowledge. And I have not been here since 1999, but to my knowledge there has been maybe one event that was longer than an hour, and that was 3 hours. But the total amount of time since 1999——

Senator CARDIN. So you are satisfied with your technology? You think you have the right technology? You are satisfied with your tracking systems now and you think everything is okay?

Mr. SHEPARD. We constantly improve our technology. We are subject to 3 million attempts a day to hack into the patient database, and we successfully repel them all. So we are never satisfied with our technology, but we do maintain 99.99 percent up-time. We disagree with the USDS analysis of our systems.

Senator CARDIN. I understand you may feel that you have restrictions by law that you cannot do certain things, but then you should try to change those laws if the system is not working right. What I do not understand is, I have heard so many examples here of mistakes that need to be corrected, whether they are surgical mistakes, whether they are testing mistakes, whether they are shipping mistakes or matching mistakes, and they are not being corrected.

Why are you not proactive in working with us if laws need to be changed so that we can get a higher efficiency on making these organs available?

Mr. SHEPARD. We would be happy to work with the committee and anyone who is interested in legislation that would improve the safety of the system.

We work directly in a peer review process with OPOs and transplant hospitals for any—either an incident, and many of our incidents, nearly half of our incidents that are reviewed by our peer committee, are self-reported.

Senator CARDIN. Self-reported is the way it should be. That is a good thing to have self-reporting.

Mr. SHEPARD. Yes.

Senator CARDIN. Dr. Locke, who retaliates against people who are making—you mentioned the intimidation factor about making reports. Can you just shed a little more light on that as to what is happening out there?

Dr. LOCKE. I personally have had people come up to me and make comments. We submitted—I signed a letter, along with the members of Region 3, related to some of the emails that were unsealed that disparaged our population in the southeastern United States. And I submitted that letter to UNOS, along with other colleagues from Region 3, and had two different board members approach me and suggest that I should not have done that, and that that was inappropriate. And so that makes it very challenging. That is just one example.

I have had other colleagues who feel that they have been blocked from being on committees and other things. And we have all been silenced at our region meetings on more than one occasion when we have spoken up about what we think is not appropriate.

We have been told "that's something that you can't vote on," that you can't present data, that only they control the data that can be presented. And certainly, we are members of the OPTN, and the purpose of those meetings is to be able to have representation and have dialogue about what we think is going well and what is not going well. And it is incredibly proscribed, and we are routinely silenced.

Senator CARDIN. Well, thank you for coming forward. I appreciate it.

Thank you, Mr. Chairman.

The CHAIRMAN. Thank you, Senator Cardin. And I also want to note this important question you asked, Senator Cardin, about all the mistakes that are taking place. As far as I can tell, there is a pretty serious operation for keeping them secret. The committee was forced to issue a subpoena to obtain information from UNOS on the number and nature of safety events that were reported to it.

So this whole question that Senator Cardin is talking about, about additional transparency in dealing with mistakes, I think is very much on point, and I thank my colleague for raising it.

Next in order of appearance will be Senator Portman.

Senator PORTMAN. Thank you, Mr. Chairman.

And, Mr. Shepard, I am going to follow on some of the questions that Senator Cardin raised. Twenty-eight hundred Ohioans are on the transplant waiting list right now; you probably know that. And according to the information obtained by the committee, nationally in a 7-year period at least 249 transplant recipients have developed diseases from infected organs, and at least 70 of these patients have died.

One of those troubling cases was in Ohio. The recipient came for a routine follow-up and was informed that he had accidentally received a transplant from a donor with cancer. Tragically, it was not on the initial report, and the recipient had a 3-week period when he did not even know. But the donor had a brain tumor, and that was on the pathology report that was not available, for some reason. So this recipient has now been told he is likely to die within 3 years.

There are four organ procurement organizations in Ohio, OPOs, and they all do lifesaving work, but we need to give them better tools to ensure that lives are not lost, and we do not have additional tragic situations like this one due to testing failures.

Can you tell us, Mr. Shepard, what more UNOS can do to ensure that these 2,800 Ohioans we talked about awaiting transplants do not receive infected organs?

Mr. SHEPARD. Yes, Senator; thank you. UNOS has created, in their operation of the OPTN, a Disease Transmission Advisory Committee, which also includes CDC. So, in addition to the peer review committee, which is studying the specific techniques, the specific operations that may need to be improved or changes that OPO or a transplant hospital might need to make in practice, the disease transmission committee actually reviews transmissions and ensures rapid communication between OPOs and all the recipient transplant hospitals. So, if one transplant hospital were to find that they had received an infected organ, there is a quick communication chain back through the rest of the organs that were recovered from that donor. And we continue—that committee routinely provides guidance, most recently offered on COVID. They offered quarterly guidance as new information came out about COVID.

Senator PORTMAN. You said earlier there is no regulation of these OPOs. Again, there are a lot of great ones that save lives every day, but others obviously fall short of the goal. So you are saying that there is a monitoring of this, and information provided, but there is no assurance that these best practices, as an example, would be followed, even on disease.

Is that true?

Mr. SHEPARD. If you are asking whether UNOS can prevent an OPO from operating, or from being an OPO, then the——

Senator PORTMAN. Not prevent them, but require them to do something. You do not have the ability to require them——

Mr. SHEPARD. The peer review process has significant persuasive authority, but all the payment authority and all the certification and decertification authority lives at CMS.

Senator PORTMAN. So you do not have the ability to require that they do things. A lot of suggestions have come out in the context of this report. It has been recommended by the University of California that we should automate data entry. They indicate that 85 percent of data entry is automated in other health-care records, and these should be automated. Right now, an individual is required to enter the data manually, which costs time and allows for error, human error. Do you agree with that?

Mr. SHEPARD. We absolutely agree that data entry should be automated. Sixty-five percent of UNOS's forms are available to be electronically filled out for APIs, and more than 200 transplant hospitals and OPOs are using electronic APIs now to automatically deliver data to UNOS.

Senator PORTMAN. Does OPTN require that?

Mr. SHEPARD. OPTN does not require them to use the API.

Senator PORTMAN. We also hear that upgrading technology at

OPTN will protect it from cyber-attacks that could be the difference between life and death for people. Do you have a response to that?

Mr. SHEPARD. I am sorry, Senator?

Senator PORTMAN. Do you believe you are protected from cyberattacks?

Mr. SHEPARD. We never are satisfied with our protection from cyberattacks, but we do know that we are attempted to be hacked into more than 3 million times a day and have not yet been successfully hacked, but we continue to upgrade those protections on a regular basis.

Senator PORTMAN. Do you think there should be tracking of organs in transit?

Mr. SHEPARD. I think that is a very beneficial thing. UNOS provides an optional service that a quarter of OPOs use. Many OPOs also use other commercially available trackers to do that. There is not a single requirement to use a particular system.

Senator PORTMAN. So the 21-percent discard rate, I understand, has a lot to do with the transporting of organs, and the lack of tracking is part of the problem. In one report, organs were 15 times more likely to be lost or damaged than your luggage when taken through an airport.

Could that be possible?

Mr. SHEPARD. I have not seen that number, and we will get you—I would certainly be surprised.

Senator PORTMAN. That is part of what came out of this report. You talked about the app that you are developing to offer transport options. Is this app fully operational?

Mr. SHEPARD. It has been fully utilized by our organ center and is in a pilot phase with several OPOs.

Senator PORTMAN. Is that something you are going to have beyond pilot soon, so people can get best practices on transit?

Mr. SHEPARD. Yes.

Senator PORTMAN. And how about manual entry? Do you have a plan to make the network safer for patients and protect from cyber- attacks by using more automation? Is there a plan to do that?

Mr. SHEPARD. Yes. We continue to expand the number of APIs that are available. That also depends on the OPOs and hospitals making the changes to their IT systems on the other end to communicate across that bridge.

Senator PORTMAN. I did not mean to leave you out [motioning to the other witnesses]. We will have some questions for the record for you all.

And again, I thank you for holding this hearing—more importantly, for this committee and its thorough report. Thank you, Mr. Chairman.

The CHAIRMAN. Thank you, Senator Portman. Next is Senator Warren.

Senator WARREN. Thank you, Mr. Chairman.

So, in the United States, when people need an organ transplant, their lives are in the hands of one Federal contractor that our government hires to run the entire national organ donation program. Today this system is run by UNOS, which first got its contract back in 1986. In fact, UNOS is the only entity that has ever been awarded, or even bid for this Federal contract.

Now UNOS is responsible for overseeing local organ procurement organizations, or OPOs. Because UNOS's oversight is so bad, some OPOs are disasters: testing errors, lost organs, never collecting healthy organs that could have been donated. And without competition, the organ transplant system overall has become a dangerous mess. Right now, UNOS is 15 times more likely to lose or damage an organ in transit as an airline is to lose or damage our luggage. That is a pretty terrible record.

Mr. Shepard, you are the CEO of UNOS, and we have documented these problems. And you have received more than 1,000 complaints in the last decade alone.

So tell me. In the 36 years that UNOS has had the contract to run our national organ system, how many times has UNOS declared its OPO members, any OPO members, not in good standing?

Mr. SHEPARD. Two times, Senator.

Senator WARREN. Two times. So that's it. Two times. UNOS has run the program for 3 decades, and in the past 10 years it has received over 1,000 complaints. At least 249 recipients have developed diseases from infected organs after a transplant; at least 70 people have died from those diseases. And you looked the other way when one of your members was part of an illegal kickback scheme that eventually sent an OPO executive to Federal prison. So 36 years, a list of deadly problems, a kickback scheme, and yet UNOS has only twice declared one of its members, quote, "not in good standing," a designation that is so toothless that it does not even require the OPO to pause its operations.

So let me get one other piece of data out here. Mr. Shepard, how many times has UNOS put an OPO on probation?

Mr. SHEPARD. I do not know right off the top of my head, but it is not a large number.

Senator WARREN. It is not large. In fact, it is three. Three times in 36 years. Look, this is not oversight. This is sitting on your hands while people die. And UNOS has been allowed to look the other way because it has never faced any competition.

Finally, HRSA, the Federal agency that awards your contract, is now heading into this contracting cycle that stakeholders have said must break up the monopoly for the first time ever. But faced with the prospect of accountability in the past, UNOS has demanded tens of millions of dollars to hand over the archaic technology sysem that it developed with taxpayer funding.

UNOS has even threatened to walk away and illegally continue to operate the organ transplant system without a contract.

So, Mr. Shepard, can you commit that UNOS will not in any way attempt to hijack the United States' transplant system during a transition to future contractors?

Mr. SHEPARD. UNOS would never make an attempt to take any actions regarding a transplant system that would harm patients. And in fact, the discussion that has come to light in the USDS report was our attempt to assure HRSA that, despite coming very close to the negotiating deadline, we would not turn the system off and walk away from patients, even if bureaucratic paperwork pushed us beyond——

Senator WARREN. So you are not going to walk away and turn the system off? You are also not going to demand millions of dollars for a system that was developed at taxpayer expense?

Mr. SHEPARD. The system has been paid for in part by taxpayers. Approximately 10 percent of the budget of this contract is taxpayer-funded. The rest of that is paid by hospitals when they list patients. The government has not, over the years, paid for the software.

Senator WARREN. So you are still planning to get millions of dollars for the system? That is what you want to do? Sell it back to the government, if you do not get this contract?

Mr. SHEPARD. The contract allows the government to purchase the software from——

Senator WARREN. At what price? I mean, we have obviously a monopoly on both sides here.

Tell you what: we will go into the pricing. I just want to be careful about my time.

I will just be clear. You should lose this contract. You should not be allowed anywhere near the organ transplant system in this country, and if you try to interfere with the process of turning the contract over to someone who could actually do the job, you should be held accountable for that.

There are a whole lot of reforms that are needed in the system, but this is a good place to start. Patients and families deserve better than they are getting right now from UNOS.

Thank you, Mr. Chairman.

The CHAIRMAN. That last sentence sums it up: patients and families deserve better.

Senator Young?

Senator YOUNG. For many years, I have taken an active, personal interest in the organ donation system. I had a very good friend I served with in the U.S. Marine Corps. His name was David McFarland. I have gotten to know his wife, Jennifer. We called him "Gunny McFarland." I reconnected with Gunny McFarland when I moved back to Indiana after service in the Marines, and he died waiting on a heart. And that was a really powerful experience for me.

So, when I was elected to the U.S. House of Representatives, I resolved to do whatever I could to bring more organs into the system. I came to find out there was seemingly very little I could do. I scrutinized an existing system that was highly opaque, and that really frustrated me. I think it is frustrating to a lot of Americans. In recent years, as some of my colleagues have indicated, there have been a number of complaints submitted to UNOS—1,118. Less than 40 percent of those were referred for additional review. Of that small number, only 1 case, 1 case out of 1,118 complaints, resulted in probation. It is either a very impressive record of success, or it is a very low record of probation.

My strong suspicion is that more of these complaints are indeed valid and should result in probation. Two of these complaints have led to a designation of a member being "not in good standing."

There have been multiple documented incidents of OPO poor performance, serious allegations ranging from illegal financial arrangements to testing failures resulting in patient deaths.

I am going to ask for a really short explanation. Maybe, Mr. Shepard, you can provide it. Please explain why UNOS very rarely uses the probation and member "not in good standing" ratings?

Mr. SHEPARD. Thanks, Senator. The reason would be that the primary tool for UNOS to promote improvement is the peer review process that is established in our regulation and in our contract. It calls for us to be the confidential coaching and best-practice arm, in contrast to the regulatory and financial oversight rules that CMS provides.

Senator YOUNG. Okay. And yet we still have a large gap between the need for organs and the number of organs that are brought forward. It does not seem like we are rewarding success. It does not seem like we are holding people accountable for falling short of success.

Once an OPO is designated "not in good standing"—Senator Warren referred to this; it is toothless. It does seem toothless to me. I will give you an opportunity, Mr. Shepard, to disabuse me of that notion, and indicate for me what penalties or sanctions are actually placed on an OPO when they are designated "not in good standing."

Mr. SHEPARD. The statute does not give UNOS any authority to offer sanctions like that. The certification, decertification, payment authorities belong entirely to CMS. The UNOS statute does not give us the ability——

Senator YOUNG. So it is toothless, in that sense?

Mr. SHEPARD. It is designed to be, by regulation and contract— it is designed to be a quality improvement process, in contrast to the oversight process operated by a Federal agency.

Senator YOUNG. Okay. What corrective actions must occur for the OPO to get back in good standing?

Mr. SHEPARD. It depends on the situation. A member not in good standing is generally in an environment where multiple things have gone wrong, where there seems to be not simply an incident. An organization that has a strong culture can recover from an incident. An organization that has more systemic issues is likely to be a member not in good standing.

Senator YOUNG. Is there a formal audit or a review process in place to ensure OPOs and other OPTN members are complying with appropriate rules and policies?

Mr. SHEPARD. Yes. A member not in good standing goes through monthly meetings with the MPSC peer committee for usually 2 or 3 years to come off of that standing. All OPOs and transplant centers are reviewed routinely.

Senator YOUNG. Okay.

On the topic of failing to perform like the American people would expect the system to perform, I would like to turn to reports of donor organs that are lost or delayed in transport, and an apparent lack of ability to solve or even improve this issue.

To what extent does UNOS currently track the status of all the organs in transit at any given time?

Mr. SHEPARD. UNOS does not coordinate transportation or track organs in transit. We do provide a service that OPOs can use to use GPS trackers. Some OPOs use ours, and some use other commercially available products.

Senator YOUNG. So why is it that—and how does UNOS plan to optimize organ delivery if you do not have a 100-percent visibility into where they are at any given time?

Mr. SHEPARD. I think that the GPS products that we offer, and that other people offer, are valuable. They do help in the delivery of kidneys—only kidneys travel unaccompanied. So this is a kidney issue. But I do think the GPS trackers are valuable, and I think that is why you have seen more OPOs using them.

Senator YOUNG. My son can order a pair of shoes, or a toy, and get a pretty good sense of where it is at a given period of time. This is lifesaving, of course, in so many instances. So it seems like that ought to be locked in.

So okay; well, we will continue—I know that the chairman and ranking member have made this a real priority, and my colleagues, many of them have been dialed into the importance of this issue for some time, and others are beginning to get energized and animated about it. And I am encouraged by that.

So we will keep fighting on behalf of our constituents. Thank you, Mr. Chairman.

The CHAIRMAN. We will. And thank you for your participation.

Before we go to Dr. Cassidy, just very quickly, colleagues, I want to make a point so that it is clear for the record.

Mr. Shepard has said twice, with respect to this whole question of the power to decertify an OPO, that CMS has the power to do it. UNOS also has the power to refer an OPO for decertification under the OPTN final rule. That has been done exactly once.

So I just wanted it understood with respect to making sure the committee knows what is really going on with respect to decertifying OPOs.

Dr. Cassidy?

Senator CASSIDY. Mr. Shepard, before I go on to some of the other stuff, I just would like to ask procedurally: according to committee staff, they have on multiple occasions sought documents relevant to the committee's inquiry, and you were not cooperative; that records were not given; that after the committee issued a subpoena to UNOS on February the 3rd, UNOS continued to withhold relevant information from the committee without asserting a recognized constitutional, Federal statutory, or Federal common law privilege, et cetera.

Finally, information was given with redactions. But these redactions were not of patients, it was not HIPAA-compliant. It was of senior OPO employees, time zones, addresses, and other contextual information.

Now first, why was UNOS refusing to respond to subpoenas? And why were you stonewalling and, by all accounts, hiding information from the committee?

Mr. SHEPARD. Thanks, Senator. We did not refuse the subpoena. In fact, we explained that because of the peer review protection of the evaluation process, the MPSC process, that it required a subpoena to open that box——

Senator CASSIDY. So the subpoena was given, and then you continue to withhold information from the committee without asserting a recognized right to do so. So what happened there?

Mr. SHEPARD. We provided redacted documents ——

Senator CASSIDY. So the redactions included senior OPO employees. That hardly seems on a doc—you know, the hospital administrator is not someone to be redacted if the patient is going to be redacted.

So why were you redacting senior OPO employees?

Mr. SHEPARD. Because the participation—the full and frank participation in our peer review process is what we believe leads to a full understanding of an adverse event. We asked the committee staff if redacted versions would allow them to understand how our oversight worked, and what had happened in these events. They said, "no." And we submitted documents that were unredacted.

Senator CASSIDY. Now, next. You mentioned the transport system. I think a lot of what is going on here is—as you mentioned earlier, almost ironically it seems—continuous improvement, quality improvement. But it seems as if that has been lacking in UNOS. I am a doc. I am a liver specialist. I had a lot of patients who died from lacking transplants because of a lack of organs.

I have worked among poor patients, and I had a lot of patients who died, just like Dr. Locke, who were Black, with renal failure who could not get transplanted. And so the remarks of your board member are particularly insulting to the patients for whom I cared for many years.

And I had a sense of indignation, and Dr. Locke shares my indignation. I don't know if you allowed her to continue to serve on your board. It is amazing that she would have been, after revealing such prejudice.

With that said, my Louisiana OPO tells me that they asked UNOS for a tracker; that they did not hear back; that they emailed more. "We need more trackers." They did not hear back. Seven weeks later they get an organ, a kidney. They ship it. It gets lost in transit because they do not have a tracker, and eventually it expires.

Now if this is a continuing quality, whatever, improvement process, and they are relying upon you—they say their emails were not being answered.

Now what kind of breakdown do we have in a system where emails are not being answered, much less where the trackers are not being sent, which results in a kidney being lost and therefore a patient going without the transplant?

Mr. SHEPARD. Senator, I am not aware of that situation. It is disturbing. It is certainly something I will look into. I know the leadership of the OPO, and I certainly wish, if they had had trouble getting an answer——

Senator CASSIDY. Well, they said they emailed the organization twice. And Dr. Locke has this specific incident in her testimony, so apparently it was known outside of Louisiana. So it just seems like a failure of the organization.

What case would you make for UNOS continuing to have the contract that CMS would award? What would give us confidence that there will be a change in direction where there is a responsiveness to emails like "I need a tracker," and then the obvious failure when the tracker does not come, and an organ is lost and the patient does not get her transplant? What case could you make?

Mr. SHEPARD. I believe that by bringing together the transplant and donation community, UNOS has a unique understanding of how organ donation and transplant works. I do not understand the particular situation, and I certainly find that as troubling as you do. But I also think that UNOS has a long track record of promoting increases in transplantation, equitable transplantation. We have a public equity tracker that says that, once listed, rural patients and African American patients are transplanted at very similar rates to other patients. It is getting to the wait list that is the real equity challenge. UNOS has a long track record of success. And, while I think that we can improve, and we do every day, I do think that it is a strong organization that has served patients well.

Senator CASSIDY. We heard a lot of testimony today, and committee reports that suggest that that is not the case.

With that, I yield.

The CHAIRMAN. Thank you very much, Dr. Cassidy. And they are very important questions. And I am just going to walk everybody through what we have turned up with respect to transportation of organs, because this is a major focus of the committee's investigation.

We asked about it. UNOS told us, and I quote, "It does not collect transportation data on a national systematic basis." That strikes me as a showstopper kind of response. UNOS doesn't track its donated organs' arrival at transplant centers? How in the world can we give people confidence if the organization that runs this says that?

It turns out UNOS only tracks the shipment handlers themselves. Four percent of organ shipments—even in this very small sample, dozens of organs are thrown away each year after transportation.

UNOS does not know if the other 96 percent of shipments are just as bad because they do not ask. UNOS has not made any policies on safe organ transportation, and OPOs are not required to report these issues. And when complaints about transportation failures are made, UNOS does not even reply.

So, Dr. Locke, you have been outspoken about this whole area with respect to the deficiencies in the operation. Tell us a little bit more about organ transplant problems, and what your response from them has been when you have reported problems with transportation?

Dr. LOCKE. Thank you, Senator. Obviously, people have described that we have about a 25-percent kidney discard. So, one in four. If you look at numbers last year—these are rough numbers—it would be about 8,000 kidneys. And really, I think in some ways these were kind of a victim of entrenched and cumbersome allocation algorithms that are very ordinal. We have to go sort of in order, when data clearly have shown that introduction of multiple simultaneous expiring offers would result in more efficient placement of kidneys, and this would decrease our cold ischemia time. Also I think it reflects a failure of transportation logistics. So, if you take UNOS's organ center, they have a very rigid system, for example, for finding flights, and lack either an ability or interest in thinking outside the box.

So, for example, if there are no direct flights from California to Birmingham, AL, instead of looking for a flight from San Francisco to Atlanta, understanding that a courier could then pick it up in Atlanta and drive it the 2 hours, they instead put it on a flight from SFO to Birmingham via Atlanta and allow it to go to a cargo hold over night where it literally is rotting, if you will, and so we are putting extra cold ischemia time on, waiting to catch the flight to Birmingham the next morning——

The CHAIRMAN. Let's make sure everybody gets this. You are saying you have seen instances of something being put in cargo hold when it is very likely to rot?

Dr. LOCKE. That is correct. So, if the kidney arrives after 10 p.m. at the Atlanta Airport, it goes to cargo hold. We discovered that and made calls to the airlines ourselves, and after several calls, the airlines—of course they were mortified, not understanding that that was what was happening, and actually had their manager meet our courier, and we were able to get the kidney out of cargo hold. But this went on before we figured out what was happening. Because essentially, they fly it in. It sits in cargo hold. It comes out the next morning to catch the next flight.

Instead of thinking outside the box—if we just get it to Atlanta, it is driveable to Birmingham. And those hours make a big difference.

The CHAIRMAN. That sounds way too logical for what UNOS has been up to.

So please go ahead.

Dr. LOCKE. So I think, from our perspective, one of the things that we really want to understand is why have we not engaged experts in applied mathematics to really optimize our matching algorithms and organ placement? And why haven't we really engaged experts in logistics around transportation?

I mean, I think of the FAA, for example; what a remarkable entity, the fact that every day thousands of flights across the U.S. are in the air at the same time and don't crash into each other. And they know exactly where a given plane is. And it happens almost seamlessly every day.

We should be able to do the same thing for our transplant system, for our organs.

The CHAIRMAN. As I said, too logical.

Ms. Brockmeier, UNOS has developed this organ tracking system. Do you all use it? And I am curious what you think of it.

Ms. BROCKMEIER. Senator, thank you for the question. Senator, we did use and participate in the beta pilot through UNOS and made the decision to not move forward using their product and have sought a commercial alternative.

The CHAIRMAN. And why was that?

Ms. BROCKMEIER. Part of the issues were some service-related issues, the lack of the interconnectivity that we wanted, to be able to facilitate a more expedited visual tracking for the organ.

The CHAIRMAN. Was the tracking technology low-quality?

Ms. BROCKMEIER. Yes, sir.

The CHAIRMAN. I will have some additional questions, but my time is up.

Senator Grassley?

Senator GRASSLEY. We are done.

The CHAIRMAN. Okay.

Mr. Shepard, in your statement to the committee today, you highlighted how people who work on the organ transplant network's board and committees come from all corners of the transplant system. You noted that this diverse group of people is essential to making difficult policy decisions for the transplant network, and how effectively the system works to protect patients.

Yet the way you describe these people and the peer review process in the documents you provided to the committee was very different. So I would like to enter into the record two emails that you wrote. Here is how you described the principal transplant oversight committee in one of your emails produced to the committee.

You said, and I quote, "Allowing the committee to fill these jobs increases the community's belief in the validity of the documents," end quote. You go on to say, and I quote, "It is like putting your kid's artwork up at home. You value it because of how it was created rather than whether it is well done. Only in this case, we persuade ourselves that it is well done anyway."

One more. In this email you describe the organ transplant network that you are in charge of as nothing more than, and I quote, "an overgrown homeowners association."

Now, when you compare the organ transplant network you oversee to an overgrown homeowners association, doesn't that call into question the effectiveness of the oversight and governance process used by the organ transplant system that you are saying works so well?

[The emails appear in the appendix beginning on p. 188.]

Mr. SHEPARD. Senator, I don't recall those particular emails, or the context——

The CHAIRMAN. They are yours.

Mr. SHEPARD. I assume that they are, sir.

The CHAIRMAN. They are yours, Mr. Shepard, and they are central to your belief, as you try to tell us, that everything is hunky dory; that you have confidence in the people.

You just wrote a bunch of emails that go 180 degrees in the other direction.

Let me turn now to the issue with respect to information technology. So the principal function of UNOS is to manage the electronic database and to keep track of organ donations, and match them to people on the transplant waiting list.

The technology that is used here is woefully out of date. The government report entitled "Lives Are at Stake: The Government's Role in Modernizing the OPTN" concluded that UNOS lacks sufficient technical capabilities to modernize their systems, which the current system requires. Instead of a modern, integrated cloudbased system, the UNOS system requires manual information updates at every stage. UNOS's transplant computers have crashed for a total of 17 days, with one February 2021 outage lasting 3 hours. When asked by our investigators, Mr. Shepard said improving the systems to meet industry standards was not a priority for UNOS, "because it is not like air traffic control."

Mr. Henry, I think you are still with us, and we are glad that you are. These organs are very perishable. As somebody who received a lifesaving transplant, my guess is you believe every minute counts when you are on the transplant waiting list?

Mr. HENRY. Yes, absolutely. And like everyone else, we have read the USDS reports. We have read The Washington Post reports from earlier this week. And the IT services have been, in our opinion, inadequate for quite some time. The Patient Affairs Committee, our leadership, has voiced their concerns about the IT systems for quite some time, without much of a response.

The CHAIRMAN. Mr. Henry, excuse me. How long have you been voicing your concerns about how outdated the IT systems are?

Mr. HENRY. I am speaking in this instance about Patient Affairs leadership. I have been recently appointed as a representative for the Patient Affairs Committee this year. So as far—I have read through a lot of the emails and background information, and spoken with leadership about these issues, including the IT services, and that is what I am referring to as far as our concerns about the IT systems being voiced but not addressed.

The CHAIRMAN. Okay.

Mr. HENRY. So you are correct, Senator Wyden. Every minute counts; every second counts. When we hear about down time as a result of IT issues, those are lives that are potentially lost. Patients die while IT systems are down.

So again, heartbreaking issues that we feel should be addressed.

The CHAIRMAN. So, Ms. Brockmeier, again because you are on the front lines, tell us your experiences with UNOS systems. And let's talk, for example, about something like DonorNet. Why has that not been modernized?

Ms. BROCKMEIER. The response, Senator Wyden, that we were provided when the committee that I was chairing asked repeatedly about improvements was that there wasn't bandwidth within the UNOS IT department to address those problems.

The CHAIRMAN. So they just did not have current technology?

Ms. BROCKMEIER. I cannot say what garnered their response, but that was their response.

The CHAIRMAN. If you don't have bandwidth for something that is a priority, that says your technology is not up to date.

All right, let's go next to OPO failure rates. Again, like everywhere in our society, there are performers that do well and some that do not. But the range of performance of organ procurement organizations is massive. The high-performing OPOs successfully recover and transplant four times as many organs as the poorly performing OPOs. After several years of debate on how to improve the performance of the subpar OPOs, the Centers for Medicare and Medicaid Services adopted a rule setting performance standards for the OPOs.

When measured against these standards, more than one-third of the 57 OPOs are failing—not 1 or 2, but 22.

Ms. Brockmeier, a lot of people in the OPO community oppose the CMS rule, including UNOS. When you see a large number of OPOs that are failing to meet the standard, I guess you can understand why.

Your OPO is not one of them. Do you think the measure is a step in the right direction for holding OPOs more accountable?

Ms. BROCKMEIER. Yes, Senator Wyden. Our organization went on the record very early on in strong support of the proposed metrics. While they may not be perfect, they are certainly an improvement over what we had had year-to-date.

The metrics are designed in such a way that everyone can accomplish that. We can all be Tier 1 performers. It takes a dedicated effort, the right staff, the appropriate training, and resourcing to ensure that your OPO is able to respond every time the phone rings to ensure all the organs are recovered.

The CHAIRMAN. All right.

Let's talk for a moment about the boards that are supposed to be overseeing these, because it looks to me like there is a serious conflict of interest here. And I will send this to Ms. Brockmeier, and perhaps you would like to get to it as well, Mr. Friedman.

The Organ Procurement and Transplantation Network—which is the formal title of the organ network that operates under Federal contract administered by HHS—and UNOS, which is the contractor that operates the network and controls information about the network, have the same boards of directors, despite efforts by the government to separate them.

That means the people who look out for the best interests of UNOS's multimillion-dollar nonprofits are the same people who look out for the interests of the entire organ transplant network. It sure sounds like a conflict to me.

Ms. Brockmeier, Mr. Friedman, UNOS claims the two boards must be the same. Okay, that is their claim. They have to be the same. And there is no need for the board of the OPTN to be independent from the board of the government contractor that runs it. Why shouldn't the network have an independent board—an independent board that can make its own judgments about whether the contractor is performing adequately?

Your thoughts, Ms. Brockmeier and Mr. Friedman?

Ms. BROCKMEIER. Yes, Senator Wyden, I think there should be an independent board. I think the division of the responsibilities of the board, and the inherent way that they are structured do pose conflicts. It would be like if you had an organization that was a supporting organization, you would want to hold it accountable for its performance. And the current structure really limits that opportunity.

The CHAIRMAN. Mr. Friedman?

Mr. FRIEDMAN. Chairman Wyden, actually HRSA and CMS, they actually changed board complexity for OPOs, requiring non-transplant individuals. And the same thing can be employed here as well.

As we make organ allocation changes, people win, people lose. And what we have done in this country, through the efforts of this board, is really allowed individuals to express their opinion at the board level, and the executive board level, that were based more towards their own individual needs. And this has to change. And that is why I, at our Region 3 meetings, continuously recommend that we separate that out and allow the membership of UNOS— this is a membership-driven organization—to bring us up to speed so that we have transparencies, and so that we regain the trust of our providers, our hospitals, our OPOs, the patients, and the donor families. We cannot lose that trust, and I fully support you as the chairman of this, to enact that immediately. That can be part of the contract.

The CHAIRMAN. We are just trying to determine if we have any Senators on the way. Let me ask our Republican colleagues. And we do. We do not? Thank you for your participation in this.

We are very pleased a strong advocate of patients, Senator Casey, is here. And let's let him get settled, and then we will go to him for his questions. And then I have a couple of other areas that we need to look at briefly.

Senator Casey, are you all set?

Senator CASEY. Mr. Chairman, thanks very much. I wanted to start by thanking you for the hearing and for the work that you and the ranking member have done in conducting this important investigation.

This is a subject area that obviously does not get nearly enough attention in Washington. Not so in the context of this hearing and the work that was done by this committee and the staff. All of their good work should be held up for commendation.

I also want to say I know I am late for the hearing, so I know I may have missed some of the engagement and some of the answers to questions. So if my questions are redundant, or duplicative, I apologize for that in advance.

I come to this issue not just in the context of a public official and a member of a committee, but also in a very personal way. My father was the beneficiary of a double organ transplant in June of 1993, a heart and liver. Not many, at the time, 61-year-olds had been the beneficiary of that kind of transplantation. In fact, when he had it, I was told he was one of only—or I should say there had been, I think, only six in the Nation at that point, and four of those six were dead. So his chances were not great. But thankfully, he came through it and was able to live 7 more years, almost to the day. So we were blessed and fortunate.

About a hundred separate things had to go right for him not to die before receiving that double organ transplantation. So we are grateful for that.

But I guess I wanted to focus on the—I guess the last two recommendations that call for both transparency and accountability for the chain of custody and the transport of organs. We know that thousands of Americans are anxiously awaiting these lifesaving, life-changing operations, and waiting for that call to save the life of a family member.

So I guess I wanted to start with Dr. Locke in terms of both transparency and accountability. How would a greater degree of both, a greater degree of transparency and a greater degree of accountability, improve the transplant system?

Dr. LOCKE. I think, quite simply, it would result in more lives saved. If you think about the three sort of areas that UNOS is supposed to oversee, greater transparency and accountability around policy would have led us to address, for example, gender disparities in liver allocation much sooner.

So in 2002, the model for end-stage liver disease was introduced, and we knew fairly quickly on that that created huge gender-based disparities in allocation because serum creatinine, one of the measures incorporated in MELD, does not reflect kidney function in women as well as it does in men. It is just this year that we finally updated the model to address that, some 20 years later. So that is a policy example that should have been addressed much sooner. And there were multiple cries from the community to do so.

If you think about transportation—I gave an example a minute ago: having a UNOS organ center that is really more flexible in their ability to sort of figure out logistics, instead of thinking about trying to get a kidney from San Francisco to Birmingham, and only looking at flights that get you all the way to Birmingham, and having the kidney go from San Francisco, to Atlanta, getting there so late that it gets stuck in cargo hold overnight like lost luggage, where it has increased cold time and is literally rotting until it can get on a plane the next day.

And then, as the surgeon getting the kidney, you have to make the decision, can I use this? Is it going to be okay? Is there too much time? Am I going to put the patient at risk for a primary nonfunction? Or should I go for it? Versus having the ability to get that kidney to Atlanta, have a courier pick it up and drive it to Birmingham, and save about 12 hours of cold time. Those things really matter.

And if you think about IT, something as simple as having a system where we can more easily put in unacceptable antigens—this was a debate for many years. So for context, we list unacceptable antigens in the system, and it allows us to better match kidneys so that, when someone comes up on the match run, we have a high probability that they will be a good tissue match.

Well, that took forever. And we could not really get our unacceptable antigens in. So routinely, people get offered kidneys that are not going to be a match, and you have to get to all of those before you can get to the person that they really should go to.

Those are simple examples. But if we could really have transparency and accountability around those kinds of things, we could save more lives.

Senator CASEY. Thanks very much. That is compelling. And I think for those of us who are concerned about the work of a committee like the Finance Committee being done, this kind of an investigation being done, of course a report and investigation study is only as good as the implementation of it.

I'm sorry; I guess I would turn to you, Mr. Shepard, and, just having heard from Dr. Locke about the benefits of both increasing accountability and transparency, would you commit to implementing—and you may have already been asked this, so I may be redundant, and I'm sorry if I am—but would you commit to implementing the bipartisan recommendations with regard to both transparency and accountability when it comes to organ transplantation?

Mr. SHEPARD. We are always looking, Senator, for ways to improve the process, and I look forward to receiving and reading the committee's recommendations on how to do that. I cannot commit to them because I have not seen them yet.

Senator CASEY. You have not seen the recommendations? Well, I hope that part of the follow-up of the work of the committee can be that kind of engagement with you and others, because we live in a world now where we can use technology and all the innovations that our economy presents to virtually have instantaneous retrieval of goods—everything from ordering food to ordering groceries or goods online. And the idea that we cannot have in place some of the practices and procedures and pathways to move organs faster, I hope would be something that would be the subject of history, as opposed to where we are headed in the future.

But I look forward to talking to you more about it.

But, Mr. Chairman, thanks very much for your time, and I know I am over, and I appreciate the work you have done.

The CHAIRMAN. Thank you, Senator Casey, chairman of the Aging Committee, which has a great interest in these topics as well.

I need to make another correction to something Mr. Shepard said, and we are going to get close to wrapping up, unless any other Senators on the committee are here.

Mr. Shepard told Senator Warren that only 10 percent of UNOS funds come from taxpayer money and the rest comes from fees paid by transplant centers who add patients to the list. But the fact is, Medicare is the largest payer of the fees, for example for kidneys. So we are talking about inefficiency. Inefficiency that puts patients at risk, and certainly taxpayer dollars are used to cover some of these practices.

So we have been at it for a couple of hours, and this has certainly been an ominous portrayal that you all have made. We have heard about organs with tire tracks. We have heard about organs left behind to spoil in airports. We have heard about reprisals against people who try to speak the truth about what is going on. We have heard about the culture of secrecy that dominates UNOS. We have emails that in effect have Mr. Shepard ridiculing employees he says that he counts on. And we have gone through some of the details with respect to the transportation system. And probably the best way I would describe it is, it is not even a system.

It just sounds like it is confusing, at best, if not bedlam.

So we heard testimony from witnesses today. And certainly, according to witnesses representing OPO transplant center patients, it is obvious that there are serious problems in the organ procurement and transplant system. And it is not keeping up with the demand for organs. Patients die every day while they wait.

The committee is going to continue its investigation. We have already looked at over 1,100 safety complaints filed with UNOS. They provide example after example of patient deaths and nearmisses after people have been selected from the list for transplant. One-third of the Nation's organ procurement organizations failed to meet even the minimum standards—the minimum standards—set out by the agency that certifies them to operate.

One in four kidneys recovered for transplant is never transplanted. The Federal experts on information technology say that the network's IT systems are not up to the task and that UNOS, the contractor that operates them, simply does not have the technical capability to update them.

Now, the testimony from UNOS, which is the organization that has run this for decades, is unrepentant. We have not heard anything resembling, "You know, we learned this and this over the last decade. We should have done that, but we are going to get it fixed soon." According to Mr. Shepard, things have never been better.

That is really what we have heard today. We have had the contract, claims Mr. Shepard, and we are doing fine, and people should be satisfied with us. The patients and the families, the physicians, basically are sending a very different message, that the situation is dire. The organization responsible for fixing it says there really is not anything to fix.

So we have certainly found in our investigation thus far that there is a lot to fix. So we are going to continue the investigation. The committee will be looking more closely at the role of Federal agencies—the Centers for Medicare and Medicaid Services, HRSA—that are charged with overseeing the system, and we will be looking at that. And the Federal contract that UNOS has had for decades is up for renewal, and this is an opportunity to fix things.

And on this committee, in a bipartisan way, we are determined not to miss this opportunity to get this fixed. Thanks to Senator Grassley, Senator Cardin, Senator Young, for their interest. They have been working with the committee for a long time. This is not a partisan issue. This is a national issue.

And, as we have touched on repeatedly over the course of the afternoon, patients waiting for organs, and families of donors, deserve better. And we are going to stay at it until they get those fixes.

And let me also note, procedurally, that members have 14 days to submit any questions or statements for the record. I want to thank our witnesses—Mr. Henry, who has patiently been out there giving us good information from cyberspace—for their patience.

The Finance Committee is adjourned.

[Whereupon, at 4:28 p.m., the hearing was concluded.]

Appendix

Additional Material Submitted for the Record

Prepared Statement of Diane Brockmeier, R.N., BSN, MHA, President and CEO, Mid-America Transplant

Chairman Wyden, Ranking Member Crapo, and members of the committee, my name is Diane Brockmeier, and I am the president and CEO of Mid-America Transplant, the organ procurement organization (OPO) serving eastern Missouri, southern Illinois, and northeastern Arkansas. Thank you for the opportunity to submit a written statement.

I joined Mid-America Transplant in 1986 as a registered nurse talking to families about organ donation on the worst days of their lives. These donor families, and the organ transplant recipients whose lives they save, remain at the forefront of my thoughts every day.

At our organization, we follow the ethos of "every donor, every time." Our clinical team is committed to giving donors and their families the care they deserve and stewarding their gifts to patients desperately in need. Mid-America Transplant depends on the broader national transplant system, administered by UNOS, to accomplish this work.

From 2018 to 2020, I served as a board member for the Organ Procurement Transplantation Network (OPTN). As an OPTN Board Member, I concurrently served on the UNOS board. My board experience revealed that UNOS's actions are often not aligned with its fundamental vision—a lifesaving transplant for everyone in need.

But change is possible; these problems can be corrected. It is critical that we urgently address patient safety, update the archaic IT system, remove conflicts to ensure good governance, and return the focus of the OPTN to providing high-quality care and exceptional system performance to *all* patients, both donor patients and transplant wait-list patients.

We need to urgently address patient safety.

Each organ lost due to system failure or provider failure has a consequence to the thousands of patients waiting for a transplant. Furthermore, a discarded organ fails to honor the heroic gift from a selfless donor and compounds the family's sense of loss.

Errors and adverse events do happen in organ procurement and transplant, just like in any other field of health care. However, unlike the rest of health care, we have few, if any, mechanisms to protect patient safety and prevent adverse events. Specifically:

- There are no clinical training, licensure, or certification standards required for OPO staff, even those operating in matters that directly affect patient care.
- There is no public adverse event reporting required of or by UNOS when patients are harmed, organs are lost, or the quality of patient care is unsafe.

UNOS lacks urgency and accountability around identifying and remediating the preventable loss of organs and addressing poor quality patient care. The process by which errors are reported and reviewed is woefully inadequate. Errors are not disclosed to the broader transplant community preventing practice improvement. In this environment, who is looking out for patients? Who is being held accountable for poor quality care? No OPO has ever been decertified, regardless of its performance or safety record.

While decertification falls to the Centers for Medicare and Medicaid Services (CMS), the entire system relies on member compliance from the OPTN. UNOS has failed to align its efforts to ensure patient safety at the system level. It is a decision with tragic and deadly consequences.

We must update an archaic technology system at UNOS.

As OPOs, we are required to work with UNOS's technology—DonorNet—every day. DonorNet is outdated, difficult to use, and often slow to function when every minute counts. Manual entry subjects it to error, and OPO and transplant center staff are not empowered with the right information when time is crucial.

I served in leadership roles on the OPO Committee from 2017–2022. Committee members and industry leaders voiced repeated requests to address the need for DonorNet improvements. Year after year, these requests were consistently met with the response that UNOS IT did not have the bandwidth to address this work.

The limitations of UNOS technology are delaying and denying transplants to patients dying on the wait list. Poor technology impacts the disturbingly high kidney discard rate in the United States; where one in four never makes it to a patient for transplantation.[1]

Consider:

- UNOS policy requires use of their Organ Center for national kidney placement. The Organ Center is highly inefficient, although UNOS does not report data about the Center's effectiveness. At our OPO, we have consistently observed that the Organ Center is rarely successful at placing kidneys and often discards kidneys after failed placement attempts leaving many OPOs aware they are better off not using it at all.[2],[3]
- Critical time is lost due to the inefficiency of DonorNet—wasting time on offers that will not be accepted and delaying or denying a transplant. Of course, an available organ should be offered to patients on the list in sequence. However, far too much of matching—particularly on harder to place organs from older donors—is left to individual OPOs and transplant programs to find each other despite, rather than facilitated by, UNOS technology.[4]
- UNOS has millions of data points that could, and should, facilitate faster, more efficient organ placement, providing the centers and OPOs with real-time information

---

[1] Available at: https://optn.transplant.hrsa.gov/about/committees/kidney-transplantation-committee/; OPTN Kid ney Transplantation Committee Meeting Summary, June 24, 2022.

[2] Noreen, SM, Klassen, D, Brown, R, et al. Kidney accelerated placement project: Outcomes and lessons learned. *Am J Transplant.* 2022; 22: 210–221, doi:10.1111/ajt.16859.

[3] Mohan, S and Scheid, JD (2022), Accelerating deceased donor kidney utilization requires more than accelerating placement. *Am J Transplant.* 2022; 22: 7–8. *https://doi.org/10.1111/ ajt.16866.*

[4] Doby, BL, Ross-Driscoll, K, Yu, S, Godwin, M, Lee, KJ, Lynch, RJ. Examining utilization of kidneys as a function of procurement performance. *Am J Transplant.* 2022; 22: 1614–1623, doi:10.1111/ajt.16985.

- Board members are kept in the dark about critical matters, and are marginalized, particularly if they have views that differ from UNOS leader- ship. As a board member, I do not recall the subject of the Senate Finance investigation being raised by UNOS leadership.
- Preparatory small group board member calls were conducted prior to the board meetings to explore voting intentions on upcoming issues. If the board member was not in agreement with the opinion of UNOS and board leader- ship, follow-up calls were initiated. Fellow board members reported feeling pressured to vote in accordance with UNOS and board leadership.
- Conflicts in the current structure, combined with the actions of UNOS leadership, have led to a deeply concerning perception that speaking out can lead to exclusion from critical decision-making, or worse—retaliation.
- After I left the board, I was disturbed to see UNOS leadership lobbying *against* Federal regulations for OPOs which would drive transparency, ac- countability, and improve performance.

to increase transplants. Leveraging this rich data source is a national imperative to improving patient outcomes.

- Mid-America Transplant intentionally identifies surgeons who accept kidneys that have been declined many times. These are lifesaving options for those patients. In May 2022, one of these patients was number 18,193 on the list. Relying on DonorNet alone, that kidney never would have been placed, and a chance to save a life would have been wasted.
- It is worth noting that when an OPO goes out of sequence to place an organ that would otherwise be thrown away, UNOS requires an explanation. However, when organs are never recovered or placed at all, UNOS remains silent. Organ Procurement Organizations are never penalized for discarding an organ. Conversely, they are penalized for placing organs out of sequence.

We must remove conflicts to ensure good governance.

Serving on the board of the OPTN automatically assigns membership on the UNOS board. How can you fairly represent the country's interests and a contractor's interests at the same time?

I implore the committee—along with CMS and HRSA—to ensure those who speak out in support of system reform are not penalized. Patients deserve a transparent, accountable system that works on their behalf.

We must refocus on patients.

To protect patients, I urge Congress and the administration to:

- Separate the OPTN functions into different contracts so patients can be served by best-in-class vendors,
- Immediately separate the boards of the OPTN and the OPTN contractors,
- Require public disclosure of all potential conflicts for the contractor and board members, and
- Ensure that patients are safeguarded through open data from both the OPTN and OPOs.

Inaction by UNOS causes real harm to patients. This harm is measured in how many patients die waiting for a transplant. Your immediate action on this matter will save lives. Thank you.

Appendix A: Morning Consult Opinion Piece in Support of the Opo Rule, October 13, 2020

Organ Donation Can Save More Lives Through Reform

By Ginny McBride and Diane Brockmeier

Last December, the Department of Health and Human Services proposed new regulations to reform the U.S. organ donation system. It would accomplish this by creating objective criteria by which to evaluate the government contractors, called organ procurement organizations, who are charged with recovering transplantable, lifesaving organs from deceased donors. These bipartisan reforms could save countless lives. It's important the Trump administration finalize them now.

As CEOs of two OPOs, this is an issue we have followed closely, and we applaud these measures as long overdue.

Our constituents are the more than 100,000 Americans currently waiting for a lifesaving transplant, with 33 dying every day for lack of an organ. Given that COVID–19 can cause organ failure, reform is even more urgent today than it was a year ago. HHS estimates that its proposal will mean an estimated 5,000 to 10,000 more lifesaving organ transplants every year.

Central to the problem is that, historically, the government has not used objective criteria to evaluate OPO performance. OPOs are allowed to self-interpret and self- report our own performance data. As a result. no OPO has ever lost its government contract, even as wildly variable performance across OPOs has led to unnecessary deaths for patients in need of transplants.

Compounding the problem is that all OPOs operate as geographic monopolies, which means we have neither regulatory nor competitive pressure to provide high service to patients. And while there may be legitimate reasons for at least some monopolism (*e.g.,* potential donor families should not have two OPOs competing for their attention), the trade-off must be increased transparency and oversight.

HHS's proposal, rightly, promises to implement much-needed accountability measures, with real consequence for our counterparts that fail to meet them—including replacing OPOs who simply do not get the job done. In response, many OPOs have responded with aggressive lobbying campaigns to block these proposed reforms by confusing the issue or proposing unworkable alternatives.

But the more future-minded OPOs, like ours, are embracing change. HHS's new proposal signals something potentially game-changing for patients: allowing the highest performing OPOs to replace those who have proven themselves incapable of serving their communities. To the extent that an OPO is not able to rise to the challenge of a high standard, the focus of our attention and energy must be on better serving patients on the national wait list, not on protecting specific OPOs.

This, of course, is threatening for OPOs who have grown a bit too comfortable. Some of our colleagues have tried to paint any changes as destabilizing and unprecedented, positing that it will lead to situations in which areas of the country do not have OPOs at all. But this is simply not grounded in HHS's proposal, which explicitly states that "our goal is to ensure continuous coverage of an OPO service area in the event an OPO is decertified."

There were originally 128 OPOs, and after decades of consolidations there are now 58 OPOs; never has this process been disruptive. Forcing OPOs to continually earn their contracts is a patient-centric accountability mechanism, ensuring that OPOs operate with the urgency befitting the life-and-death consequences of this work.

Additionally, many OPOs have argued that the standard for OPO performance HHS has proposed is "arbitrary." But the more important question is whether the improvements HHS seeks to drive are realistically achievable, and we believe unequivocally that they are; HHS data show the difference between the best and worst OPOs is almost 500 percent. Put another way, some OPOs recover 4 or 5 times as many organs as their peers.

So if we accept that higher performance is possible—and we understand that it would also be lifesaving—realizing these gains is not simply a policy question, but a social imperative. As patient advocates have argued, and with which we wholeheartedly agree, "In a chronically underperforming system, patients should fear a perpetuation of the status quo, not a disruption of it."

It's time that HHS unleashed the best weapon it has against the life-threatening organ shortage: OPOs who have already proven themselves motivated and capable. HHS should finalize its proposal as urgently as possible, trusting the best among us to rise to that challenge. Any weakening of HHS's proposed standard will—definitionally—result in lives lost, which is directly antithetical to our mission. Patients deserve nothing less.

Ginny McBride is the CEO of OurLegacy, a Florida-based OPO. Diane Brockmeier is the CEO of Mid-America Transplant, which serves parts of Missouri, Illinois, and Arkansas; she also is the past president of the Association of Organ Procurement Organizations.

Appendix B: RFI Response with Other Proreform CEOs to CMS Re. Opos, February 1, 2022

To: Administrator Chiquita Brooks-Lasure, Centers for Medicare and Medicaid Services
From: Diane Brockmeier, Mid America Transplant Virginia McBride, OurLegacy
Patti Niles, Southwest Transplant Alliance
Kelly Ranum, Louisiana Organ Procurement Agency
Matt Wadsworth, Life Connection of Ohio
Janice Whaley, Donor Network West
Jennifer Erickson, Federation of American Scientists

The FAS Organ Procurement Organization Innovation Cohort is committed to using data science and transparency to accelerate improved patient outcomes and to inform ongoing, data-driven policy development.

The seven organ procurement organizations that are leading in opening up their data include: Donor Network West, Life Connection of Ohio, LiveOn New York, Louisiana Organ Procurement Agency, Mid-America Transplant, OurLegacy, and South-west Transplant Alliance.

During a transformative period in the organ procurement industry, the Innovation Cohort will help shape the future of organ recovery in America, improving OPO practice and informing OPO policy. Most importantly, the Innovation Cohort will strive toward new heights of operational excellence in order to increase organ transplants in an effort to best serve the public, organ donors, donor families and patients waiting for transplants.

The FAS Organ Procurement Organization Innovation Cohort has publicly committed to:

1) Transparency: public sharing of data/analysis in order to set a standard to which all OPOs can be held;

2) Accountability: support for the OPO final rule, and any efforts to move up implementation date so all parts of the country can be served by highperforming OPOs as soon as possible in 2024; and
3) Equity: commitment to analyzing/publishing data to ensure all parts of community served.

Reducing disparities—p. 68599

1) Are there revisions that can be made to OPO CfCs to reduce disparities in organ transplantation?

Given bipartisan congressional leaders have called for accelerations of reforms of the donation and transplant ecosystem as an "urgent health equity issue" exacerbated by the COVID pandemic, we call on CMS to make the public disclosure of all OPO process data a requirement of the OPO CfCs immediately.

To reduce disparities in organ transplantation, it is critical to enforce the final rule as quickly as possible, and to update CfCs:

- The metrics contained in the final rule, are already best suited to measure OPO performance and hold OPOs accountable to the highest performance and to the idea of pursuing every donor and organ every time to save as many lives as possible.
- It is critical that the final rule be:
  - Enforced as quickly as possible. moving up the implementation date so that all parts of the country can be served by high-performing OPOs;
  - Not be revised in a way that dilutes or distorts its impact.
    - ✓ CMS should maintain its earlier correct judgment disallowing both race-based adjustments (which could harm patient outcomes) and zero donors (which could allow for gaming of metrics).
    - ✓ To have evidence of effective and equitable service, CMS should make all OPO process data publicly available.
  - It is undeniable that a number of the questions raised in the RFI could be answered or resolved if all OPO process data were required to be made public, giving regulators the opportunity to understand and identify where performance gaps and inequitable service and outcomes exist.
  - This data-driven transparency would ensure all OPOs are accountable to the highest levels of operational excellence, and would offer opportunities to design interventions to address particular gaps in service.

OPO metrics/performance—p. 68601, 68602, 68603

1. Independent of CMS's specific outcome measures, what other metrics or attributes reflect a model or highest performing OPO?; 2. What are quantitative or qualitative indicators of excellent performance and how can CMS incorporate these with outcome measures when assessing OPOs for recertification purposes?; 3. Should CMS consider additional metrics, such as those that measure equity in organ donation or an OPO's success in reducing disparities in donation and transplantation, and how should this be measured?; 4. Are there ways to scale, or

rate, performance of other (new) factors that CMS may consider in assessing OPO performance? 5. Can the OPO CfCs address the issue of organs that are lost during transport to a transplant program?

In answer to the above questions, CMS should look for evidence of effective and equitable service as seen in open and transparent OPO process data.

The OPO Innovation Cohort is committed to transparency, accountability, and equity, and is already taking steps to make these commitments a reality through its collaboration with the Massachusetts Institute of Technology to make de-identified process data publicly available.

This level of transparency should be required of all OPOs. This addresses the questions above as well as a range of questions related to OPO operational practices (e.g., organ tracking and lost organs; operational differences between high- and low- performing OPOs; standardization of definitions and practices; the potential impact of organ recovery centers; best practices regarding automated referrals, and so on).

Competition—68601

Are there additional factors or criteria that CMS should consider when determining which OPO should be selected for an open service area? 2. Should CMS consider other performance measures when selecting an OPO for an open DSA?; 3. What would be the anticipated impact from consolidation or expansion of the OPO community? Would consolidation or expansion of OPOs facilitate increased competition and improved performance or have a negative impact? 4. Any other helpful information that could inform potential changes to the current recertification and competition processes.

Appreciating the principles of the Biden Executive Order on Competition, the FAS OPO Innovation Cohort agrees with bipartisan congressional leaders that given COVID makes reform an "urgent health equity issue," all parts of the country deserve to be served by high-performing OPOs as soon as possible.

As CMS considers elements for competition, transparency, accountability, and equity are critical. In addition to overall donor and recovery rates, through requiring all OPO process data to be publicly available, CMS will have evidence of an OPO's ability to equitably serve all donors in a designated service area (including by race/ ethnicity), as well as improvements over potential, and transparency of key financial and organizational data to understand capacities to best serve OSAs (including transparency in any conflicts that may exist in an OPO's governance structure).

The FAS OPO Innovation Cohort has already committed to these principles, and extending these practices to all OPOs via CfCs can allow CMS to best evaluate OPOs as they compete for serving an underserved community.

For example, publicly available OPO process data via CfCs will allow CMS to consider evidence of effective and equitable treatment of donor patients/families (e.g., no disparities in response rates/times based on race/ethnicity).

The anticipated outcome of both increased competition as well as replacing lower performing OPOs with higher performing OPOs would be more lives saved. See:

- The Bridgespan Group guidance on how CMS can oversee and implement the DSA competition process in a manner that is pro-patient and foregrounds racial equity;
- OPO CEOs in the news:
    - Diane Brockmeier and Ginny McBride in Morning Consult: "HHS's new proposal signals something potentially game-changing for patients: allowing the highest

performing OPOs to replace those who have proven themselves incapable of serving their communities. To the extent that an OPO is not able to rise to the challenge of a high standard, the focus of our attention and energy must be on better serving patients on the national wait list, not on protecting specific OPOs . . . forcing OPOs to continually earn their contracts is a patient-centric accountability mechanism, ensuring that OPOs operate with the urgency befitting the life- and-death consequences of this work."

- o Patti Niles in The Dallas Morning News: "The performance gaps seen in the OPO community would not be acceptable in any other sector of health care. There is no reason to accept them in the life-and-death context of organ donation. Many organ procurement organization leaders are on the record in favor of reform. We have worked together with patient groups, doctors, researchers, senior Obama and Trump administration officials, philanthropies and bipartisan members of Congress to get this right Lives are at stake. Patients deserve better. Our communities deserve better. We must do better."

Oversight—p. 68601

5. Are the current CMS requirements for a governing body and advisory board adequate for OPO governance? Have OPOs included additional board positions or structures beyond what is required by CMS to improve operations? What structure best serves accountability, and efficient and effective organ procurement?

The FAS OPO Innovation Cohort believes the principle of transparency should apply throughout the entire ecosystem, and that it is critical for CMS to:

- Release information related to OPO performance quickly and in an understandable way so that boards are aware and can exercise fiduciary responsibilities;
- Require transparency of potential conflicts of interest throughout the entire donation and transplantation ecosystem as a top priority, following the transparency commitment of FAS OPO Innovation Cohort.

Appendix C: RFI Response with Other Pro-Reform CEOs to HRSA Re. OPTN, May 2022

To: HRSA Administrator

From: Diane Brockmeier, Mid-America Transplant Ginny McBride, OurLegacy

Kelly Ranum, Louisiana Organ Procurement Agency Matt Wadsworth, Life Connection of Ohio

This letter Is in response to a Request for Information (RFI) regarding the contract to operate the national Organ Procurement and Transplantation Network (OPTN). Each of our organ procurement organizations (OPOs) supports HRSA's stated objectives of:

- Increasing accountability in OPTN operations, Including board governance, financial structures, data transparency, and policy development;

- Enhancing the usability and performance of the OPTN IT system and related tools; and
- Strengthening equity, access, and transparency in the organ donation, allocation, procurement, and transplantation process.

With the above objectives in mind, key recommendations for HRSA to reform the OPTN in such a way that best serves patients, focusing on core competencies and removing conflicts, include:

- Ensure patient-centered governance of the OPTN, separating the OPTN board from any contractor(s) serving OPTN functions; and
- Revise the OPTN contract so that it subdivided into areas where the OPTN contractors can provide critical and expert functions:
  - Policy: reforming OPTN governance (above) is critical to de-conflicting policy. Policymaking by an OPTN contractor should then be transparent, fueled by openly available data, aided by experts in government and the wider community, and with all potential conflicts publicly known and acted on accordingly.
  - IT: the IT components of OPTN operations be outsourced by HHS in ways that are independent of, but complimentary to, the rest of the OPTN contract
    - ✓ The Office of the National Coordinator (ONC) at HHS should work with the tech contractor on matters critical to national/health IT and organ donation/transplantation, including exploring better use and/ or integration of hospital EMRs.
  - Organ placement and shipping: these should be separate from existing OPTN contract, with best in class options available for OPOs to opt into as appropriate.

Note: the Membership and Professional Standards Committee should cease its activities to evaluate OPO performance and conduct peer review, with OPO oversight being the purview of CMS, instead of fractured between CMS and OPTN.

- All of the above functions—both from HHS and OPTN contractors—should have strengthening equity, access, and transparency at their core, including ensuring all de-identified data are publicly available to best serve patients, and enable continuous innovation and improvement.

A. OPTN Technology—IT System: (A.1-4)

We are acutely aware OPTN technology lags significantly behind other technology platforms because our OPOs use it every day. As citizens of the U.S. we enjoy the use of numerous corporate IT platforms to perform the most basic functions of life. These platforms have been developed by enterprising companies whose survival relies on capturing market share. Ease of use, convenience and continuous innovation are among the most prized factors. Companies compete against each other to satisfy and retain customers. Poor performers do not survive.

Companies succeed because they prioritize continuous, rapid IT system improvement because IT is a core function. The current OPTN contractor has not positioned itself to provide state-of-the-art service and does not view evolving technology as a priority. The OPTN Board of Directors and committees and the current contractor's board and committees lack the needed expertise to make the necessary changes because the OPTN Bylaws restrict the involvement of individuals who could expand its capabilities. From an IT perspective, the current OPTN contractor is slow and reactive.

It is our recommendation that the IT components of OPTN operations be separated from the monolithic OPTN contract by HHS In ways that are Independent of, but complimentary to, the rest of the OPTN contract. HRSA could require any other OPTN contractors to incorporate the services of the independent technology provider into its workflows. That independent contractor should be answerable to and benefit from digital service experts within the govemment— including HHS and the ONC—who can competently exercise oversight on behalf of patients and taxpayers.

The flow of information among OPOs, donor hospitals, transplant programs and the OPTN in support of successful donation and transplantation, while constant, remains fractured. Donor hospitals and transplant hospitals utilize their own electronic health record systems. OPOs and transplant programs utilize customized, built-to-purpose databases that interact with the OPTN only to transfer donor, candidate and recipient data that are, for the most part, not used for the critical functions of organ matching, offer and acceptance. The OPTN database operates in a one-way fashion in which members provide data but very little information is provided directly to them in return, and the entire process is hindered by the current OPTN contractor's inability to deploy APIs.

The use of multiple databases to operate a network dependent on timely and accurate communication to achieve maximum performance is not efficient. The OPTN technology contractor should be working toward seamless integration from hospital EHR to OPTN database. The rules of engagement with the OPTN database should be changed so OPOs are no longer required to maintain an additional database to collect and store donor information. OPOs should be able to transfer donor clinical information directly from the hospital EHR to the OPTN database for the purpose of communicating donor evaluation information and organ allocation. OPOs should be able to enter and extract data from the national database utilizing their own internal capabilities, aided by APIs, rather than pay for an expensive database "middleman." Additionally, there should be mutually agreed upon national OPO datasets that can be used for research and analysis purposes (see earlier response to CMS RFI on data transparency). Data availability and transparency are key to improving organ procurement. The database should be managed by the OPTN technology contractor in a way that prioritizes data transparency. The current OPTN contractor has not proven capable of this function.

Historically, motivation for the OPTN to accelerate improvements to its technology platform have come from outside the OPTN. Pressure to create DonorNet came from HRSA. More recently, calls to implement a GPS system to track organ movements went unheeded by the OPTN until media accounts exposed the lack of a systematic method to protect vulnerable organs while in transit Incorporation of technology requirements into a single OPTN contract has not sufficiently served the needs of OPOs, and the noncompetitve monopoly structure has relieved all pressure from the current OPTN contractor to keep current with even basic technology standards, creating risks to patient safety and data security. HRSA must create opportunities to incorporate a wider array of contractors to serve technology needs, including by opening the pool to the widest range of innovative applicants. There are numerous U.S. companies with the ability to track and deliver packages. It would serve the interests of organ sharing better if one of those companies could establish a national organ shipping system that would monitor the progress of all shipments in real time on behalf of OPOs that opt in.

B. Data Collection Activities: 1. Describe how you would/how vendors could develop performance metrics and benchmarks for the organ donation, procurement, allocation and transplant system, including through expert consultation, subcontracting, and engagement with transplant candidates, transplant recipients, organ donors and their families about the metrics they value. 2. Describe how you would/ how vendors could structure data collection and reporting mechanisms for the system: a. To report OPTN performance metrics including process, outcome, and patient engagement measures. b. To establish OPTN member performance benchmarks. c. To capture patient and donor demographics, including race, ethnicity, language, and socioeconomic factors. d. To create public OPTN national, regional and local performance dashboards. e. To track long-term patient outcomes and health and non-health-related factors that contribute to outcomes.

C. CMS recently finalized new, objective OPO regulations which we supported along with patient groups, bipartisan congressional leaders, and equity advocates. The performance measures recently published by the CMS are already having substantial influence on OPO performance. One case in point is the Arkansas Organ Recovery Agency (ARORA), an OPO which had never recovered organs from more than 77 deceased donors in a single year. Because of leadership changes driven by years of underperformance, a new executive director achieved 108 deceased organ donors in 2021. It seems unlikely this leadership change would have occurred without external pressure from CMS to change course.

HRSA, and other HHS entities, must establish national goals in collaboration with leading experts external to the OPTN but can use the donation and transplantation community as sources of data, information and insights. Additionally, all deidentified OPTN data should be publicly available to allow for oversight, innovative research, and donation/transplantation stakeholders to improve patient outcomes based on data.

Additionally, we and the aforementioned groups have advocated for HHS to publish OPO process data (see CMS RFI response), which will not only inform best practices for OPO management, but help inform policy considerations at the intersection of multi-stakeholders, including in regards to best practices and thoughtful regulation related to donor hospital referrals and organ discards. Regardless of whether HHS takes on some of these responsibilities directly (including potentially through an Office of Organ Policy), or outsources them to an external vendor, all metrics and benchmarks should be informed by transparent process data, in line with international best practice standards.

(d) OPTN Finances

The OPTN board and any OPTN operational contractor board must achieve complete separation. The OPTN board, populated mostly by transplantation professionals, does not have the expertise or background to oversee a financial, technological, human resources, customer service enterprise. UNOS's performance as the OPTN contractor bears this out. Its ability to keep pace with technological advances has been in question for many years, as evidenced by board and OPTN members who are frustrated at the time it takes to implement policy changes. The current board does not have the background enabling it to build wider corporate relationships enabling it to achieve strategic goals. The OPTN community has suffered as a result. UNOS's current strategy of using one board to serve two purposes must be abandoned. Any new contractor boards should commit to develop an independent operational plan that focuses on human resources needs, financial strategies, corporate IT objectives and other strategies to enable goal achievement that allows for HHS to meet its objectives for the transplant community. The OPTN board and staff should be financed by OPTN registration fees. Because both the OPTN board and the contractor operational board would be in accountability relationships with HRSA, they both would report on successes and barriers in meeting the strategic objectives of the OPTN. This reporting process could be extended to all elements within HHS with a stake in the operations of the OPTN to ensure alignment of goals and communication transparency. Ideally, NOTA should be updated, including to create a financing structure that aligns incentives for any OPTN contractors with the actual goals of HHS and patients in mind, which is to constantly increase transplant availability through improved stakeholder performance, something which is not accomplished in the current financing structure.

Any donation and transplantation clinician who is a member of the OPTN board and employed by an OPO or transplant hospital is in a conflict of interest when voting on certain OPTN policies. And since at least 50 percent of the board meets this criterion (because of OPTN final rule requirements for board composition), a method of addressing the conflict must be identified. Currently, conflicts are self- reported, narrowly defined, and not disclosed. One strategy specific to organ allocation could be that policies are voted on by non-OPO and transplant program members. This leaves patients, donor families, trade organizations (which would each get a single vote to represent each industry) and other non-allied members to vote. Board members would be prohibited from lobbying the patients and donor families to gain their votes. However, the best and most sustainable strategy would be to eliminate inherent conflicts entirely through subdivision of the OPTN contract. For example, organ allocation could be handled by a separate contractor with no financial or other business relationships to the stakeholders with a vested interest in the outcome of organ allocation policy.

D. Increasing Organ Donation and Improving Procurement: 1. Describe how you would/how vendors could structure, finance and staff an OPTN board of directors independent of membership of the OPTN operational contractor's board of directors.

1. Describe the conflict of interest policies you would/vendors could implement to ensure independence of the OPTN board of directors. 3. Describe the reporting mechanisms you would/vendors could utilize to hold operational contractors' accountable tor system performance and outcomes. 4. Describe the additional factors and process steps you would/vendors could take to ensure effective operations of such an independent board of directors.

The OPTN contractor should no longer be actively engaged in supporting OPO performance improvement activities. There should not be contract activities to support OPO performance and the Membership and Professional Standards Committee should cease its activities to evaluate OPO performance and conduct peer review. Neither of these activities has resulted in immediate and sustained donation increases and the OPTN has permitted some severely underperforming OPOs to continue practicing rather than make referrals to the HHS Secretary to decertify the underperformers. The MPSC began evaluating OPO performance many years ago at a time when CMS's OPO performance standards were vague and Incapable of identifying poor performers. At HRSA's request, the OPTN and SRTR stepped in to develop measures that would identify low performing OPOs. Despite having a set of standards, the OPTN has done little to positively impact the number of donors and organs transplanted. This inability came into stark relief in 2003 when HRSA launched the breakthrough collaboratives and, with almost no assistance from the OPTN except data analysis support, achieved unprecedented donation increases. Any funding to improve OPO performance could be better spent and allocated through a formal CMMI process of the best available data-driven options. The OPTN could then stay focused on evaluating OPOs for compliance with OPTN policies, such as following official OPTN allocation processes.

CMS is already demonstrating with its new performance outcome standards that, despite the OPTN's 20-year history of OPO performance evaluation and improvement activities, more than a third of OPOs are failing. The Scientific Registry of Transplant Recipients (SRTR) data used by the OPTN MPSC to evaluate OPOs also seem ineffective in identifying poor performance. Therefore, it has been extremely ill-structured for the OPTN, rather than CMS, to have unique visibility into the day-to-day issues necessary for CMS to exercise such oversight responsibility. Given this, HHS should reabsorb all OPO oversight functions from the OPTN.

If, as alluded to earlier, HHS publishes full process data, this will help generate a multitude of solutions for remediating OPO performance failures during the course of a contracting cycle. For example, with specific deficiencies identified. including issues related to diversity, equity, and inclusion, OPOs will be able to engage external partners (including partners both traditionally within and outside of the OPO industry) to implement data-driven solutions. Such process data, in line with international best practice for data transparency, should include: whether OPOs are appropriately staffed to serve their communities; data about referral and request outcomes based on potential donor and family race; and other issues that could identify any deficiencies in any OPOs' service of communities of color. Using these data, HRSA could then also partner with multiple organizations to develop strategies to improve equity in organ donation at a systems-level.

A. Organ Usage: 1. Describe how you would a vendor could support the OPO performance Improvement activities to decrease discarded organs and further increase the use of organs. 2. How can OPTN organ matching activities be modified to decrease non-usage (discards) of procured organs? 3. Describe the steps you would/ vendors could take to improve transparency around the organ matching and acceptance process for transplant candidates, transplant recipients, other affected patients, organ donors and family members served by the OPTN.

The most effective way to discourage OPOs from recovering organs is to ensure they don't get transplanted. This is the biggest problem facing the OPTN. From an OPO perspective, the OPTN is unintentionally enabling organ discards because organ allocation policies, particularly kidney allocation policies, prioritize how candidates are ranked on the waiting list rather than ensuring a transplantable kidney is implanted into a compatible recipient The balance between ensuring equity in candidate selection and ensuring viable organs are transplanted has been lost. This is partly because the people driving kidney allocation policy development (the OPTN Kidney Committee) are predominantly transplant professionals. There are no OPO voices advocating for better kidney utilization during the policy development phase. Discard rates are also influenced by an OPOs inability to get an offer to a program willing to use the kidney in a timely manner. High KDPI kidneys are "at risk" from the moment of aortic crossclamp. But they aren't treated with sufficient priority. OPOs, or the Organ Center, must use precious time to wade through offers to transplant programs that rarely, if ever, use high KDPI kidneys. Kidney filters only do so much. Rather than rely on voluntary engagement of transplant programs to filter offers, high KDPI kidney allocation should prioritize the programs with a track record of using them.

Much of the problem also results from the frictionful and otherwise insufficient UNOS technology system over which organ offers as made, leading to calls from the House Appropriation Committee for HHS to promote competition for the IT component of the OPTN contract for this explicit reason.

Honoring donors and donor families by ensuring their kidneys are transplanted is our national obligation. Anything less is a disservice to those who have donated.

Not every OPO agrees that handing kidneys to the Organ Center for the purpose of national placement is an effective means of getting kidneys transplanted. OPOs generally are not confident that placement will occur when relying on the Organ Center. The Organ Center's organ placement outcomes are not widely shared and OPOs deserve to be better informed about the likelihood of their organs being placed and should have a choice about whether to ask the Organ Center for assistance. OPOs are more invested than the Organ Center in placing organs because we know the families who have donated them and we will work to get them placed. Unfortunately, current OPTN policy makes this difficult.

But there could be a different option to place difficult organs. Because transplant programs and OPOs are relying more frequently on staffing and operational support from third parties or call centers, it may be possible to create an organization whose sole purpose is to place kidneys. This organization could be operated under a separate section of the OPTN contract but receive financial support from OPOs that would be willing to utilize it (e.g., a fee-for-service, which would be optional for OPOs and applied on an opt-in, voluntary, case-by-case basis). The objective would be to place high KDPI kidneys faster. Such an organization could quickly learn which centers are more inclined to transplant certain organs and collaborate with the host OPOs to develop a placement strategy. We must develop an increased level of national urgency to place the kidneys OPOs have successfully made available. It is our experience that transplant programs do not feel urgency when a kidney is at risk. But the OPOs feel that risk very acutely. Perhaps it is time to move away from the Organ Center concept and toward a more independent process.

1. Describe how you would/vendors could incorporate, to the full extent permitted under applicable law, the NASEM report's recommendations on increasing racial, ethnic, professional, and gender diversity on the boards and committees responsible for developing OPTN policies. 2. Describe how you would/vendors could engage with experts in quality improvement and stakeholder collaboration in executing OPTN deliverables. Page 6 of 7. 3. Describe what you would/vendors could include in their code of business ethics and conduct for the entity that holds this contract to ensure the highest standards of conduct and integrity are observed. 4. What other improvements to OPTN operations and policy development processes can and/or should be incorporated into the OPTN contact?

B. OPTN Operations and Policy Development Improvements

We support NASEM's recommendation that improvements to the OPTN's policy- making process to increase racial, ethnic, professional and gender diversity on the OPTN's board and committees are urgently needed. This can be accomplished by increasing or changing the number or type of medical/scientific members or public members and permitting them, via the OPTN bylaws, to serve on committees and the board. HRSA and the OPTN should actively recruit membership of organizations with expertise in health-care delivery to DEI communities. HHS should also clearly articulate its goals, as well as to foster a dynamic in which any OPTN contractor(s) understand that they will likely lose their contract should they fail to meet these goals.

Many OPTN members are losing confidence in the OPTN policymaking process. It seems that significant time and resources are devoted to changes that make only small, incremental differences in the number of organs donated and transplanted.

Many policies are also perceived to be tainted by the conflicts of interest inherent in the current OPTN structure, which again underscores the need for HHS to subdivide the OPTN. Although OPTN policies are developed by members, their impact is felt far beyond OPTN membership. Their ability to success is dependent on factors also beyond the membership of the OPTN. If the OPTN is to improve its success it is essential that we allow those societal factors that can affect our success be part of the policy development process. And to do that, we must re-examine that process, specifically our public comment process. Currently, the OPTN is reliant on commenters coming to regional meetings or depositing feedback on a website to obtain public feedback. To build trust in our system, we must consider how we can more actively engage influential communities to help us understand how we can do better. OPTN policies aren't just medical policies, they are public trust policies. The OPTN must build a community that is willing and capable to provide honest feedback. And we must have a public comment process that honestly and transparently incorporates that feedback so participants feel heard and valued. We strongly support the involvement of organizations such as the National Academy of Public Administration to assess the OPTN's current policy making process and advise on strategies to diversify how its development is influenced.

Additionally, given how critical DEI is to all aspects of a high-functioning organ donation and transplantation system. all OPTN contractors should include DEI expertise within its core leadership and DEI metrics as part of its transparent reporting.

Creating strong foundations for the policy making process is what will drive how the OPTN ensures its code of ethics and integrity is maintained. Many perceive the OPTWs integrity has suffered and it is our belief that this is because the policy- making process lacks transparency and accountability.

Questions Submitted for the Record to Diane Brockmeier, R.N., BSN, MHA
Questions Submitted by Hon. John Barrasso

Question. As a doctor for over 20 years, I've seen how complex and fragile the organ procurement and transplant system in the United States is. A single, seemingly minor mistake can cascade into the loss of the most important thing of all— a human life. That's why we need to make sure those involved in the procurement and transplant system are held accountable so patients—our constituents—are afforded the opportunity for a longer, healthier life.

The committee's report highlighted multiple shortcomings in the U.S. Organ Procurement and Transplantation Network (OPTN). Specifically, it documented instances over the past years where OPOs' clear mistakes were not elevated within United Network of Organ Sharing (UNOS) to the appropriate staff, or the same mistakes were repeated with seemingly inadequate corrective action, investigation, oversight, or guidance from UNOS. This suggests a part of the problem could be systemic organizational failure.

What regulatory or legislative actions could be taken to enhance accountability and performance within the OPTN, especially within UNOS or other potential OPTN contract recipients?

Answer. I thank Senator Barrasso for this important question, and I appreciate how the Senator's experience as a physician brings attention to what is at stake: the lives of patients.

As I testified, to protect patients, I urge Congress and the administration to separate the OPTN functions into different contracts so patients can be served by best- in-class vendors; immediately separate the boards of the OPTN and the OPTN contractor; require public disclosure of all potential conflicts for the contractor and board members; and ensure that patients are safeguarded through open data from both the OPTN and OPOs.

Inaction by the current OPTN contractor, UNOS, has caused real harm to patients; the harm is measured in how long patients wait, and how many patients die waiting for a transplant.

I agree with the bipartisan Senate Finance Committee recommendations (released on August 3, 2022) that the OPTN monopoly needs to be broken up. Having one entity—UNOS, or any singular OPTN monopoly contractor—is not serving patients.

Question. The committee report briefly discussed how the legal requirement that the OPTN contract be awarded to only one entity may deter bidding and competition from other potential contract recipients. Similarly, the report suggests that the OPTN's responsibilities could be better carried out through multiple contracts with entities specialized in one function, like IT or compliance.

What are the advantages and disadvantages of the current OPTN contract that allows only one entity to operate the Network?

What potential trade-offs exist between having only one contract entity versus multiple specialized entities?

Answer. Per my response above, it is critical to break up the OPTN contract and ensure transparency and accountability in the procurement, administration, and competition of the contract moving forward. In my opinion, the current OPTN contract structure does not permit competition, and through this lack of competition, innovation is stifled, suboptimal practice is calcified, and opportunities to improve are lost through the failures of UNOS leadership.

Question. This committee has obviously been hard at work trying to identify shortcomings in the organ procurement and transplantation system over the past couple years. Also within the past couple years, the Trump administration proposed and the Biden administration finalized the OPO final rule. This rule established new performance metrics for OPOs as well as helped promote more frequent oversight and competition among OPOs.

Are there other regulatory or legislative actions Congress or the administration should take to ensure the OPTN is performing to its maximum potential for patients and providers?

Answer. I reiterate my support for the bipartisan recommendations released by the committee on August 3, 2022. As stated in my answers above, I believe that the most important steps Congress and HHS can take are to separate the OPTN functions into different contracts so patients can be served by best-in-class vendors; immediately separate the boards of the OPTN and the OPTN contractor; require public disclosure of all potential conflicts for the contractor and board members; and ensure that patients are safeguarded through open data from both the OPTN and OPOs.

Questions Submitted by Hon. Todd Young

Question. Are there minimum standards and/or training at Organ Procurement Organizations (OPOs) set in Federal regulations or by the OPTN? If not, should there be? What is being done to make sure everyone is performing at their best at OPOs?

Answer. I believe this is a critical issue facing our industry and our transplant system, and I am grateful for the opportunity to describe what can be done to support improvement and increased patient safety at OPOs.

Under current regulations and OPTN policies, there are insufficient standards for OPO provider qualifications and inadequate safety monitoring and protections for patients. OPOs provide clinical care to critically ill patients, and those patients deserve highly qualified clinical providers. Right now, standards in Federal regulations, CMS audits, and OPTN policies do not require that all clinical care provided to donor patients is provided by licensed or certified health-care workers. To ensure patient safety, to protect quality of patient care, and to increase OPO performance, regulations must be revised to include a minimum standard of licensure/certification and a minimum training requirement for any OPO staff who provide clinical care to donor patients.

In my response, I will describe the current state of requirements, and also provide recommendations for actions legislators and regulators can take to address insufficiencies.

First, as the Senator references, the Code of Federal Regulations does contain language that references qualifications of organ procurement organization (OPO) staff. The regulation reads in full:

42 § 486.326 Condition: Human resources.

All OPOs must have a sufficient number of qualified staff, including a director, a medical director, organ procurement coordinators, and hospital development staff to obtain all usable organs from potential donors, and to ensure that required services are provided to families of potential donors, hospitals, tissue banks, and individuals and facilities that use organs for research.

a) Standard: Qualifications.
   1) The OPO must ensure that all individuals who provide services and/or supervise services, including services furnished under contract or arrangement, are qualified to provide or supervise the services.
   2) The OPO must develop and implement a written policy that addresses potential conflicts of interest for the OPO's director, medical director, senior management, and procurement coordinators.
   3) The OPO must have credentialing records for physicians and other practitioners who routinely recover organs in hospitals under contract or arrangement with the OPO and ensure that all physicians and other practitioners who recover organs in hospitals with which the OPO has agreements are qualified and trained.

b) Standard: Staffing.
   4) The OPO must provide sufficient coverage, either by its own staff or under contract or arrangement, to assure both that hospital referral calls are screened for donor potential and that potential donors are evaluated for medical suitability for organ and/or tissue donation in a timely manner.

   5) The OPO must have a sufficient number of qualified staff to provide information and support to potential organ donor families; request consent for donation; ensure optimal maintenance of the donor, efficient placement of organs, and adequate oversight of organ recovery; and conduct QAPI activities, such as death record reviews and hospital development.
   6) The OPO must provide a sufficient number of recovery personnel, either from its own staff or under contract or arrangement, to ensure that all usable organs are recovered in a manner that, to the extent possible, preserves them for transplantation.

c) Standard: Education, training, and performance evaluation. The OPO must provide its staff with the education, training, and supervision necessary to furnish required services. Training must include but is not limited to performance expectations for staff, applicable organizational policies and procedures, and QAPI activities. OPOs must evaluate the performance of their staffs and provide training, as needed, to improve individual and overall staff performance and effectiveness.
d) Standard: Medical director. The OPO's medical director is a physician licensed in at least one of the States or territories within the OPO's service area or as required by State or territory law or by the jurisdiction in which the OPO is located. The medical director is responsible for implementation of the OPO's protocols for donor evaluation and management and organ recovery and placement. The medical director is responsible for oversight of the clinical management of potential donors, including providing assistance in managing a donor case when the surgeon on call is unavailable.

In the text of 42 § 486.326, OPOs are only held to a standard of "sufficient number of qualified staff" under the regulation. The definition of "qualified" is left to the interpretation of the OPO. Such ambiguity in the regulatory text allows for an unacceptable level of variability in training, credentialing/licensing, and verification of qualifications in OPO staffing.

In my opinion as an OPO CEO and critical care nurse, I believe that CMS should define the term "qualified" for any OPO role that includes patient clinical care and interaction with patient health data. An unqualified or underqualified OPO staff person with a role in direct patient care and/or clinical evaluation of health information presents a safety risk to potential donor patients and transplant waitlist patients who rely on the safe, effective procurement of organs.

Right now, some OPOs hire non-licensed health-care workers, or non-health-care workers, in roles with direct patient care. This is permissible under the current regulatory environment. And, since neither CMS nor the OPTN contractor collect information about the number of OPO employees with clinical responsibilities or patient care interactions, our system does not have a way to quantify what lax standards for training and qualification may lead to in terms of adverse events, safety issues, or quality of patient care.

For example, at Mid-America Transplant, we require that any staff member with patient interaction and/or clinical care responsibilities for in our Organ Recovery Center is a registered nurse with a minimum of 2 years of critical care experience. Our definition of "qualified" is based on 3 decades of organizational data and clinical care delivery. Our independently run Donor Care Unit has made this a more salient issue; when donor patients are moved to our facility, outside of a hospital, it is imperative that our team of care providers have a rich experience basis, clinical discernment, and the ability to address a wide range of clinical challenges.

We know that potential donor patients (1) are critically ill with multi-system dysfunction; (2) are unable to personally advocate for their care, due to their condition; and (3) may provide lifesaving organs for transplant only if provided appropriate, safe, evidence-based donor management and monitoring in the course of clinical care at our facility, or in our partner hospitals.

The stakes for the care OPOs provide could not be higher. And, as more OPOs open organ recovery centers outside of hospitals, the qualifications, abilities, and experience level of OPO staff becomes more relevant to quality of care. When a donor patient is in an OPO recovery center, there is no way to rely upon other health-care providers and expertise that would be available in a hospital. A highly qualified OPO workforce is not just an issue of quality, but also safety, for the donors, OPO, transplant centers, and potential organ recipients.

I also wish to direct the Senator to the section of the CMS audit that covers OPO personnel. The relevant text is below:

State Operations Manual Appendix Y from CMS QSOG/CCSQ Part I—Survey Protocol for Organ Procurement Organizations

E. Task Three—Personnel Record Review and Interview (Rev.)

This task covers requirements of the CfC on Human Resources (§ 486.326).

The surveyor should use the organizational chart and/or staff list of OPO staff to select a sample of full-time and contract personnel. Request the personnel records for the selected sample. The personnel interviews and personnel file reviews should cover all staff positions. Review a minimum of five employee files for the clinical and family support staff at the OPO including contract employees in those positions. Expand the sample as necessary based on other survey findings.

1. Personnel Review
   - I. Review the personnel records of OPO employees and contract employees to ensure that the OPO is meeting all requirements in the OPO CfCs at § 486.326.
     - (i) Review current licensure records, orientation records, position description, performance evaluations, conflict of interest evaluations, and training records for the staff.
     - (ii) Verify that the staff are licensed and/or registered in their State.
     - (iii) Verify that orientation and periodic in-service training are provided to the staff.
2. Confirm that the OPO verified prior to recovery that recovery surgeons were currently credentialed.
3. Review the file for the OPO medical director to verify that he/she is currently licensed as a physician in one of the States within the OPO DSA or as required by State or local law. The position description for the medical director clearly delineates his/her roles and responsibilities for implementation of the OPO's protocols for donor evaluation and management and organ recovery and placement.

Under this language, a CMS audit checks for current licensure and certifications held by a sample of 5 staff members. The audit does not verify whether *all* staff members with patient care or patient health record evaluation responsibilities are licensed or certified. The audit also does not define which licenses or certifications are acceptable.

CMS can remediate this problem by modifying the Task Three Personnel Review to include:

- The roles of staff members with direct patient care and/or clinical evaluation of patient health records.
- The number of staff that occupy these roles at the OPO.
- Require a threshold for licensed/certified health-care workers who occupy roles with direct patient care and/or clinical evaluation of patient health records.

There are OPTN policies that reference the requirement that "licensed health-care workers" complete certain tasks or hold certain responsibilities (see: OPTN policy 3.3, 5.8, 14.5). *However, all but one of these OPTN policies reference transplant center activities.* The only reference to OPO qualifications is in OPTN policy 2.14.B, which reads: "Review the OPO's internal policies, procedures, and protocols to verify that it has a written protocol(s) that includes: Definition of qualified health-care professionals to perform the pre-recovery verification [of organs]."

The current OPTN contractor does demonstrate understanding that having qualified health-care workers is important for the care provided by transplant centers. I cannot explain to the committee why the contractor has neglected to ensure that donor patients are cared for by qualified health-care workers, and that the only time at which a qualified health-care professional is necessary for an OPO role under OPTN policy is *at the time of verifying the organ being allocated for transplant.*

An OPO can decide, as an organization, that a person without medical training, without a relevant license or certification (R.N., LPN, paramedic, respiratory therapist, APP, etc.) can occupy a role that requires the ability to evaluate patient health information, make clinical determinations, and even provide clinical care to patients. The OPO would remain in compliance with 42 § 486.326, pass the associated CMS audit requirements, and adhere to current OPTN policy as long as their staffing remained "sufficient" and their own internal employee training declared the person as "qualified."

I cannot speak for anyone else, but I can speak for myself and my family: I would not want a person who is not a licensed or certified health-care provider to perform a physical examination, or evaluate my medical records, or perform a medical procedure on me or someone I love. OPOs provide clinical care to patients. Patients, even those at the end of their lives, deserve high quality, safe, and dignified clinical care performed by highly trained, licensed or certified, health-care workers. Congress, and CMS, must act on this issue in order to ensure patient safety, and increase quality of care provided by OPOs.

Question Submitted by Hon. Maggie Hassan

Question. In 2019, the National Council on Disability (NCD) released a report finding that people with disabilities are often excluded as organ transplant candidates due to their disabilities. Does your organization have a policy that covers organ transplant access for individuals with disabilities?

Answer. As an organ procurement organization (OPO), Mid-America Transplant does not have a direct role in evaluating and listing patients for transplantation. Instead, our work is with potential donor patients who are referred to our OPO by hospitals.

Our OPO strongly supports equitable access to transplantation for people with disabilities. Although our own practice is with potential deceased donor patients, instead of potential transplant recipients, we have ensured in our clinical processes that no potential deceased donor patient may be excluded from consideration for organ, eye, and tissue donation due solely to disability.

Our team has provided high-quality, compassionate care to deceased donor patients with documented disabilities and their families. We believe that equitable access to care for people with disabilities should be a goal for both organ procurement and transplant center providers. People with disabilities who are able to be organ donors should receive equitable, safe, high quality care from all organ procurement organizations. We believe that people with disabilities who have become deceased organ, eye, and tissue donors have provided a lifesaving gift, and should be honored and recognized for the legacy they create as donor heroes.

Question Submitted by Hon. Bill Cassidy

Question. Section 413.408 of CMS Proposed Rule 1752 sought to clarify that when a donor is transferred from a certified transplant center (CTC) to an Organ Procurement Organization Recovery Center, the CTC would be allowed to count the organs recovered at the OPO center in their cost report. This portion of the proposed rule has not been finalized by CMS. What is your view on this proposed change?

Answer. I feel very strongly that the CTC should be allowed to count the organs on their cost report that are recovered at OPO Recovery Center. The recognition and incentive for CTCs, who are also donor hospitals, to identify, refer, and provide early clinical management for the potential donor patients remains imperative to increasing the volume of donors and transplantable organs. Currently, the financial barrier placed on the CTCs who transfer their cases to OPO ORCs handicaps growth and cost savings. The location where the organs are excised, which is the defining statement today for how this count is determined, is contained in an instruction line on the cost report at the CTC. This action in the donation process is not the driver of increased supply of organs, and as such, should not serve as the financial incentive for donation.

Equally concerning is that this methodology for organ counting provides tremendous financial benefit for organ recovery centers based at CTCs, as some OPOs have adopted. The drain on the CMS trust fund has increased as donor patients are transferred from many outside hospitals to the CTC, where all the organs can be counted based on this instruction line. This serves as an additional revenue stream for the CTC and while this practice has certainly been deemed appropriate, leaving the financial barrier in place for independent ORC transfers from CTCs does not seem to be in the best interests of increasing lives saved through transplantation.

These two distinct actions appear to be in conflict. I urge the committee, and CMS, to consider what can be done to address this financial conundrum while ensuring we are all good stewards of CMS dollars. Allowing the CTCs to define success as "where the potential donor patient was identified and declared dead" would equalize the incentive to aid in increasing the transplantable organ supply.

Questions Submitted by Hon. Rob Portman

Staff Requirements

Question. In your opening statement you mentioned that there are not any clinical training, licensure, or certification requirements for OPO staff. It is my understanding that CMS has standards from 2005 relating to OPO practitioners and states that OPO staff must be qualified and trained. Clearly this ambiguity has been an issue.

Could you elaborate on the requirements that you think should be mandatory for OPO staff?

Answer. I believe this is a critical issue facing our industry and our transplant system, and I am grateful for the opportunity to describe what can be done to support improvement and increased patient safety at OPOs.

Under current regulations and OPTN policies, there are insufficient standards for OPO provider qualifications and inadequate safety monitoring and protections for patients. OPOs provide clinical care to critically ill patients, and those patients deserve highly qualified clinical providers. Right now, standards in Federal regulations, CMS audits, and OPTN policies do not require that all clinical care provided to donor patients is provided by licensed or certified health-care workers. To ensure patient safety, to protect quality of patient care, and to increase OPO performance, regulations must be revised to include a minimum standard of licensure/certification and a minimum training requirement for any OPO staff who provide clinical care to donor patients.

In my response, I will describe the current state of requirements, and also provide recommendations for actions legislators and regulators can take to address insufficiencies. First, as the Senator references, the Code of Federal Regulations does contain language that references qualifications of organ procurement organization (OPO) staff. The regulation reads in full:

42 § 486.326 Condition: Human resources.

All OPOs must have a sufficient number of qualified staff, including a director, a medical director, organ procurement coordinators, and hospital development staff to obtain all usable organs from potential donors, and to ensure that required services are provided to families of potential donors, hospitals, tissue banks, and individuals and facilities that use organs for research.

a) Standard: Qualifications.
    1) The OPO must ensure that all individuals who provide services and/or supervise services, including services furnished under contract or arrangement, are qualified to provide or supervise the services.

2) The OPO must develop and implement a written policy that addresses potential conflicts of interest for the OPO's director, medical director, senior mangement, and procurement coordinators.
3) The OPO must have credentialing records for physicians and other practitioners who routinely recover organs in hospitals under contract or arrangement with the OPO and ensure that all physicians and other practitioners who recover organs in hospitals with which the OPO has agreements are qualified and trained.

b) Standard: Staffing.
1) The OPO must provide sufficient coverage, either by its own staff or under contract or arrangement, to assure both that hospital referral calls are screened for donor potential and that potential donors are evaluated for medical suitability for organ and/or tissue donation in a timely manner.
2) The OPO must have a sufficient number of qualified staff to provide information and support to potential organ donor families; request consent for donation; ensure optimal maintenance of the donor, efficient placement of organs, and adequate oversight of organ recovery; and conduct QAPI activities, such as death record reviews and hospital development.
3) The OPO must provide a sufficient number of recovery personnel, either from its own staff or under contract or arrangement, to ensure that all usable organs are recovered in a manner that, to the extent possible, preserves them for transplantation.

c) Standard: Education, training, and performance evaluation. The OPO must provide its staff with the education, training, and supervision necessary to furnish required services. Training must include but is not limited to performance expectations for staff, applicable organizational policies and procedures, and QAPI activities. OPOs must evaluate the performance of their staffs and provide training, as needed, to improve individual and overall staff performance and effectiveness.

d) Standard: Medical director. The OPO's medical director is a physician licensed in at least one of the States or territories within the OPO's service area or as required by State or territory law or by the jurisdiction in which the OPO is located. The medical director is responsible for implementation of the OPO's protocols for donor evaluation and management and organ recovery and placement. The medical director is responsible for oversight of the clinical management of potential donors, including providing assistance in managing a donor case when the surgeon on call is unavailable.

In the text of 42 § 486.326, OPOs are only held to a standard of "sufficient number of qualified staff" under the regulation. The definition of "qualified" is left to the interpretation of the OPO. Such ambiguity in the regulatory text allows for an unacceptable level of variability in training, credentialing/licensing, and verification of qualifications in OPO staffing.

In my opinion as an OPO CEO and critical care nurse, I believe that CMS should define the term "qualified" for any OPO role that includes patient clinical care and interaction with patient health data. An unqualified or underqualified OPO staff person with a role in direct patient care and/or clinical evaluation of health information presents a safety risk to potential donor patients and transplant waitlist patients who rely on the safe, effective procurement of organs.

Right now, some OPOs hire non-licensed health-care workers, or non-health-care workers, in roles with direct patient care. This is permissible under the current regulatory environment. And, since neither CMS nor the OPTN contractor collect information about the number of OPO employees with clinical responsibilities or patient care interactions, our system does not have a way to quantify what lax standards for training and qualification may lead to in terms of adverse events, safety issues, or quality of patient care.

For example, at Mid-America Transplant, we require that any staff member with patient interaction and/or clinical care responsibilities for in our Organ Recovery Center is a registered nurse with a minimum of 2 years of critical care experience. Our definition of "qualified" is based on 3 decades of organizational data and clinical care delivery. Our independently run Donor Care Unit has made this a more salient issue; when donor patients are moved to our facility, outside of a hospital, it is imperative that our team of care providers have a rich experience basis, clinical discernment, and the ability to address a wide range of clinical challenges.

We know that potential donor patients (4) are critically ill often with multi-system dysfunction; (5) are unable to personally advocate for their care, due to their condition; and (6) may provide lifesaving organs for transplant only if provided appropriate, safe, evidence-based donor management and monitoring in the course of clinical care at our facility, or in our partner hospitals.

The stakes for the care OPOs provide could not be higher. And, as more OPOs open organ recovery centers outside of hospitals, the qualifications, abilities, and experience level of OPO staff becomes more relevant to quality of care. When a donor patient is in an OPO recovery center, there is no way to rely upon other health-care providers and expertise that would be available in a hospital. A highly qualified OPO workforce is not just an issue of quality, but also safety, for the donors, OPO, transplant centers, and potential organ recipients.

I also wish to direct the Senator to the section of the CMS audit that covers OPO personnel. The relevant text is below:

State Operations Manual Appendix Y from CMS QSOG/CCSQ Part I—Survey Protocol for Organ Procurement Organizations

E. Task Three—Personnel Record Review and Interview (Rev.)

This task covers requirements of the CfC on Human Resources (§ 486.326).

The surveyor should use the organizational chart and/or staff list of OPO staff to select a sample of full-time and contract personnel. Request the personnel records for the selected sample. The personnel interviews and personnel file reviews should cover all staff positions. Review a minimum of five employee files for the clinical and family support staff at the OPO including contract employees in those positions. Expand the sample as necessary based on other survey findings.

1) Personnel Review
   I. Review the personnel records of OPO employees and contract employees to ensure that the OPO is meeting all requirements in the OPO CfCs at § 486.326.
      (i) Review current licensure records, orientation records, position description, performance evaluations, conflict of interest evaluations, and training records for the staff.
      (ii) Verify that the staff are licensed and/or registered in their State.

(iii) Verify that orientation and periodic in-service training are provided to the staff.

2) Confirm that the OPO verified prior to recovery that recovery surgeons were currently credentialed.
3) Review the file for the OPO medical director to verify that he/she is currently licensed as a physician in one of the States within the OPO DSA or as required by State or local law. The position description for the medical director clearly delineates his/her roles and responsibilities for implementation of the OPO's protocols for donor evaluation and management and organ recovery and placement.

Under this language, a CMS audit checks for current licensure and certifications held by a sample of 5 staff members. The audit does not verify whether all staff members with patient care or patient health record evaluation responsibilities are licensed or certified. The audit also does not define which licenses or certifications are acceptable.

CMS can remediate this problem by modifying the Task Three Personnel Review to include the roles of staff members with direct patient care and/or clinical evaluation of patient health records; the number of staff that occupy these roles at the OPO; and require a threshold for licensed/certified health-care workers who occupy roles with direct patient care and/or clinical evaluation of patient health records.

There are OPTN policies that reference the requirement that "licensed health-care workers" complete certain tasks or hold certain responsibilities (see: OPTN policy 3.3, 5.8, 14.5). However, all but one of these OPTN policies reference transplant center activities. The only reference to OPO qualifications is in OPTN policy 2.14.B, which reads: "Review the OPO's internal policies, procedures, and protocols to verify that it has a written protocol(s) that includes: Definition of qualified health-care professionals to perform the pre-recovery verification [of organs]."

The current OPTN contractor does demonstrate understanding that having qualified health-care workers is important for the care provided by transplant centers. I cannot explain to the committee why the contractor has neglected to ensure that donor patients are cared for by qualified health-care workers, and that the only time at which a qualified health-care professional is necessary for an OPO role under OPTN policy is at the time of verifying the organ being allocated for transplant.

An OPO can decide, as an organization, that a person without medical training, without a relevant license or certification (RN, LPN, paramedic, respiratory therapist, APP, etc.) can occupy a role that requires the ability to evaluate patient health information, make clinical determinations, and even provide clinical care to patients. The OPO would remain in compliance with 42 § 486.326, pass the associated CMS audit requirements, and adhere to current OPTN policy as long as their staffing remained "sufficient" and their own internal employee training declared the person as "qualified."

I cannot speak for anyone else, but I can speak for myself and my family: I would not want a person who is not a licensed or certified health-care provider to perform a physical examination, or evaluate my medical records, or perform a medical procedure on me or someone I love. OPOs provide clinical care to patients. Patients, even those at the end of their lives, deserve high quality, safe, and dignified clinical care performed by highly trained, licensed or certified, health-care workers. Congress, and CMS, must act on this issue in order to ensure patient safety, and increase quality of care provided by OPOs.

Declined Organs

Question. You noted in your opening statement that time is wasted by organs being declined and that your organization has been successful at identifying surgeons that accept kidneys that would otherwise be declined.

Can you explain the differences in why some surgeons are more willing to accept organs for transplant that would otherwise be declined?

Answer. Our system's transplant center metrics—those produced by the Scientific Registry of Transplant Recipients—monitor and grade even minute areas of transplant center practice, such that half of transplant centers are rated as "aggressive" or "not aggressive" in their organ acceptance practices in a given year.1 Emphasis on flagging transplant center practice means that much of our information about discarded or utilized organs is, as a system, related to transplant centers, not OPOs.

In contrast, only 1 in 5 OPOs received a similar, definitive message from SRTR on their organ procurement performance over the same period.1 We can, as a system, improve organ utilization, but we must understand all of the drivers of under-utilization of organs at both transplant centers and OPOs, and create standards for donor management, organ offers, and allocation practice across OPOs.[5,6,7,8]

Little data exists about why some OPOs appear to be more successful at allocating organs to transplant centers that accept them.[8] What I can tell you is that our OPO has navigated our own way to increasing utilization of organs, and that efforts made by the current OPTN contractor to improve organ acceptance have not just been unhelpful, but have actually worsened the problem.[9]

Additionally, I can share that from Mid-America Transplant's own experience, not all OPOs allocate organs in the same way, with the same staffing model, or with the same emphasis on making every donor organ offer as amenable to acceptance or consideration by surgeons. There is significant variation between OPOs in how organs are described in organ offers, allocated, and even how they are procured and transported to transplant centers. Some of us have dedicated allocation staff who are trained to maximize utilization. Some of us have a dedicated process to establish relationships with transplant centers outside of our area that are

[5] Doby, B.L., Ross-Driscoll, K., Yu, S., Godwin, M., Lee, K.J., and Lynch, R.J. (2022). Exam- ining utilization of kidneys as a function of procurement performance. *American Journal of Transplantation: Official Journal of the American Society of Transplantation and the American Society of Transplant Surgeons, 22*(6), 1614–1623, *https://doi.org/10.1111/ajt.16985.*

[6] Lentine, K.L., Fleetwood, V.A., Caliskan, Y., Randall, H., Wellen, J.R., Lichtenberger, M., Dedert, C., Rothweiler, R., Marklin, G., Brockmeier, D., Schnitzler, M.A., Husain, S.A., Mohan, S., Kasiske, B.L., Cooper, M., Mannon, R.B., and Axelrod, D.A. (2022). Deceased Donor Procure- ment Biopsy Practices, Interpretation, and Histology-Based Decision-Making: A Survey of US Kidney Transplant Centers. *Kidney International Reports,* 7(6), 1268–1277, *https://doi.org/ 10.1016/j.ekir.2022.03.021.*

[7] Giorgakis, E., Ivanics, T., Khorsandi, S.E., Wallace, D., Burdine, L., Jassem, W., Mathur, A.K., and Heaton, N. (2022). Disparities in the Use of Older Donation After Circulatory Death Liver Allografts in the United States Versus the United Kingdom. *Transplantation,* 106(8), e358–e367, *https://doi.org/10.1097/ TP.0000000000004185.*

[8] Cannon, R.M., Nassel, A.F., Walker, J.T., Sheikh, S.S., Orandi, B.J., Lynch, R.J., Shah, M.B., Goldberg, D.S., and Locke, J.E. (2022). Lost potential and missed opportunities for DCD liver transplantation in the United States. *American Journal of Surgery,* 224(3), 990–998, *https:// doi.org/10.1016/j.amjsurg.2022.05.001.*

[9] Schold, J.D., Mohan, S., Huml, A., Buccini, L.D., Sedor, J.R., Augustine, J.J., and Poggio, E.D. (2021). Failure to Advance Access to Kidney Transplantation over Two Decades in the United States. *Journal of the American Society of Nephrology: JASN, 32*(4), 913–926. Advance online publication, *https://doi.org/10.1681/ASN.2020060888.*

less risk averse in their organ acceptances. Some of us see that this variation between how OPOs work leads to longer case times, longer times to organ acceptance, and what can be a very inefficient system of communication between surgeons and OPOs. All of these issues could, and should, be addressed by a functional OPTN contractor. To date, UNOS has not.

Prepared Statement of Barry S. Friedman, R.N., BSN, Executive Director, AdventHealth Transplant Institute

Chairman Wyden, Ranking Member Crapo, Senator Grassley, and members of the committee, on behalf of AdventHealth, I am honored to be extended the opportunity to provide testimony on the current state of organ transplant policy in the United States. My testimony reflects more than 30 years of health care/transplant experience and my direct leadership involvement in the United Network for Organ Sharing (UNOS) and the Organ Procurement Transplantation Network (OPTN), including the UNOS board of directors and the Membership Professional Standards Committee. I also proudly served 30 years in the United States Air Force—including two tours of duty during Operation Iraqi Freedom.

I currently serve as the executive director for the AdventHealth Transplant Institute, one of the busiest transplant centers in the Nation, having performed more than 4,000 transplants. Our survival rates are among the highest in the country, making us one of the most highly-sought adult and pediatric multi-organ transplant programs in the United States. We were the first hospital in central Florida to successfully perform a heart transplant. Today, we offer a wide range of transplant options, including, heart, kidney, lung, liver, pancreas, and blood and marrow. We are also home to a comprehensive living donor kidney program.

As the executive director of the Institute, I take very seriously our sacred duty to the families and patients who entrust us with the gift of life to provide organs for transplant. It is our duty to be good stewards of these organs, honoring the faith of these families and the health of our communities. I offer testimony specifically on UNOS/OPTN oversight of transplant policy, data and interoperability challenges, and opportunities to improve transplant equity across the Nation.

Unos's Oversight of Transplant Policy

Families in need of a lifesaving organ have no option but to trust the organ tranplantation system that is in place. Unfortunately, that system has failed many awaiting organ transplant due to lack of oversight and accountability. An organ is the greatest gift someone can give and yet, we have created a system that does not result in the good stewardship of that gift. Approximately 23 percent of kidneys procured from deceased donors are not used and discarded, resulting in preventable deaths.[10]1 It is our responsibility to address this issue.

[10] How to Decrease the Discard Rate of Donated Organs, The American Society of Nephrology, *https://www.sciencedaily.com/releases/2017/10/171005190255.htm.*

Avoidable Organ Loss

Organ transportation is a process left to each federally designated organ procurement organization (OPO) to implement. OPOs currently develop their own relationships with transportation couriers, relying on them to engage with airlines, charter flights, ground transportation and Federal agencies to facilitate transportation. If an organ leaves the OPO's custody, OPOs and transplant centers are solely dependent on airline personnel to move organs on and off commercial flights in an expedited manner. In many cases, organs must connect from one flight to another, leaving airline personnel responsible for transfers. Neither OPOs nor couriers have control of an organ upon surrendering it to the airlines. While anyone can now track where their Amazon or FedEx package is, there is currently no consistent way of tracking organs.

The OPTN recently broadened kidney-sharing policies with the goal of increasing the number of organs available. However, this policy is being instituted in an environment where the kidneys may be unescorted and unprotected during transit, making them more vulnerable to discard. This problem has been exacerbated due to industry staffing shortages caused by the pandemic and flight delays. There are occasions when we try to put the organs on charter flights, however, there are not enough charter flights available and the costs are significantly higher. When the transplant community raised these issues to UNOS at the regional meetings, UNOS staff stated that UNOS was not responsible for providing this service and that it was "out of scope for discussion."

Many news articles have promoted the use of GPS tracking during organ shipments.[11,12,13] UNOS developed an organ-tracking system to pilot with OPOs and transplant centers. However, staff from the UNOS Organ Center did not participate in organ tracking. There were no built-in warnings when an anticipated check point was not met. Further, the system depended on recycling the GPS trackers for repeated use, which was difficult if not impossible to do. Due to these challenges, we opted out of the UNOS tracking system and are now working with a different courier company that uses less expensive and higher quality trackers which can be discarded and monitor shipments in real time.

To address these organ transportation issues, this committee should recommend the following:

1) Promote increased transparency by requiring the reporting of all organ loss and "near misses" due to transportation issues. UNOS has a safety reporting system; however, our program has reported these near misses with no feedback or follow-up to the safety report submission.
2) Establish a national organ shipping system that would monitor the progress of all shipments (e.g., aircrafts, ground transport, train transportation) in real time on behalf

[11] For All Transplant Programs: The UNOS Organ Tracking Beta Test. UNOS, 2021, *https:// unos.org/news/labs-organ-tracking-beta-test/.*

[12] How BrickHouse Security's GPS Tracking Helps the National Kidney Registry Save Lives. Fierce Healthcare, 2010, *https://www.fiercehealthcare.com/healthcare/transplants-transformed-how-brickhouse-security-s-gps-tracking-helps-national-kidney.*

[13] How Lifesaving Organs for Transplant Go Missing in Transit. Kaiser Health News, 2020, *https://khn.org/news/how-lifesaving-organs-for-transplant-go-missing-in-transit/.*

of OPOs and transplant centers that opt in. This could be done through a partnership with a third-party organization that actually has expertise in this.

3) Require all OPOs to utilize GPS technology to transport unaccompanied organs. GPS tracking should be constantly monitored by either OPO staff or a contracted service.
4) Require the development of safety standards for courier and airline companies to follow when transporting human organs for transplant.

Inferior Data Availability and Interoperability

Data availability and transparency are key to improving organ procurement, UNOS has not proven capable of this function. OPTN technology lags significantly behind other technology platforms. In daily use by our transplant center, we have found the current OPTN IT contractor to be slow and reactive, one that does not provide state-of-the-art service and does not prioritize being technologically current. This contributes to a fractured flow of health IT between OPOs, donor hospitals, transplant programs, and UNOS with significant data interoperability challenges. During regional meetings, this issue was raised and even though transplant centers voted for a resolution, UNOS called these concerns "sentiments," and they were not given serious consideration.

I also believe there is a conflict of interest related to the management of IT functionalities by UNOS, as the IT tools that they offer transplant centers come with an additional cost despite these being essential for the safely management of organs.

To help improve the availability and useability of data, Congress should:

1) Separate the IT components of UNOS operations from the broader OPTN contract with HHS.
2) Authorize and require OPOs and the OPTN to participate in Health Information Exchanges.
3) No longer require OPOs to maintain additional, separate databases with donor information, instead allowing them to transfer donor information directly from hospital EHRs to the OPTN database.

Ineffective Organ Screenings

UNOS is not effectively screening organ offers so they can be quickly directed to transplant programs. Rather, UNOS asks transplant centers to voluntarily opt out of certain organ offers via an organ offer filtering process. History has repeatedly demonstrated that transplant programs desire to be informed of every organ available, even if they would never transplant it. Thus, they have a poor track record of voluntarily filtering offers. As a result, OPOs must waste valuable time making organ offers to centers that will never accept them. Time wasted equates to prolonged cold ischemic time, which equates to lost transplant opportunities. It is a vicious cycle that disadvantages patients on the waiting list. Thus far, UNOS refuses to adopt a more "placement friendly" philosophy. Additionally, while UNOS is proposing to increase their patient registration fees, they are not offering any increase in value or improvements in their processes.

Due to the limited expertise that UNOS has in the placement of organs, it would be best if they were no longer responsible for developing organ placement practices. In the early years of UNOS, the placement of organs was stellar. If UNOS cannot perform this task, we recommend high-performing OPOs and transplant centers be partnered with technology and artificial intelligence experts using predictive models about organ utilization. Prioritizing organ offers to the centers most likely to use them will drive change in transplant center organ acceptance practices.

The UNOS policymaking process lacks transparency. Currently, OPTN board members concurrently serve as the board members of UNOS, which creates a conflict of interest that contributes to the lack of transparency. The board then further delineates with an executive board, where closed-session decisions are made and sent out to the transplant community for implementation. UNOS has formed many committees throughout the years to develop policy changes. However, these committees are formed in a vacuum; there is no call for nominations and no data shared with the transplant community to explain the rationale behind a given policy change. A perfect example of this is the recent organ allocation change of policy where a geography committee was formed; this policy resulted in the inequitable distribution of organs and higher kidney discard rates.

UNOS requires transplant centers to pay a registration fee for adding patients to the OPTN wait list to receive an organ transplant. Since 2021, these fees have increased from $926.00 to $990.00 in 2022; UNOS has proposed to increase the registration fees to $1,044.00 in 2023. These are additional costs that go into the Medicare cost report, costing the Federal Government more money, with little transparency as to why. Transplant center leaders in the past have not been given a reason for these increases.

There is no representation from patient advocacy groups or experts in quality measurement and improvement. The OPTN should be required to ensure that all populations, including ethnic minorities and persons with disabilities, are represented in the transplant policy development process. Finally, there should be representation of organizations, like the National Quality Forum, that have experience in quality measurement. Failure to make these changes will result in the continued development of inequitable policies and practices that do not result in measurable quality improvements.

Overall and most importantly in this equation, we are jeopardizing the trust to our most precious resource—organ donors and their families and the recipients of those organs.

We applaud the Senate Finance Committee for listening and learning today and thank you for providing the United States of America the opportunity to maintain the stellar clinical care for our patients who require lifesaving organ transplants.

Questions Submitted for the Record to Barry S. Friedman, R.N., BSN
Questions Submitted by Hon. John Barrasso

Question. What regulatory or legislative actions could be taken to enhance accountability and performance within the OPTN, especially within UNOS or other potential OPTN contract recipients?

Answer. First, I would like to endorse the bipartisan findings of the Senate Finance Committee's August 2022 investigation into the Nation's organ transplant system.[14] My recommended actions to be taken align with that report's recommendations, particularly: removing barriers to competition; increasing the pool of potential bidders by clarifying that the OPTN functions described in NOTA and subsequent amendments may be operated by more than one contractor; and promoting innovation in all OPTN functions (e.g., policy development, compliance and patient safety mentoring, IT infrastructure, coordinating transport of organs, etc.) as the best qualified entities with distinct skill sets could compete for contracts for these functions.

In order to enhance accountability, Congress should require that any entities managing the OPTN:

- Establish a public comment process for stakeholders to suggest innovations and new methods to improve the system. The goal of this suggestion is to improve the level of trust between any OPTN contractors and OPTN member institutions during the policy development process. Currently, OPTN members are encouraged to submit written comments regarding policies under development. However, unlike the Federal public comment process, the OPTN is not required to respond publicly and in writing as to the OPTN committee's response to each comment and whether/why the comment was adopted or rejected. If OPTN committees were to engage in this process it would improve the accountability relationship among the committees, any OPTN contractors and the members. A similar process could be implemented at OPTN member regional meetings in which comments could be provided during discussion, catalogued by contractor staff, and provided to committees for review and written response. This process would help foster transparency and create an environment for self-improvement within the OPTN. These written summaries could also help establish a record of issues brought to the OPTN and how they were addressed.
- Develop a feedback loop in the decision-making process, allowing members to quickly share any opportunities for improvement or refinement of a policy after a change. Currently there is not a rapid response process available to OPTN members when a policy change creates unintended consequences or is not achieving the intended effect. The only rapid response mechanism available to OPTN members is the patient safety portal but this suggestion is not consistent with the portal's current purpose. Members become frustrated when occurrences happen and there is nowhere to catalogue events that provide needed insights about the "real-world" implications of a policy change. The absence of a feedback loop perpetuates distrust between members and the OPTN/contractor and discourages opportunities for rapid course corrections when required.
- Promote increased transparency by requiring the public reporting of all organ loss and "near misses" due to transportation issues. There is currently no OPTN policy requiring members to report the failure to transplant organs. Organ loss can result from:
    - Insufficient efforts to match an organ with a candidate;

---

[14] A System in Need of Repair Hearing Report. The United States Senate Committee on Fi- nance (August 3, 2022), *https://www.finance.senate.gov/imo/media/doc/UNOS%20Hearing%20Memo.pdf.*

- o Insufficient efforts to optimize organ function prior to placement attempts;
- o A turndown in the donor operating room leading to a non-transplantable organ;
- o Mishandling the organ acceptance/candidate notification process; and
- o Lateness/damage/loss during transportation.

Current OPTN data vastly underreport the incidence of organ loss during transportation, which has resulted in a lack of urgency from the OPTN to address the issue. Although UNOS has a safety reporting system, which could be deployed for the purpose of documenting organ loss or near loss, there is no public reporting, feedback, or follow up to members when the system is used. Because problems submitted by OPOs and transplant centers go unaddressed, there is no incentive for members to report occurrences. This is a glaring omission in need of rapid correction.

In order to enhance performance, Congress should:

- Require the establishment of a national organ shipping system that monitors the progress of all shipments (e.g., aircrafts, ground transport) in real time on behalf of OPOs and Transplant Centers that opt in. This could be done through a partnership with a third-party organization with demonstrated logistics expertise. This logistics system could be awarded via contract, with operational fees paid for by OPOs and transplant programs that utilize it. Responsibility for tracking and trending logistics problems would lie with the system; it would also be accountable for developing relationships with national commercial airline carriers to support better treatment of organs while in transit.
- Require that all OPOs utilize GPS technology to transport unaccompanied organs. GPS tracking should be constantly monitored by either a contracted service, the OPO, or the Transplant Centers.
- Require the development and adoption of safety standards, with involvement of the Federal Aviation Administration, for OPOs as well as courier and airline companies when transporting human organs for transplant. The lack of safety standards for the management of organs results in them being often handled as any ordinary piece of merchandise.
- Separate the IT components of the OPTN contract so that a third-party with expertise in this area can manage this function.
- Require OPOs and the OPTN participate in Health Information Exchanges.
- Encourage automated exchange of data between OPOs and hospital electronic health records (EHRs) for the purpose of potential organ donor referral and evaluation. This process would allow hospitals to have an electronic notification option so that clinicians don't have to cease their work to make donation referrals. Further, all OPOs should have the technological capability to receive these referrals electronically.
- Ensure that any OPTN contractor(s) develop and maintain Application Programming Interfaces (APIs) that automatically provide required data to the OPTN and ease access of data for researchers/ other contractors, stakeholders, and outside organizations. OPTN and transplant program databases should no longer be the mechanism through which data are provided to the OPTN. The This will allow for better access to OPTN data and operations information (e.g., data generated during the process of making and

receiving organ offers) so efficiencies can be created to decrease the number of discarded organs.

Question. What are the advantages and disadvantages of the current OPTN contract that allows only one entity to operate the network?

Answer. I strongly encourage Congress to ensure the OPTN contract can be opened to multiple contractor bids, particularly by separating out the IT function from the rest of the contract. Having a single entity manage the entire OPTN contract puts all the decision-making power into the hands of one organization, making it more difficult to hold it accountable to Federal oversight agencies, OPTN members or the patients it is intended to serve. In the current environment, policy-making becomes self-serving to the needs and capabilities of the contractor rather than what is in the best interest of recipient and donor patients. For example, when UNOS was tasked by the Federal Government to create an IT system, they built it but did not seek feedback on what capabilities members needed or what the price point of using the technology should be. Because the current OPTN contractor is not, per se, an IT company, the choice of technologies it adopts cannot be rapidly altered to keep up with industry advances. Consequently, the OPTN's current IT infrastructure is inefficient, outdated and inadequately serves patients and OPTN members. Implementing even small changes to the system takes months to years to accomplish, as illustrated by several sources.[15]

UNOS also determines the transplant candidate registration fees with little input or transparency beyond a small subset of board members as to how those fees will be used or why they are necessary. Currently, members have no other choice but to pay whatever rate is set by UNOS with no explanation. Registration fees have increased from $926.00 in 2021 to $990.00 in 2022 and UNOS has already proposed to increase the registration fees to $1,044.00 in 2023. These price hikes are then reflected on the Medicare Cost Report, costing the Federal Government more money, with little transparency as to why they are necessary. Additionally, the Senate Finance Committee noted the issue of UNOS double charging transplant centers (and ultimately payers, including Medicare) for each wait-listed patient—charging a fee once as the OPTN and once as UNOS. UNOS fees are also not subject to contractual controls from HRSA, allowing UNOS to spend taxpayer dollars for self-benefit and entrenchment, rather than to benefit patients.

When one organization is tasked with fulfilling so many different functions, it can essentially become an expert at nothing, contributing to inefficiencies. For example, UNOS currently requires information from our providers that they have already been provided but fail to retain in a way that allows ongoing use. When transplant programs hire a new physician that comes from another transplant center, the physician has to resubmit all their cases and certifications to UNOS despite having already provided the same information to UNOS from their previous transplant center. Even though these physicians have worked for other member transplant centers and have previously submitted all the same cases and certifications, they must resubmit that same information in its entirety when they move facilities. Because UNOS does not fear the loss of its OPTN contractor responsibilities, it does not have any sufficient incentive to build efficiencies into an outdated process.

---

[15] National Library of Medicine. Restructuring the OPTN contract to achieve policy coherence and infrastructure excellence, *https://www.ncbi.nlm.nih.gov/pmc/articles/PMC6494733/*.

Question. What potential trade-offs exist between having only one contract entity versus multiple specialized entities?

Answer. I believe that one organization operating in today's health care and technology environment cannot achieve the operational quality required to fulfill all aspects of the OPTN contract. If another singular organization were to replace UNOS, similar issues would eventually arise. There are many aspects to organ procurement and transplantation, including identifying organs, transporting organs, tracking organs and quality improvement, to rely on a single contractor to achieve high performance levels. It would be very difficult for one sole organization to deliver the best quality on every aspect or to be an expert in all these functions.

To ensure the greatest quality, entities could submit bids to fulfill one or more responsibilities of the OPTN. The best organization equipped for that responsibility should be granted a contract. For example, a technology-focused organization would be better suited to develop a national system of automated, electronic notifications for organ donation than a company with limited IT capabilities.

I believe that multiple organizations could achieve functionality together provided there is engaged and collaborative oversight by Federal entities. Involving multiple contractors in OPTN operations is not a new concept. In 2000, HRSA chose for the first time to award the Scientific Registry for Transplant Recipients (SRTR) to an entity other than UNOS and while it took time to adapt to the changes, UNOS did collaborate with the SRTR. This arrangement has benefitted the donation and transplantation community, particularly around data transparency. It is not unreasonable to expect that if the existing OPTN contractor (or any future OPTN contractors) were awarded only a portion of current OPTN contracted responsibilities, cooperation and collaboration with other entities would develop.

Question. Are there other regulatory or legislative actions Congress or the administration should take to ensure the OPTN is performing to its maximum potential for patients and providers?

Answer. Congress or the administration should ensure that there is more meaningful engagement from UNOS with patient advocacy groups, as well as experts in quality measurement and improvement. The OPTN should be required to ensure that all populations, including racial/ethnic minorities and persons with disabilities, are represented in the transplant policy-development process. Further, the OPTN should ensure that the voices of patients and donor families who volunteer on OPTN boards and committees are heard and their priorities for better service/resources for patients are acted upon.

Next, Congress should require for the OPTN board and any contractor boards to be separated. This would help prevent any conflict of interest, enable the OPTN board to focus on service to patients, and allow members to provide feedback more openly to contractors.

Congress or the administration should also ensure that all organizations that are managing the OPTN follow security guidelines to protect member data. UNOS requires significant information about our transplant centers and practices. Now, more than ever, it is critical that this information be protected. Managing organizations should be required to follow security requirements to ensure that patient data is protected.

Question Submitted by Hon. Maggie Hassan

Question. In 2019, the National Council on Disability (NCD) released a report finding that people with disabilities are often excluded as organ transplant candidates due to their disabilities. Does your organization have a policy that covers organ transplant access for individuals with disabilities?

Answer. AdventHealth Transplant Institute adheres to guidelines set up by HHS and the U.S. Public Health Service (USPHS) to determine who is qualified to receive an organ. AdventHealth maintains policies addressing how we provide equitable care to patients with disabilities across our system. AdventHealth Transplant Institute evaluates every patient's intellectual and adaptive functioning in a clear, evidence-based and systematic manner. If a patient's disability hinders their ability to receive an organ, we do everything in our power to provide special accommodations for them. For example, having someone available to support the patient through the transplant process is a requirement in being a candidate for an organ. If someone does not have anyone or cannot support themselves, AdventHealth Transplant Institute would help find them a caretaker so they could meet the criteria to receive an organ transplant.

Prepared Statement of Calvin Henry, Region 3 Patient Affairs Committee (PAC) Representative, Organ Procurement and Transplantation Network (OPTN)

Chairman Wyden, Ranking Member Crapo, and members of the committee, my name is Calvin Henry, and I serve on the OPTN Patient Affairs Committee as the Region 3 Representative for the southeastern U.S. and the U.S. territory of Puerto Rico. I am also a double lung transplant recipient of 9½ years and have spent much of that time as a dedicated patient advocate in direct support of organ transplant candidates and recipients, as a community advocate for organ donation, and as a strong proponent for system-wide improvements and transparency throughout the organ procurement and transplantation process. It is a privilege to be invited here today to share my thoughts regarding the current state of this system.

I would like to share with the committee a bit of my experience navigating the transplant system in order to get wait-listed and then receive a transplant.

Fifteen years ago, I was diagnosed with a terminal lung disease that was later identified as scleroderma and informed that my only option for survival was to receive a double lung transplant. I was told, however, that I was unlikely to receive one and that I should just begin making end of life preparations. I quickly moved on to another practitioner who subsequently made the referral for me.

The several years after that initial diagnosis were perilous. On three separate occasions, I nearly lost my life due to the adverse effects of the disease. First, during the early progression of my disease, I traveled to a high elevation destination without the realization that my scarred lungs could not process oxygen at a sufficient rate in order for me to adequately breath. A local doctor who checked my symptoms found that I had a blood oxygen level of 53 percent and noted I likely would have suffered from a stroke within that same day without immediate care.

Secondly, during year 3 of my 5-year journey to transplant, I went into respiratory arrest primarily due to the weakened lungs during a medical procedure and had to be resuscitated. Finally, just a few months before the transplant, I was hospitalized with a lung infection so widespread that it required hospitalization for a period of time that was 2 weeks longer than my post-transplant stay. The medical team later informed me that clearing the infection may not have been possible if I had sought treatment 8–12 hours later than I did. I've also had more instances of a collapsed lung than I would care to remember.

During this period, I was also diagnosed with achalasia. This is a disorder characterized by the inability of the esophagus to properly move food and liquids into the stomach. I was told after going through the evaluation process that this disorder disqualified me from receiving a transplant at my State's only lung transplant program since the risks of my surgery outweighed the benefits of receiving donor lungs. The rejection I received from that program launched a solo effort, without transplant program assistance, to locate another program that would take me on as a patient. Over the next several months I reached out to one program after another, slowly losing hope as each new month brought a new letter of rejection in the mail until I eventually found a program by happenstance while traveling out of State for work.

Several things stood out to me during this experience: the absence of a basic standard of care from the specialty physician who did not give a referral to an appropriate transplant hospital so that I could receive follow up care, the void in guidance to an appropriate transplant hospital when my first-choice program disqualified me from theirs which left me ill-informed and on my own, and the lack of clarity as to which programs would automatically exclude me as a potential candidate based on my medical complications.

When finally wait-listed, patients also do not have the visibility to know which organ offers are declined on their behalf. This lack of visibility disenfranchises the patient from the decision-making process and deprives us of opportunities to receive a life-saving transplant. These gaps in care and guidance are opportunities for improvement. We need a system that works for patients, is easily navigable, and is unambiguous.

The specific circumstances of my own experience may be unique but the consistent difficulties in accessing transplant services are all too common. I was fortunate that I had the means, including access to good insurance, that allowed me to travel to another State to receive care. That is not always the case. Many studies highlight the disparities and inequitable access to transplant services that disproportionately harm Black people and people of color who do not have the resources to access transplant in these circumstances.

This committee has previously highlighted that organ donation system failures are an "urgent health equity issue."[16] Consider the numbers for kidney failure[17] — Hispanic Americans are 1.5 times more likely to experience kidney failure than White Americans; Black Americans are 3 times more likely; and Native Americans are 4 times more likely. Yet we also know Black people and people of color are less likely to receive transplants. One particularly troubling piece of data: organ procurement organizations (OPOs) have massive disparities amongst recovery rates of donors of color across the country. Axios highlighted a tenfold disparity[18] of Black recovery rates between OPOs across the country. Since same ethnicity

[16] https://www.finance.senate.gov/chairmans-news/bipartisan-bicameral-members-of-congress- commend-federal-efforts-to-reform-organ-donation-system-urge-acceleration-of-rules-impact-.

[17] https://opodata.org/equity/.

[18] https://www.axios.com/2021/11/09/organ-donation-recovery-worse-people-of-color.

matches are more likely, Axios[19] was clear about "why [that] matters: Fewer Black donors correlates to fewer Black recipients, which has led to more Blacks dying on the organ transplant wait list."

As a transplant recipient, I am committed to taking the best care of my organ as possible. Not only is it a necessity for my health, safety, and best long-term outcome success, but I also consider it an almost sacred duty. It is the bare minimum for me to be the best steward possible to show the proper respect and honor for my donor. Patients resoundingly agree on this point.

It is troubling to see, then, that we as Americans are asked to donate our organs but our OPOs do not appear to be the best stewards of the organs that we are donating. It is heartbreaking that thousands of recovered organs each year are not used while thousands more are not recovered at all. In addition, 23 percent of kidneys are wasted that could have made a significant dent in our transplant wait list and saved lives.

Here is some additional data that is equally troubling:

Thirty-three[20] Americans die every day for lack of a transplant, while thousands of organs go unrecovered and not transplanted every year. That number includes both patients dying on the wait list and the removal from the wait list of those who have died from being too sick to transplant.

The federally funded deceased donor potential study showed the U.S. may be recovering as few as one in five[21] potential organ donors.

To make this shocking status quo real: 28,000[22] organs go unrecovered each year, including: 17,000 kidneys; 8,000 livers; 1,500 hearts; and 1,500 lungs.

For scale, according to the chief of transplant at Vanderbilt[23] who testified at the House Oversight hearing last year, if the system were fully functioning, there would be no waiting list for livers, hearts, or lungs within 3 years, and the kidney wait list would be dramatically reduced.

According to data released by the Centers for Medicare and Medicaid Services this April, the majority[24] of organ procurement organizations are failing to miss performance standards; again, which translates into thousands of organs unrecovered each year.

Research has documented that often Black families receive differential treatment from OPOs. As former Surgeon General Dr. Ken Moritsugu[25] noted: "Often, mis-allocation of OPO resources means OPOs do not respond to all donation cases, or do not properly train and support their front-line staff. The impact of this, unsurprisingly, falls disproportionately on families of color." When I have personally spoken at donor remembrance ceremonies or other events in my community these same anecdotes supporting Dr. Moritsugu's research have been shared with me. Similar anecdotes have been shared with me by mainly Spanish-speaking families who have had the hurdle of language barriers that are difficult to clear.

---

[19] https://www.axios.com/2021/11/09/organ-donation-recovery-worse-people-of-color.

[20] https://www.washingtonpost.com/opinions/many-die-waiting-for-organs-the-trump-administration-could-help/20 2007/31/77e3a102-dfd6-11e9-b199-f638bf2c340f_story.html.

[21] https://optn.transplant.hrsa.gov/media/1161/ddps_03-2015.pdf.

[22] https://www.bridgespan.org/bridgespan/Images/articles/reforming-organ-donation-in-amer- ica/reforming-organ-donation-in-america-01-2019.pdf.

[23] https://www.youtube.com/watch?v=TnKo8Q-Hemk&t=2748s.

[24] https://qcor.cms.gov/main.jsp.

[25] *https://opodata.org/equity/.*

Senators, the leaders and several of my colleagues on the OPTN Patient Affairs Committee asked me to submit a letter (Appendix A) for the record. I have joined them. Among their messages to you:

Antiquated technology and an apathetic culture cause patients to languish with incomplete and often incorrect information, and leave people to die every day on the list. OPTN PAC members have raised these points often with UNOS leadership, and have seen our calls for reform ignored. We have been aghast at the absolute failure of UNOS to operate the practice and business of transplant, and to acknowledge—much less effectively serve— patients who are waiting and dying on the organ wait list. . . .

The alarming revelations in The Washington Post . . .[26]11 [including] covering for failures of organ procurement organizations; and lack of cooperation with the government, even devolving to UNOS having "threatened to walk away," lead us to believe that UNOS has proven itself incapable of functioning as the OPTN.

We ask that you ensure that the Federal Government makes the fast-approaching contracting OPTN cycle competitive for the first time since the original OPTN contract was awarded in 1986, opening critical functions up to best-in-class innovators across the country; and we implore you to ensure that UNOS does not hold patients hostage in the process."

Senators, I urge you all to act to ensure that we make better use of the organs that are donated, to ensure that health equity issues with Black people and people of color are addressed, and that the glaring technology issues causing patients harm are quickly remedied.

I thank you for your time.

Appendix A: UNOS Hearing Pac Letter, August 2, 2022

Dear members of the Senate Finance Committee,

As the leaders of the OPTN Patients Affairs Committee (PAC), we are reaching out to share our experiences on the committee that we believe indicate a systemic failure of UNOS to serve patients as the OPTN. This is all the more urgent in light of investigative reporting from The Washington Post.[27]

Antiquated technology and an apathetic culture cause patients to languish with incomplete and often incorrect information, and leave people to die every day on the list. OPTN PAC members have raised these points often with UNOS leadership, and have seen our calls for reform ignored. We have been aghast at the absolute failure of UNOS to operate the practice and business of transplant, and to acknowledge— much less effectively serve—patients who are waiting and dying on the organ wait list.

On July 28th, in preparation for the upcoming August 3rd Senate Finance Committee hearing into UNOS, PAC leaders received an email from UNOS CEO, Brain Shepard, referring to your investigation, in which he makes four assertions that UNOS has shared with the committee.

We wish to correct the record for your urgent consideration.

[26] https://www.washingtonpost.com/health/2022/07/31/unos-transplants-kindeys-hearts- technology/.
[27] https://www.washingtonpost.com/health/2022/07/31/unos-transplants-kindeys-hearts- technology/.

Shepard: "Our IT system remains safe, secure and routinely meets and surpasses Federal standards"

The Washington Post[28] reported "The system for getting donated kidneys, livers and hearts to desperately ill patients relies on out-of-date technology that has crashed for hours at a time and has never been audited by Federal officials for security weaknesses or other serious flaws."

We hope the committee asks UNOS how many patients have died due to the inability to match organs during downtime, as well as other technological inefficiencies such as data error due to manual entry, as well as how many patient life-years have been lost due to delays in organ transportation. That said, given the lack of transparency in the UNOS tech system, it is difficult to imagine anyone at UNOS could answer this question with any confidence.

Shepard: "We have worked together as a community to improve the transport of organs with innovative, evidence-based products."

The UNOS transportation record on organs is woefully—and fatally—inadequate, as outlined by investigative reporting from Kaiser Health News[29] —as well as cases brought before the Senate Finance Committee. Put simply, UNOS operates as an antiquated, closed system that keeps out external innovators that could help patients with better tools and services.

Shepard: "Our committees and staff are proud to work collaboratively with all members to serve as partners in improvement."

PAC members have often sought—and not received—clarity on how patient input is used. When PAC takes clear positions (such as the need to fast-track proposed changes to using eGFR results to list people of color), UNOS has refused to act. Compare this to a recent UNOS fast track process that addressed a hardware defect in a mechanical heart that went through in less than a month. Black patients deserved this kind of speedy remedy when eGFR was proven to have racial bias. We also note Washington Post[30] reporting that UNOS's policy making processes have been so divisive that they have "spark[ed] open conflict" among OPTN members.

Shepard: "The system we are all so honored to be a part of just surpassed 41,000 transplants in 2021, while continuing to expand equitable access to transplant."

UNOS obscures its underperforming record behind recent increases in organ donation rates that have resulted from tragic spikes in opioid overdoses, gun deaths, and car accidents, including as second-order effects of the COVID pandemic, not from UNOS's own performance. See the former U.S. Chief Data Scientist making this point in MedPage,[31] and research in the Journal of the American Medical Association[32] finding that, after controlling for public health trends and scientific advancements which have increased the size of the donor pool, organ donation rates have not even kept pace with population growth.[33]

The alarming revelations in The Washington Post[34] (antiquated technology; covering for failures of organ procurement organizations; and lack of cooperation with the government, even devolving to UNOS having "threatened to walk away") lead us to believe that UNOS has proven itself incapable of functioning as the OPTN.

---

[28] *https://www.washingtonpost.com/health/2022/07/31/unos-transplants-kindeys-hearts- technology/.*

[29] https://khn.org/news/how-lifesaving-organs-for-transplant-go-missing-in-transit/.

[30] https://www.washingtonpost.com/national/health-science/liver-transplant-rules-spark- open-conflict-among-transplant-centers/2019/05/16/91b37f84-781c-11e9-bd25- c989555e7766_story.html.

[31] https://www.medpagetoday.com/opinion/second-opinions/98363.

[32] https://jamanetwork.com/journals/jamasurgery/article-abstract/2771051.

[33] https://bloomworks.digital/organdonationreform/assets/PDF/donation-increase.pdf.

[34] *https://www.washingtonpost.com/health/2022/07/31/unos-transplants-kindeys-hearts- technology/*

We ask that you ensure that the Federal Government makes the fast-approaching contracting OPTN cycle competitive for the first time since the original OPTN contract was awarded in 1986, opening critical functions up to best-in-class innovators across the country; and we implore you to ensure that UNOS does not hold patients hostage in the process.

We urge you to continue with your oversight and institute urgent reforms that will literally result in lives saved.

Signed, Garrett Erdle
Chair, OPTN PAC
Living Kidney Donor, Alexandria, VA

Molly J. McCarthy Vice Chair, OPTN PAC
3-time Kidney Transplant Recipient, Redmond, WA

Chris Yanakos
Former Member of OPTN PAC

Living Liver Donor, Caregiver and Donor Family Member, Pittsburgh, PA

Steve Weitzen
Region 2 Representative, OPTN PAC Heart Recipient, Randolph, NJ

Calvin Henry
Region 3 Representative, OPTN PAC Lung Recipient, Dacula, GA

Lorrinda Gray-Davis
Region 4 Representative, OPTN PAC Liver Recipient, Yukon, OK

Julie Spear
Region 8 Representative, OPTN PAC Donor Family Member, Boulder, CO

Eric Tanis
Region 10 Representative, OPTN PAC Liver Recipient, Highland, IN

Questions Submitted for the Record to Calvin Henry Questions Submitted by Hon. John Barrasso

Question. This committee has obviously been hard at work trying to identify shortcomings in the organ procurement and transplantation system over the past couple years. Also within the past couple years, the Trump administration proposed and the Biden administration finalized the OPO final rule. This rule established new performance metrics for OPOs as well as helped promote more frequent oversight and competition among OPOs.

Are there other regulatory or legislative actions Congress or the administration should take to ensure the OPTN is performing to its maximum potential for patients and providers?

Answer. Opinions are mine only and do not reflect OPTN policy or views.

1) Pass the Living Donor Protection Act (S. 377/H.R. 1255).
2) Require UNOS, as the OPTN contractor, to work with Organ Procurement Organizations (OPO) and transplant centers to expand transplants performed under the HIV Organ Policy Equity (HOPE) Act (Pub. L. 113–51).
3) Require UNOS, as the OPTN contractor, to begin work to require transplant centers to implement informed, shared decision making with transplant candidates when considering organ offers.
4) Require UNOS, as the OPTN contractor, to collaborate with OPOs in evaluating OPO personnel makeup to ensure that they appropriately represent the demographics of the patients and communities that they serve.
5) Allow research pilot studies to determine if providing incentives can increase

U.S. Organ Donor Availability

Because of the depth of supporting material available, it is challenging to fully detail these proposed actions within this response from my viewpoint as a transplant recipient and patient advocate for the past decade, so I will briefly state what I think are the pertinent points. I welcome the opportunity to clarify or further discuss these in greater detail. These proposed actions address goals of reducing the donated organ non-use rate and increasing the number of transplants performed while improving access and equity in transplant.

1) Pass the Living Donor Protection Act (S.377/H.R.1255).

The organ donation and transplant community has long advocated for Congress to enact law to provide protections for living organ donors. Bipartisan legislation has been introduced to Congress in successive sessions over the past 25 years in order to accomplish this goal. In the absence of Federal guidance, at least 28 States have enacted law to protect living organ donors and improve the number of transplants performed but these laws are not all consistent or comprehensive; my State of Georgia being the latest to pass such a law earlier this year. Only 8 more of your Senate colleagues are needed for cosponsor in order to push a standardized and comprehensive bill forward to a historic vote in the Senate. Passing this bill would not only be a lifesaving aid for many living donors, recipients, and their families in navigating the transplant process, I also believe it would help improve living donor rates by removing disincentives to the donation process. I ask that you urge your colleagues to action in cosponsoring and subsequently passing this bill.

2) Require UNOS, as the OPTN contractor, to work with the Organ Procurement Organizations (OPO) and transplant centers to expand transplants performed under the HIV Organ Policy Equity (HOPE) Act (Pub. L. 113–51).

Approximately 240 HIV+ transplants have been performed under the HOPE Act, but currently less than 15 percent of the approximately 250 U.S. transplant centers perform these organ transplants.[35] Expansion of transplants performed under this act can save many more lives per year per the latest recommendations from the HHS Advisory Council on Organ Transplantation (ACOT) and also reduce the burden on organ donor availability.[36] The council also unanimously agreed that there was cause to examine potential inefficiencies in organ procurement from HIV+ organ donors and to determine how many potential organs that could have been donated were not recovered.

3) Require UNOS, as the OPTN contractor, to begin the work to require transplant centers to implement informed, shared decision making with transplant candidates when considering organ offers.

As patients, we should have the ability to participate in the decision-making process when determining how transplantation will affect our lives. Our goals for quality of life post-transplant don't always coincide with expectations of transplant centers. Overwhelming patient sentiment supports our willingness to sometimes accept higher-risk organs that transplant centers traditionally would not consider. These transplant center practices contribute to the rate of organ non-use when organs that are considered higher-risk could have been used to satisfy unique patient needs, but are too often not used at all. Also, on average, people who die while waiting for a kidney transplant had 16 kidney offers that were ultimately transplanted into other patients.[37] CMS rules may also need to be addressed in order to support transplant centers when accepting higher risk organs.

4) Require UNOS, as the OPTN contractor, to collaborate with OPOs in evaluating OPO personnel makeup to ensure that they appropriately represent the demographics of the patients and communities that they serve.

I shared in my August 3rd testimony that it has been my experience that OPOs do not consistently treat all organ donors in the same manner.[38] Also, surveys of organ donor attitudes have shown that Black, Hispanic, Native American, and other historically disadvantaged populations are willing to become organ donors, yet OPOs often do not take steps necessary to recruit these donors. I believe UNOS should collaborate with OPOs and use best industry practices to ensure that OPO personnel makeup throughout the entire organization, and especially within executive leadership, is representative of the community demographics that it serves. Precedence exists to show that having such a structure in place can rapidly improve organ donation rates, especially in these historically disadvantaged populations.

---

[35] https://www.finance.senate.gov/chairmans-news/bipartisan-bicameral-members-of-congress- commend-federal-efforts-to-reform-organ-donation-system-urge-acceleration-of-rules-impact-.

[36] OPTN. Transplant centers approved for Hope Act. *https://optn.transplant.hrsa.gov/media/ex3bmasx/hope-act-hospitals.pdf* (accessed October 3, 2022).

[37] U.S. Department of Health and Human Services Recommendations 66 through 67. *https:// www.hrsa.gov/advisory-committees/organ-transplantation/recommendations/66-67* (accessed September 19, 2022).

[38] Husain, S.A., K.L. King, S. Pastan, R.E. Patzer, D.J. Cohen, J. Radhakrishnan, and S. Mohan. 2019. Association between declined offers of deceased donor kidney allograft and outcomes in kidney transplant candidates. *https://jamanetwork.com/journals/jamanetworkopen/fullarticle/2749266* (accessed October 12, 2022).

5) Allow research pilot studies to determine if incentivizing organ donation can increase U.S. organ donor availability.

We discussed in this recent hearing that the demand for donated organs continues to increase and outpace the supply available to provide lifesaving transplantation, and I believe that newer approaches should be considered when determining methods to increase the organ supply since current and long-standing practices are not effective in reducing the size of the organ wait list. NOTA currently prohibits both the giving and receiving of incentives for organ donation as well as research to even determine if providing incentives would be effective. Public attitudes continue to show a positive view of incentives of some type for organ donation even though transplant professional concerns regarding the commodification of organs and the potential exploitation of vulnerable populations are well documented, but recent views suggest that Federal management of incentives is viable.[39] Some States have already included forms of financial incentives in their respective living organ donor protection laws.[40] I believe that providing incentives, other than direct compensation for organs, such as deceased donor funeral costs or reimbursement of living donor medical and life insurance premiums is not only a decent act, but could significantly increase organ donor rates and it is already demonstrated that reimbursements from the National Living Donor Assistance Center (NLDAC) are insufficient.[41] Other countries that have enacted similar laws have realized a rapid increase in organ donor rates post-implementation.[42] An amendment to NOTA is required to allow HRSA funding for a research pilot program to allow for examination of viability.

Question Submitted by Hon. Maggie Hassan

Question. The Organ Procurement and Transplantation Network's 2021–2024 Strategic Plan includes priorities to help ensure broad access to transplants. That effort should include individuals with disabilities. How is the network ensuring that individuals with disabilities have equal access to organ transplants?

Answer. The OPTN does not currently have a policy addressing disabilities nor does it explicitly offer a position on whether disabilities should be removed as exclusionary criteria for transplant. This absence of policy is a barrier that helps prevent equal access to organ transplants for individuals with disabilities. The OPTN, beginning in 2017, completed a significant amount of work in resolving this topic, but was notified by HRSA in early 2019 that the Health and Human Services (HHS) Office of Civil Rights (OCR) should be the agency first issuing guidance on this topic and that the OPTN would need to halt work on publishing any

---

[39] Hearing of the Senate Finance Committee: "A System in Need of Repair: Addressing Organi- zational Failures of the U.S.'s Organ Procurement and Transplantation Network," 117th Cong. (2022) (testimony of Calvin Henry, OPTN Patient Affairs Committee). *https://www. finance.senate.gov/imo/media/doc/SenateFinance Cmte_832022_HenryCalvin_v2.pdf* (accessed September 15, 2022).

[40] HRSA 2019 National Survey of Organ Donation Attitudes and Practices: Report of Findings. 4.13 Payments and Organ Donation, Q18. Payments Would Increase Likelihood of Organ Donation. *https://www. organdonor.gov/sites/default/files/organ-donor/professional/grants-research/nsodap-organ-donation-survey-2019.pdf* (accessed September 14, 2022).

[41] S.B. 330, 2021 Biennium, 2022 Reg. Sess. (GA 2022). *https://www.legis.ga.gov/api/legislation/document/ 20212022/203236* (accessed September 27, 2022).

[42] *https://www.youtube.com/watch?v=TnKo8Q-Hemk&t=2748s.*

white papers or guidance representing the official position of the OPTN until the OCR completed their own guidance. My understanding is that the halting of this work was due, in part, to the then pending release of the Organ Transplant Discrimination Against People with Disabilities Report by the National Council on Disability (NCD) which was completed against the backdrop of increased widespread interest in this topic.[43] The OPTN subsequently sent a memo to HRSA in August 2019 summarizing the progress to date as well as recommendations to aid the OCR as they began their work on a guidance document. The OPTN is not aware of any guidance document or further developments from the OCR subsequent to this memo, but a general public Request for Information from interested stakeholders was solicited by the office in January 2021.[44]

It is my strong belief that excluding patients for organ transplantation solely on the basis of disability is discriminatory and undercuts access to health care for an already vulnerable population. Removal of this barrier is critical to the success of ensuring equitable access to transplant services and restoring trust in the transplant system. In the absence of Federal or OPTN guidance, 34 States have enacted laws prohibiting transplant programs from excluding individuals with disabilities solely on the basis of disability, recognizing the need to protect the rights afforded under the Americans with Disabilities Act, section 504 of the Rehabilitation Act, and section 1557 of the Affordable Care Act.[45] I urge the HHS and the OCR to accelerate their process in issuing Federal guidance on this matter to help ensure that equal access to transplant is available for those with disabilities.

Prepared Statement of Jayme E. Locke, M.D., MPH, Director, Division of Transplantation Surgery, Heersink School of Medicine, University of Alabama

Chairman Wyden, Ranking Member Crapo, and members of the committee, my name is Dr. Jayme Locke, and I am the director of the Division of Transplantation Surgery at the University of Alabama at Birmingham (UAB), where I also serve as the Director of the Comprehensive Transplant Institute. I have dedicated my career to serving vulnerable populations with the goal of eliminating or at least mitigating health disparities. I believe that patients should be the focus of everything we do.

At UAB, we currently have 1,022 patients wait-listed for kidneys, the majority self-identified as African American/Black. We have performed more than 10,000 kidney transplants and have performed the most living donor kidney transplants among African American/Black persons than any other program in the country. Our center is located in the southeastern United States, an area known to have one of the highest end-stage kidney disease burdens as well as communities with extreme social vulnerability—characteristics that drive demand for transplantation and reflect a limited supply.

---

[43] Organ Transplant Discrimination Against People with Disabilities, September 2019. *https://www.ncd.gov/sites/default/files/NCD_Organ_Transplant_508.pdf* (accessed September 21, 2022).

[44] OCR Seeks Information on Addressing Disability Discrimination in Health Care and Child Welfare Contexts, January 2021. *https://www.hhs.gov/about/news/2021/01/15/ocr-seeks-information-addressing-disability-discrimination-health-care-child-welfare-contexts.html* (accessed September 21, 2022).

[45] National Down Syndrome Society (NDSS). Policy and Advocacy. Organ Transplant Discrimination State-Level Legislation. *https://ndss.org/advocacy#p_health* (accessed September 30, 2022).

Transplantation was always supposed to be about the patient, but the system we operate now has almost a complete lack of ownership and responsibility—whether it is an OPO failing to show up at donor hospitals and engage families, or UNOS failing at the most basic responsibilities of getting recovered organs matched and safely to the recipients at the other side. These are the government's own contractors.

My patients, your constituents, need your help.

We know that thousands of kidneys are recovered and discarded every year, and that thousands more are never recovered at all. Discards have increased steadily and transportation errors are frequent particularly since the most recent allocation change, as the new system increased complexity, and to date UNOS has shown no ability to manage even simple logistics.

The most powerful thing to know about this is that every organ represents a life. You could argue it represents more than one life; it has a profound impact on the patient, their family, and their community. We can never forget that. Imagine having a medication you need to live being thrown away simply because someone took too long to get it to you. Your life quite literally in a trash can. Organs are no different. They too have shelf lives, and they are measured in hours.

Discarded kidneys and transportation errors may sound abstract. Let me make this negligence real for you—and please remember the disregarded donors whose families trusted us with the most sacred of gifts, and the sick and dying patients waiting for these transplants. Think of the young girl looking forward to not having to miss the prom for dialysis, the mom who wants to live long enough to see her children grow-up, the parent who needs to be able to hold down a job to provide for his/her family. The things we take for granted are the things that end-organ disease robs our patients of. Transplant is the cure—that is if the organ ever makes it to the patient.

In 2014, I received a kidney that arrived frozen. It was hard as a rock, like an ice cube you could put in your drink. The intended recipient was highly sensitized— meaning difficult to match. The only thing we could do was tell the waiting patient that, due to the lack of safeguards regarding transportation of organs, the kidney had to be thrown in the trash—the final, generous act of a donor in Maryland.

In 2017, I received a kidney that arrived in a box with tire marks on it. The box was squished, and the container inside had been ruptured (Image 1). We were "lucky" and were able to salvage the kidney for transplant. Why should luck even play a role?

This is the level of care too many kidneys receive. How does UNOS allow this?

Once the kidney is packaged and leaves, no one really knows what happens, and that is as shocking as it is unacceptable.

Consider this: for our patients in Birmingham, most of our kidneys fly through Atlanta. When they were arriving on flights after 10 p.m., they were being taken down to sit in cargo hold like lost luggage, only to be taken out in the morning when flights restarted.

But Birmingham is only 2 hours away from Atlanta by car—and delays in transplanting organs literally mean life or death. Think of cold ischemia time this way: like shelf life. Each minute, each hour, that an organ is out of the donor's body, those cells are dying, which increases risk to the receiving patient. Increased cold ischemia time can mean delayed graft function—meaning the patient requires dialysis after transplant. Delayed graft function is a known risk factor for acute rejection and reduced long-term graft survival.

When we realized what was happening with kidneys stuck in cargo hold at Atlanta airport, we called the airlines and dealt with it ourselves. I don't blame the airlines—their job is to move hundreds of thousands of people around the country each day. But where was UNOS? How did it ever let organs sit in cargo hold?

Another even simpler example: instances of UNOS saying that no flights are available, when my team has hopped on Expedia and found available flights themselves.

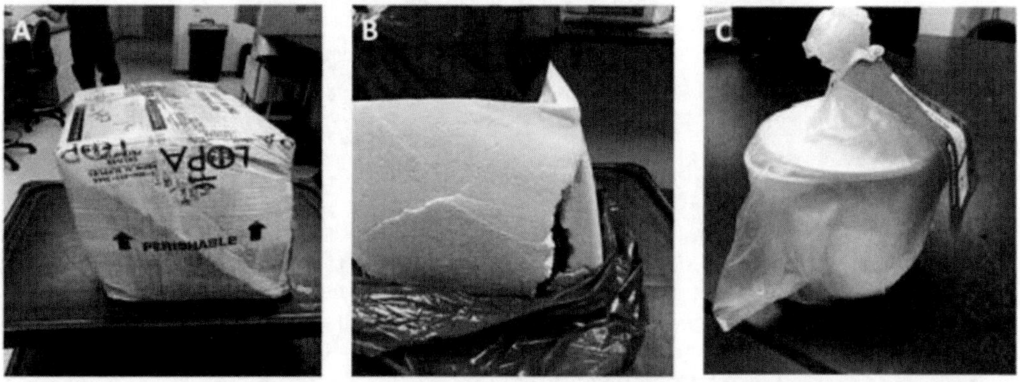

Image 1: Box as arrived to UAB. Tire marks - potentially from a luggage conveyor - were visible on the box; (B) Crushed styrofoam cooler housed inside box; and (C) Sterile bag inside white container intact but white container and external sterile bag disrupted. (Note: I understand these pictures were also shared with the Senate Finance Committee by the Louisiana Organ Procurement Agency, which similarly reported this issue at the time to UNOS.)

UNOS has failed at its responsibility for the efficient matching and distribution of organs. There are countless stories of inefficient algorithms and process that led to organs accruing unacceptably long cold ischemia times resulting in discard. In an era of same-day delivery of household goods from Amazon, the OPTN and its contractors have relied on outdated logistical systems akin to the Pony Express.

Moreover, UNOS has abdicated its duty to hold under-performing OPOs responsible for failing to convert eligible donors and manage organs on their end, and as such, have not optimized the number of organs available for transplant.

Since the frozen kidney, and the box with tire marks—I have received other kidneys that had to be discarded either due to surgical and OPO handling issues or UNOS transportation errors. But one week this May was particularly difficult.

In 1 week, I received four kidneys from four different OPOs—each with basic errors that led to the need to throw away those lifesaving organs (Images 4 and 5).

- One kidney had to be thrown away due to a botched biopsy into the kidney's collecting system, which means urine would have leaked from the kidney once transplanted;
- Another kidney had to be thrown away because the lower pole artery had been cut during procurement. That would have been fixable if someone involved in the procurement had assessed the kidney for damage and flushed it before packing, but that didn't happen; and
- Two other kidneys arrived to me blue—meaning they hadn't been flushed.

Errors happen. We all understand that. However, opacity at UNOS means that we have no idea how often basic mistakes happen across the country, nor can we have confidence that anything is being done to redress such errors so they don't keep happening.

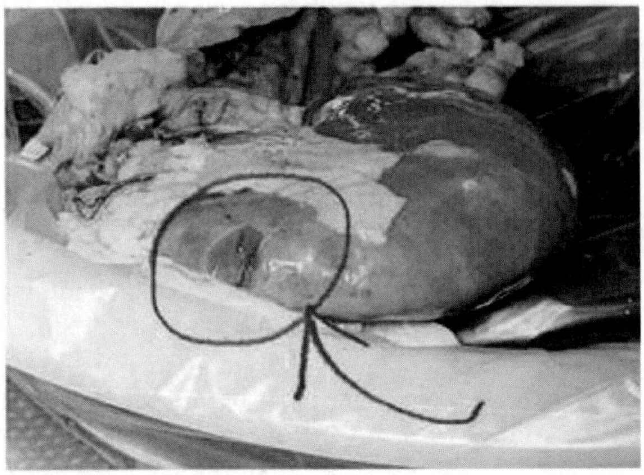

Image 4: Kidney with botched biopsy that cut into the kidney's collecting system. Collecting system injury could not be repaired. Urine would have leaked from biopsy site instead of flowing to bladder. (see red circle/arrow)

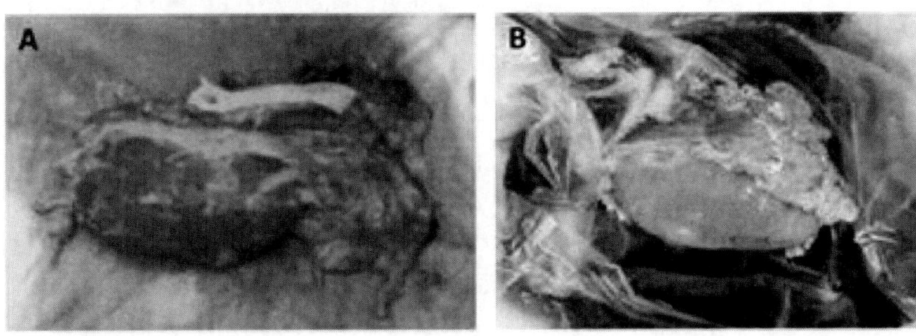

Image 5: (A) Blue kidney – unflushed; arrived from outside OPO; (B) Same kidney after having been flushed on the backtable more than 20hrs after initial procurement. Kidney was discarded secondary to high risk of primary non-function.

All I know is that in 1 week I received four kidneys—two from donors in Tennessee, one from a donor in Florida, and one from a donor in Georgia—that had to be thrown away.

What was particularly heartbreaking was that two of these kidneys were for highly sensitized African American/Black women—meaning they were the proverbial needle-in-a-haystack kidneys for patients that are hard to match. Our patients become sensitized through prior exposure to foreign tissue—previous transplant, blood transfusion, and/or pregnancy.

Women who have been pregnant—especially multiple times—are more sensitized/ harder to match, and pregnancy related sensitization contributes to both gender and racial disparities in access to kidney transplantation. So when we talk about the system being inequitable, this is a very real example of how a constrained pool of organs for transplant, and high discards, are failures that disproportionately hurt women, and women of color who are more likely to have multiple pregnancies.

Somewhere along the way we forgot why we're here—saving people's lives. We have to do better, and that includes transplant centers, too.

I know others in my field have spoken up, and more still who want to speak up. But, Senators, please know that every person I have talked to who has spoken up about system failures has told me they have been punished in some way through both micro- and macroaggressions. The very highest levels of leadership within UNOS is an insular club that has turned its back on the very patients they purport to support by ignoring their own unconscious biases, and even impugning patients behind closed doors.

For example, a UNOS board member in an email to the UNOS CEO, labeled patients from the southeastern United States as "dumb f*$#". This is not who we are as medical professionals. We are here to serve all people and in particular those who are the most vulnerable among us. We need reform now.

The solutions are clear and I am asking for your urgent help on behalf of my patients and all the other patients waiting around the country:

- Immediately separate the OPTN board from any of the boards of any contractors;
- Bring in the real experts to ensure our patients are served by the best-of-the- best in each field, separating out key functions of the OPTN: for example, policy, technology/matching, and logistics; and
- Ensure that patients are safer by holding all contractors accountable, including through public adverse event reporting and immediate redressing of problems.

One final and critical point. I can't tell you how disturbing it was to read recent reporting of the way UNOS has allegedly held the U.S. transplant system hostage. According to The Washington Post: "UNOS also 'has at times even threatened to walk away and continue operating the [transplant network] without a contract, despite the fact that it would be illegal.'"

Doing anything to jeopardize patients—including even threatening to walk away—violates a basic principle of health care. It's called patient abandonment. You simply can't do that—or even threaten to do that. I would lose my medical license for walking away from a patient.

If it is true that in any way UNOS has suggested that it might walk away, or in any way not cooperate with a transition to new OPTN contractors, that would make it an organization that cannot be responsible for taking care of lives.

There is very little in health care that has the immediate life and death stakes as organ transplantation. Please realize that every day that passes with these failing systems in place means more of our neighbors will die. My patients need the Senate to act.

Attachment: OPTN Region 3 Letter, February 23, 2022

Dear Chairman Wyden, Senator Grassley, Senator Young, and Senator Cardin, We are writing to you as Region 3 members of the Organ Procurement Transplantation Network (OPTN) about grave concerns we have about the leadership of the OPTN (current contractor, UNOS) and to express our strongest possible objection to the content of recently published email communications among OPTN leaders.

At the February 1, 2022 OPTN Region 3 meeting, several members sought to raise the issue of leadership, as a Federal judge recently unsealed deeply concerning emails from the UNOS CEO (Brian Shepard) and a then-OPTN/UNOS board member (Alexandra Glazier).

In policymaking deliberations, we note the following exchanges:

Glazier to Shepard: "The fact that some States do better than others in preventing preventable deaths and providing health-care insurance coverage and access means you're a dumb fuck for living there."

Shepard to Glazier: "Only people who have means can get a transplant. So this isn't a 'give txs to poor people argument; its a 'give txs to those of us who have to live near poor people' argument."

These exchanges are only a fraction of the concerning transgressions found in the unsealed emails, representing a serious failure of leadership and breach of trust. Irrespective of positions on any given policy, these comments are disqualifying for positions of public service. It does not represent who we are as leaders of the organ donation and transplantation community. It is equally concerning that the OPTN/ UNOS Board of Directors has failed to apologize or publicly denounce these disparaging opinions voiced by Shepard and Glazier, suggesting that these views are truly those of the OPTN. UNOS speaks often of the importance of "maintaining public trust" in the organ donation system; it is unfortunate that its executives have so flagrantly flaunted it, and, as such, must be held accountable.

At the most recent meeting, Region 3 member representatives wished to raise that (1) we believe Shepard should resign as the CEO of UNOS; and (2) that Glazier should no longer be permitted the privilege of OPTN/UNOS policymaking positions. However, we were told we could not raise this issue at the OPTN meeting as it was intended only for OPTN policy development purposes, not other matters pertaining to the OPTN or UNOS. Unfortunately, UNOS has offered no other public venues to discuss our concerns.

Having been denied the opportunity to vote on our concerns for patient welfare, we and others in the community were further stifled in our discussion by repeated statements that we should discuss our opinions "offline" with OPTN/UNOS board president Dr. Matthew Cooper. During the public meeting, Mr. Shepard and Dr. Cooper misrepresented the OPTN/UNOS board's discussions of the emails and actions we have outlined above. The continued attempts to suppress conversations about vulnerable patients and avoid accountability for reprehensible views and actions has broken our faith in UNOS's ability to self-regulate its leaders, so, instead, we are writing to you.

As you are aware, OPTN board members concurrently serve as the board members of UNOS. This creates a serious conflict of interest as, too often, the principal goal of UNOS is maintaining its status as the monopoly OPTN contractor, rather than focusing on issues that will actually help more patients and steward the use of precious donated organs. In fact, in 2018, the Government Accountability Office agreed with a directive from HRSA that the OPTN and the OPTN contractor (currently UNOS) must maintain separate boards, though, nearly 4 years later, UNOS still has not done so.

It was more than 20 years ago that Forbes called UNOS the "cartel" that's "chilling the supply of transplantable organs and letting Americans who need them die needlessly," and—in the absence of structural reform to the OPTN—this dynamic remains today.

The quashing of dissenting voices within the OPTN is both ongoing and deeply damaging to the patients we serve. If the OPTN/UNOS had proper governance, not only do we believe there would be clear leadership changes, we trust that there would be more attention—and action—on issues that cost patients their lives, rather than a primary focus on UNOS continually maintaining its monopoly hold on the U.S. organ donation system.

Thirty-three Americans die every day for lack of an available organ transplant. Please ensure that proper governance is in place to help change this.

Yours sincerely,
Keith Wille, M.D.
OPTN Board of Directors Region 3 Councilor 2020–2022
Professor of Medicine Medical Director, Advanced Lung Diseases Program University of Alabama, Birmingham, Alabama

Christopher Anderson, M.D. OPTN Board of Directors Region 3 Councilor 2018–2020

James D. Hardy Chair
Professor and Chair, Department of Surgery Chief Perioperative Services Physician Medical Director, Transplant Service Line University of Mississippi Medical Center Jackson, Mississippi

Virginia McBride, R.N., MPH OPTN Board of Directors Region 3 Councilor 2022–2024 Executive Director
Our Legacy Organ and Tissue Donation Services Maitland, Florida

Kelly Ranum
OPTN Board of Directors 2019–2021
Chief Executive Officer
Louisiana Organ Procurement Agency Covington, Louisiana

Raymond Lynch, M.D., MS, FACS
Associate Professor of Surgery Executive Director Director of Public Policy and Community Relations Emory Transplant Center, Atlanta, Georgia

Barry Friedman
Advent Health Transplant Institute AdventHealth Orlando
Orlando, Florida

Jayme Locke, M.D., MPH, FACS, FAST
Professor of Surgery Director
UAB Comprehensive Transplant Institute Chief, Division of Transplantation Arnold G. Diethelm Endowed Chair in Transplantation Surgery Birmingham, Alabama

Jonathan Hundley, M.D.
Surgical Director
Liver Transplantation Piedmont Transplant Institute Piedmont Healthcare, Atlanta, Georgia

M. Kevin Stump
Chief Executive Officer
Mississippi Organ Recovery Agency Jackson, Mississippi

Questions Submitted for the Record to Jayme E. Locke, M.D., MPH
Questions Submitted by Hon. John Barrasso

Question. As we know, OPOs are overseen by UNOS, as well as the Centers for Medicare and Medicaid Services (CMS). One would think for organizations overseen by two different entities, serious mistakes would not frequently occur. Yet, as the committee report shows, grave mistakes, like testing errors and transportation failures, still plague OPTN members and cost numerous lives.

Are there specific gaps in oversight between UNOS activities and those of CMS, and if so, can you shed some light on these?

Answer. One of the biggest gaps in our transplant system is accountability with regard to organ transport. Once the kidney has been procured and packaged and begins its journey to the transplant center where it will be transplanted, the kidney, a lifesaving organ, is reliant on the goodwill of complete strangers (e.g., airport personnel, couriers, etc) who quite likely are unfamiliar with transplantation and the need for efficient and timely transport of the gift of life. No transplant-specific entity wants to "own" the kidney or be responsible for its care for the duration of the transport process. There is no system for holding a particular entity responsible or accountable for ensuring the kidney arrives in good condition and on time (e.g., "on time" being defined as a transportation route resulting in as little cold storage or cold ischemia time as possible; decreasing cold storage time has been associated with improved patient outcomes post-transplant).

For all intents and purposes, kidneys in transit are on their own, with no metrics for delivery. This is a profound failure of the OPTN contractor.

HRSA and CMS should reform this issue with urgency, as it relates to alarmingly high rates of kidney discards in the United States. According to the most recent data highlighted at the Senate Finance Committee hearing, one in four kidneys from generous donors in America are thrown in the trash. Much of this senseless waste is due to failures of clinical standards, processes, and technology from HHS's own contractors. Given patients of color are disproportionately impacted by kidney disease, these failures impact communities of color most, and further emphasize the fact that the organ shortage and kidney discards represent an urgent health equity issue.

The government has a role to play in transparency and reform on this life-and-death issue. HHS (HRSA or CMS) should publish a lost organ reporting system— a dashboard of all kidneys recovered and not transplanted. These data are available to HHS agencies via the OPTN, and would allow for a near-real time reporting of:

1) total number of kidneys recovered and not transplanted;
2) where those kidneys originated (i.e., from which OPO);
3) where those kidneys were due to arrive (i.e., to which transplant center or State); and
4) why the kidney was discarded (e.g., clinical problems in recovery; transportation problems in delivery).

It may also be worth reaching out to the FAA to understand how this agency has so successfully collaborated with stakeholders to ensure precise times in transit. In short, we have figured out complex systems with airplanes, understanding arrival and delay times . . . and imagine if we hadn't. This should be possible with kidneys too.

Question. This committee has obviously been hard at work trying to identify shortcomings in the organ procurement and transplantation system over the past couple years. Also within the past couple years, the Trump administration proposed and the Biden administration finalized the OPO final rule. This rule established new performance metrics for OPOs as well as helped promote more frequent oversight and competition among OPOs.

Are there other regulatory or legislative actions Congress or the administration should take to ensure the OPTN is performing to its maximum potential for patients and providers?

Answer. I support the bipartisan recommendations of the Senate Finance Committee[46] to break up the OPTN monopoly, and open competition to the best-of-the-best in each field for the good of patients.

As I included in my testimony:[47] "The solutions are clear, and I am asking for your urgent help on behalf of my patients and all the other patients waiting around the country:

- Immediately separate the OPTN board from any of the boards of any contractors;
- Bring in the real experts to ensure our patients are served by the best-of-the-best in each field, separating out key functions of the OPTN; for example, policy, technology/matching, and logistics; and
- Ensure that patients are safer by holding all contractors accountable, including through public adverse event reporting and immediate redressing of problems."

The OPTN should never again be allowed to be a monopoly. Having one organization/contractor performing a vast and disparate array of functions is a mistake, leading to a situation where a single organization acts as the proverbial "jack of all trades" while being the master of none.

Separate contracts will allow for expertise, for example in allocation/mathematical modeling and transportation/logistics. What's more, for the good of patients, not only must the upcoming OPTN contracting cycle be transparent and competitive, every future cyclet should be transparent and competitive as well.

As I said in my testimony,[48] "There is very little in health care that has the immediate life and death stakes as organ transplantation. Please realize that every day that passes with these failing systems in place means more of our neighbors will die. My patients need the Senate to act."

Question Submitted by Hon. Maggie Hassan

Question. In 2019, the National Council on Disability (NCD) released a report finding that people with disabilities are often excluded as organ transplant candidates due to their

---

[46] https://www.finance.senate.gov/imo/media/doc/UNOS%20Hearing%20Confidential%20Me mo%20(FOR%20 RELEASE).pdf.

[47] https://www.finance.senate.gov/imo/media/doc/SenateTestimony_8.2.22_Written%20Final v2.pdf.

[48] https://www.finance.senate.gov/imo/media/doc/SenateTestimony_8.2.22_Written%20Final v2.pdf.

disabilities. Does your organization have a policy that covers organ transplant access for individuals with disabilities?

Answer. At the University of Alabama at Birmingham (UAB), I have transplanted patients with a range of disabilities, and similar, to their non-disabled counterparts they too have achieved a significant survival benefit from the lifesaving gift of transplantation. In short, people with disabilities should not be excluded from transplantation. A belief that my institution supports. The UAB Comprehensive Transplant Institute (CTI) does not discriminate against individuals with disabilities. Specifically, UAB CTI has a list of absolute and relative contraindications for each organ program, and neither category includes disabilities.

Question Submitted by Hon. Benjamin L Cardin

Question. Given the overrepresentation of Black Americans waiting on a kidney, do transportation problems that seem to disproportionately impact kidneys impact the disparity we observe?

Answer. Transportation problems—along with all problems that unnecessarily constrain the supply of kidneys—exacerbate disparities in access to transplantation.

As I testified before the Senate Finance Committee, highly sensitized patients are hard to match, and finding kidneys for these patients can be like finding the proverbial needle in a haystack. Our patients become sensitized through prior exposure to foreign tissue—previous transplant, blood transfusion, and/or pregnancy. Women who have been pregnant—especially multiple times—are more sensitized/harder to match, and pregnancy related sensitization contributes to both gender and racial disparities in access to kidney transplantation. So when we talk about the system being inequitable, this is a very real example of how a constrained pool of organs for transplant, and high discards, are failures that disproportionately hurt women, and women of color who are more likely to have multiple pregnancies.

Therefore, it's critical that HHS (HRSA and CMS) immediately address the kidney discard problem, which is exacerbated by a lack of clinical standards and a lack of process standards in transportation.

HHS (HRSA or CMS) should publish a lost organ reporting system—a dashboard of all kidneys recovered and not transplanted. These data are available to HHS agencies via the OPTN, and would allow for a near-real time reporting of: (1) total number of kidneys recovered and not transplanted; (2) where those kidneys originated (i.e., from which OPO); (3) where those kidneys were due to arrive (i.e., to which transplant center or State); and (4) why the kidney was discarded (e.g., clinical problems in recovery; transportation problems in delivery).

Additionally, it is paramount that we evaluate whether the government's own contractors are using the most efficient/effective modes of transportation. For example, UAB is in the southeastern United States, an area with particularly high rates of end-stage kidney disease and health disparities. It is also a region where it is harder to get flights, and where missed flights can have calamitous consequences, yet too often simpler modes of transportation—such as driving—are not consistently explored and used.

Question Submitted by Hon. Tim Scott

Question. During the hearing, our committee heard that organs in transport are 15 times more likely to go missing than customer luggage. You provided an example of an organ that was flown late at night and was placed in airport holding. Were it not for the quick actions of your team and cooperative airport staff, this organ likely would have been lost.

Are there additional process improvements that were not discussed during this hearing that should be considered with regard to organ transportation to improve transplantation rates and care outcomes?

Answer. HHS (HRSA or CMS) should publish a lost organ reporting system—a dashboard of all kidneys recovered and not transplanted. These data are available to HHS agencies via the OPTN, and would allow for a near-real time reporting of:

(1) total number of kidneys recovered and not transplanted;
(2) where those kidneys originated (i.e., from which OPO);
(3) where those kidneys were due to arrive (i.e., to which transplant center or State); and
(4) why the kidney was discarded (e.g., clinical problems in recovery; transportation problems in delivery).

It may also be worth reaching out to the FAA to understand how this agency has so successfully collaborated with stakeholders to ensure precise times in transit. In short, we have figured out complex systems with airplanes, understanding arrival and delay times . . . and imagine if we hadn't This should be possible with kidneys.

Simply put: we are not currently working with people/organizations who are experts in logistics and transportation. Whether that is the FAA or external organizations such as UPS and FedEx (as well as specialized logistics companies), transplant is too critical to be left to non-experts in logistics and supply chain issues.

Prepared Statement of Brian Shepard, Chief Executive Officer, United Network for Organ Sharing (UNOS)

Chairman Wyden, Ranking Member Crapo, and members of the committee, thank you for inviting me to discuss our Nation's organ transplant system and the role of United Network for Organ Sharing, or UNOS. I am Brian Shepard, the CEO of UNOS, the nonprofit organization which holds the Federal contract to serve as the U.S. organ donation and transplantation network.

I look forward to having a conversation with you about our Nation's diverse and thriving organ transplant system that just marked its 9th consecutive record-setting year of lifesaving transplants.

In 1984, Congress passed the National Organ Transplant Act (NOTA) to address the Nation's critical organ donation shortage and improve organ matching and placement. The law called for an Organ Procurement and Transplantation Network (OPTN) to maintain a national registry for organ matching, and specified that the network would be a private, nonprofit entity.

UNOS is proud to have been awarded the OPTN contract successively since 1986. Each contract rebid is based on a competitive process. We welcome this competitive process, and it has been our honor to serve the Nation for over 3 decades.

From UNOS's inception as a mission-based non-profit and since we began serving as the Federal contractor, we have never once taken this privilege lightly; UNOS staff, volunteers—including transplant professionals, recipients, and donor families—and others dedicate their time and expertise every day to saving lives and improving the system. Our work focuses on three main areas: developing equitable allocation policies that ensure the fair distribution of organs; maintaining the national wait list with safe, secure and modern technology; and continuing to improve overall performance.

But we do not exist in a vacuum; we convene a community of 40,000 organ donation and transplant professionals and work in concert with our Federal partners.

The OPTN contract is awarded and managed by the Health Resource Services Administration (HRSA). The Centers for Medicare and Medicaid Services (CMS), meanwhile, covers the cost for many of the Nation's lifesaving transplants and related services. Through its reimbursement programs, CMS regulates transplant hospitals, and is also charged with certifying and overseeing organ procurement organizations (OPOs).

Together, UNOS, HRSA and CMS each play important roles in ensuring both the integrity and continuity of the complex national system on which so many rely. UNOS strives to align its efforts with those of HRSA and CMS so that we all work in concert as we fulfill our respective roles, while recognizing that there will always be room for improvement.

OPTN Background

The OPTN, as described in the statute, is a membership organization. We count amongst our members physicians, patients, transplant hospitals, organ procurement professionals, living donors, donor families, professional organizations, advocates, and volunteers, all of whom make the system what it is. And that is by design.

When Congress developed the framework for the OPTN, it did so knowing that it was entrusting physicians and patients with the responsibility to make critical, medically complex policy decisions based on firsthand experience, shared values, and their ongoing participation in the organ donation and transplant process. We still agree with that prescient decision.

That is the community UNOS is so proud to represent—a community dedicated to the equitable distribution of organs no matter who you are or where you live to save as many lives as possible through transplant.

With this commitment to equity underpinning everything we do, we have seen rapid and remarkable changes in the past few years alone; changes that have expanded equitable access to transplants for candidates on the wait list, increased priority for the sickest patients on the wait list, addressed disparities by increasing transplants for historically marginalized communities, and so much more.

However, while access to a transplant once a patient has been added to the wait list is largely equitable, there are systemic shortcomings within the larger U.S. health-care system that make getting added to the wait list inequitable. We must confront this issue as a Nation and we are committed to addressing it within our purview as the OPTN.

Ours is a complex system; one that is dedicated to continuously improving, monitoring and adapting; one that involves thousands of people coming together every single day across the country in order to save lives.

It is a system Congress set in motion nearly 40 years ago, and which, thanks to the decisions and expertise of those who laid the foundation, allows us to best serve patients in need of a transplant.

Ongoing Successes

UNOS works to save lives every day, and the numbers bear out our successes in both improving the system and identifying new areas for enhancement.

In 2021, for instance, the national system made global history: for the first time in a single year, the United States surpassed 41,000 lifesaving transplants. That same year, the system also saw record numbers of liver, heart and lung transplants. These exciting milestones are the result of year-over-year increases in organ transplants for the past decade and occurred in the midst of worldwide pandemic.

Additionally, post-implementation monitoring reports show the positive impact of recent modifications to kidney and liver allocation policies. According to the 1-year monitoring report analyzing changes to kidney allocation (the most transplanted organ), we saw an ongoing increase in kidney transplants nationally, especially for historically marginalized communities, patients on dialysis, and others. This includes increases of:

- 23 percent for Black patients;
- 29 percent for Hispanic patients;
- 20 percent for Asian patients;
- 36 percent for patients with long wait-times on dialysis; and
- 63 percent for pediatric patients.

Meanwhile, the 2-year monitoring report for changes to liver allocation policy continued to show increases, with national rates increasing by 4.3 percent, including for the sickest patients, historically marginalized communities, and others.

Again, these successes have taken place in the midst of the global pandemic that imperiled access to health care. Deceased donor transplant rates dipped in March of 2020, but quickly rebounded to pre-pandemic levels by April 2020. This was the result of the collective effort of physicians, professionals and others on the front lines.

It should also be noted that these successes are not stand-alone achievements, but instead the product of years of ongoing policy development, inclusive debate, rigorous discussion, monitoring, and a commitment to continuous improvement.

While the votes to enact these policies were not unanimous, the changes were enthusiastically supported by a vast majority of Board members. Additionally, our policy development process has now been reviewed by HHS and the General Accounting Office, as well as multiple courts, and these policies are now in effect and benefitting patients across the country.

Unfortunately, an ongoing misconception is that our Nation's success in donation and transplant is due to the ongoing and tragic opioid crisis and to the prevalence of gun violence.

The national increase in transplants predates the beginning of the opioid crisis and the recent rise in violent crime. Additionally, both policy changes and technological advancements have played a role in increasing transplants. Yet there is another, more important point to be made here.

Every death is tragic. However, regardless of the manner in which a potential donor dies, the Organ Procurement Organization (OPO) is still there to counsel the family, surgeons are still there to recover the selfless donor's organs, and the transplant hospital is still there to give the gift of life to a grateful recipient.

As previously mentioned, we have seen dramatic increases in the number of transplants taking place over the past decade. We are also focused intently, not just on the number of transplants, but the equitable distribution of lifesaving organs.

The OPTN Minority Affairs Committee (MAC) has been looking at these issues for years, resulting in the policies that have helped drive increases in transplants for patients of color.

Just recently, following the efforts of a diverse workgroup made up of both patients and physicians, the OPTN Board passed a new rule requiring that all transplant hospitals must use race-neutral measures of kidney function.

Role of UNOS

With the creation of the OPTN, Congress designed a system to address the Nation's critical organ donation shortage and improve organ matching and placement. To accomplish this, Congress did not create a centralized, government-run process to determine policies impacting these life-saving actions. Instead, Congress believed that patients and physicians should lead the way. This was the correct decision then, and remains the best choice today.

Thanks to congressional foresight, we now have an OPTN with a board and committees populated by patients, physicians, living donors, donor families and patient advocates who help make policy through rigorous debate and based on their unique experiences. There are currently 26 OPTN Committees, including committees dedicated to specific organ transplant types, technology, minority affairs, patient affairs, policy oversight, safety, and others.

These experiences are essential to making difficult, complex, and often emotional policy decisions that impact the lives of thousands across the country.

So much of the ongoing discussion of our shared successes, collaborative efforts, and everything this diverse and thriving national community has accomplished is muddled by a basic misunderstanding of UNOS's role in our complex national system.

Some think of UNOS as a regulator, with codified regulatory authority and congressionally mandated powers to oversee and penalize those not in compliance.

However, based on the law Congress enacted, UNOS, in its role as the OPTN, is not a regulator.

Regulatory authority of the Nation's organ donation and transplant system rests with CMS, and the delineation of our different roles is clear, established in both statute and policy, and essential to our ongoing collaboration and alignment.

Our particular role is multifaceted, complex and essential:

- UNOS members work alongside each other as partners in improvement;
- We operate a rigorous peer review process which includes site visits, reviews, helping to develop plans of action, offering educational opportunities, and other limited oversight functions;
- We built, monitor and continuously improve the IT infrastructure that makes it possible to match donor organs with recipients in need of a transplant;
- We develop, implement, and monitor equitable organ allocation policies; and
- We serve as both a convener of the transplant community and as an advocate on behalf of the Nation's organ donation and transplant system.

Membership and Professional Standards COMMITTEE (MPSC)

The Membership and Professional Standards Committee (MPSC) is an operational committee of the OPTN. In this role, the committee maintains OPTN membership criteria, monitors OPTN member compliance with this criteria, as well as compliance with OPTN bylaws, policies, and the OPTN final rule. As needed, the MPSC takes action or makes recommendations for further action to the OPTN board of directors.

The MPSC also identifies opportunities for individual member improvement and opportunities for transplant community education, all in an ongoing effort to improve patient safety and safeguard the integrity of the transplant system.

The MPSC is made up of volunteers who reflect the transplant community at large, including physicians with expertise in each organ transplant type and OPO volunteers. Health Resources Services Administration (HRSA) representatives also participate as ex officio members.

Integral to UNOS's success in supporting continuous improvement among members and the community at large is the MPSC's confidential medical peer-review process—a vital process required by the OPTN final rule and the Federal contract that allows the OPTN to review member performance, conduct investigations, and fact-find within a confidential setting.

Confidential peer review is a common practice across the U.S. health-care system. This was driven in large part by a landmark Institute of Medicine (IOM) report from 2000, which emphasized the importance of confidential peer-review to boost performance, ensure patient safety and encourage continuous improvement.

This report led to a national sea change and spurred the adoption of confidential peer review across the health-care landscape. HHS incorporated this approach into the final rule in 2000 and this critical tool was included into the OPTN contract soon after.

The "peer review" component is essential. Clinicians and professionals on the MPSC represent all the primary disciplines involved in transplantation. This expertise makes it possible to view member actions within the proper context, including what should have been known and what actions should have been taken under any given circumstance.

Confidentiality is equally important, as it increases the possibility that OPTN members are more likely to come forward to report issues that occur at their organization. Without willing members able to provide critical information, the committee would not be able to fully assess a given event, and suggest needed improvements. Removing confidentially protections would imperil the process and may have a chilling effect on those who might otherwise report troubling behavior.

The protection afforded by confidential medical peer-review also includes the opinions, statements and deliberations of MPSC committee volunteers themselves, ensuring their participation in the process without fear of professional reprisal or litigation.

A range of actions are available if, after investigation and deliberation, the MPSC finds a member has not followed OPTN requirements. Some of those sanctions are not public, such as notices of noncompliance or letters of warning. However, if the MPSC recommends that the OPTN board of directors take an "adverse action," which includes placing a member on probation or declaring a member not in good standing, and the Board acts on the recommendation, these designations are made public.

The board may also decide a member's non-compliance with OPTN requirements risks patient health or public safety, or that the member consistently fail to improve while under an adverse action. In these cases, the Board must make an official referral to the U.S. Secretary of HHS.

This complex but essential process helps ensure the Nation's organ donation and transplant system holds itself to the highest standards, drives member improvement and makes it possible to work with our community partners to address issues and arrive at workable, patient-centered solutions, all with appropriate governmental oversight.

The MPSC works collaboratively with every member in our community as a partner in improvement, and its rigorous process ensures prompt responses and swift action if necessary.

National Academies of Sciences, Engineering, and Mathematics (NASEM) Report

UNOS has continued to pursue efforts to improve the Nation's organ donation and transplant system, increase equity, expand access, increase patient opportunities for involvement, and save even more lives.

NASEM's February 2022 report addressed many of these issues. We were pleased that their in-depth analysis recognized many of our ongoing efforts, which aligned with their recommendations and reflect work already underway within and across our community, in many instances led by, in collaboration with or made possible by the support of UNOS.

These include:

- Enhancing current educational offerings for patients;
- Emphasizing shared-decision making between patients and physicians;
- Establishing new patient-centric transplant program performance metrics that go into effect this year;
- Adjusting payment policies to incentivize the utilization of harder to place organs; and
- Increasing transparency and accountability by launching a new list of codes for transplant programs to use when they refuse an order offer.

And other efforts outlined in more detail below.

Equity

The NASEM report emphasized the importance of increasing equity in access to the national wait list, regardless of where the patient lives or who they are. We agree, and have been dedicated to this proposition since our inception, both as a condition of our own organizational values and as a condition of the law which first established the OPTN.

One recent example is the development of the "Continuous Distribution" framework, an approach the NASEM committee vigorously supported. The Continuous Distribution policy will erase hard boundaries, ensuring that no single attribute will determine if a patient gets a transplant. Importantly, this framework is also designed to be augmented over time, allowing for ongoing feedback from a wide range of stakeholders and giving patients an important seat at the table.

As mentioned earlier in this statement, the OPTN board of directors voted in June on an equity-based proposal to prohibit the use of race-based estimation of kidney health in OPTN policy.

Systemic Improvements

The NASEM Committee also made several recommendations for the OPTN and the donation and transplant community overall to improve the system. One of these was the development and adoption of national performance metrics, which we fully support. Other tools we currently offer to the public and policymakers to monitor ongoing progress are the OPTN Metrics Dashboard and the OPTN Equity Dashboard. Both can be found on the OPTN website.

NASEM also made recommendations for maximizing organ use. In its capacity as the OPTN, UNOS already has developed, tested and now offers the Kidney Offer Filters tool to transplant hospitals, which is in keeping with this NASEM recommendation. Our innovative tool, first available in January of 2022, allows kidney transplant programs to preemptively screen out offers they are unlikely to accept, reducing administrative burden, accelerating organ placement and making it easier for OPOs to find best-fit candidates quicker. We also must continue to reduce differences in practices from hospital to hospital and do our part to make sure everyone understands the organ offer review and acceptance process.

As a part of overall system improvement, NASEM also recommended that the U.S. Department of Health and Human Services (HHS) conduct an evaluation of the OPTN IT system within 1 to 2 years. UNOS welcomes this evaluation; as of this writing, one has not been conducted.

Beyond and before NASEM's recommendations, UNOS has always undertaken efforts to continuously improve the national system, bolster performance and support others within our community.

While the above efforts, projects and tools are in no way a comprehensive list of ongoing work, they do represent an accurate picture of UNOS, as a Federal contractor, responding to the needs of patients, physicians, and the organ donation and transplant community at large.

Transportation

Transportation is essential to the success of the organ donation and transplant system. Unless a recovered organ happens to be accepted by a candidate in the same hospital where the organ was recovered, the organ must necessarily be transported from the donor hospital to the transplant hospital. The vast majority of organ shipment logistics are determined between the OPO and the transplant hospital on the ground, although the OPO may request OPTN assistance in rare cases. Additionally, the OPTN has multiple policies in place that address the safety of organs in transport, particularly regarding packaging, labeling, and ultimately verifying successful delivery to the patient who accepted the organ.

Additionally, except for kidneys, most organs (hearts, lungs, livers, etc.) are transported in the company of the transplant physician who will be conducting the surgery. Disruptions are rare, but can still have a direct and serious impact on a patient in need of an organ.

Like many things within this national system, transporting an organ is extremely complex. Something as simple as a courier taking a wrong turn can delay the delivery of an organ.

That is why we have engaged in several collaborations with the community to improve the transport of organs through the development and adoption of innovative, evidence-based products to ensure patient safety.

The UNOS organ tracking service, for example, is now in use by 15 OPOs across the country and allows users to oversee organ shipments in real time. The tool provides OPOs with real-time location data, package updates and maps with easy-to- read visualizations. It also fully integrates with existing tools and systems, all in an effort to improve performance, speed, and patient outcomes.

We have also conducted a successful pilot of a UNOS Travel App, which will allow OPOs to select the best options for transporting organs. Once fully operational, the app will allow OPOs to view and select the most efficient options for shipping lifesaving organs on commercial flights. While these are all important innovations, we continue to pursue efforts to further improve the transport of donor organs.

IT Infrastructure

Our focus on continuous improvement also includes constantly enhancing our safe, secure and efficient IT infrastructure; a modernized system that we built, maintain, and enhance to ensure the highest performance on behalf of all those who have come to rely on it.

Our system is audited by both Federal authorities and third-party cybersecurity firms. We regularly meet and exceed both their standards and our rigorous Federal contract obligations. Additionally, the OPTN's Network Operations Oversight Committee (NOOC) assists the OPTN Board in overseeing a variety of essential IT functions, including organ matching and data collection.

We have spent years developing and improving our infrastructure, building and incorporating technological innovations, partnering with industry leaders, and leveraging Cybersecurity and Infrastructure Security Agency (CISA) resources to ensure robust performance and security on behalf of the communities we serve. This is why, despite more than 3 million hacking attempts each day, our system has remained safe and secure.

Our modern infrastructure was designed to make the Nation's complex allocation policies possible; an effective, one-of-a-kind approach that weds robust technological capabilities with in-depth policy knowledge and has maintained, outside of periodic scheduled maintenance, a system uptime of 99.99 percent.

While the votes to enact these policies were not unanimous, the changes were enthusiastically supported by a vast majority of board members. Additionally, our policy development process has now been reviewed by HHS and the General Accounting Office, as well as multiple courts, and these policies are now in effect and benefiting patients across the country.

Our IT developers and business analysts are experts in both technology and transplant and donation; it requires this kind of unique background to successfully and thoughtfully integrate effective technology and lifesaving policy.

A Shared Vision for the Future

Our vision for the U.S. donation and transplant system is straightforward: being able to provide a lifesaving transplant for everyone who needs one. There is still much work to do, but in collaboration with our community partners, physicians, patients, OPOs, hospitals, policymakers, advocacy organizations, volunteers and others, we are making this vision a reality. From transportation to technology, from equity to system-wide improvements, by building on the successes of our national system and our community's ongoing efforts on all fronts, we can come together around these shared goals. It is challenging and sometimes controversial; we welcome constructive debates. But when we come together, our work can literally change someone's life.

This collaborative, ambitious vision is transforming the system as we know it, building an even stronger national system we can be proud to call our own.

I would like to thank Chairman Wyden, Ranking member Crapo, and the entire Senate Committee on Finance once again for inviting me to discuss the status of donation and transplant today and what we can accomplish when we work together to further improve this lifesaving system. I look forward to your questions.

Attachments follow.

United Network For Organ Sharing (UNOS)

700 North 4th Street Richmond, VA 23219
tel: 804–782–4800
fax: 804–782–4816
www.unos.org

Memorandum

To: OPTN/UNOS Membership and Professional Standards Committee

From: Suzanne Gellner, Assistant Director, Department of Evaluation and Quality Date: July 23, 2009
Re: MPSC action following member waiver of rights to an interview

Historically, if a member waived its right to an interview for a proposed action, the department of evaluation and quality would, on behalf of the MPSC, issue the proposed sanction without further committee deliberation. It has come to our attention that this process has never been formally adopted by the Committee. Therefore, the department of evaluation and quality requests that the MPSC consider whether it would like to formally standardize this practice in all cases where a member waives its right to an interview.

According to OPTN Bylaws, Section 3.01A (3) (Interviews), except in the case of Category I potential violations, if the MPSC or MPSC/PCSC considers recommending an adverse action such as Probation or Member Not in Good Standing or is considering issuing a Letter of Reprimand, the applicant or member is entitled to an interview. OPTN Bylaws, Section 2.11 A (Procedural Rights) states that if a member waives its right to an interview, the MPSC may proceed to implement its proposed action. In order to exercise its rights to an interview before the MPSC or the MPSC/ PCSC, the member must deliver a written request for an interview to UNOS within 14 days following its receipt of the notice of the MPSC's proposed action. In accordance with Section 2.11A of the OPTN Bylaws, if the member does not deliver a written request for an interview, the MPSC may proceed to implement its proposed action.

Since 2006, the MPSC has issued seven letters of reprimand to members who have waived the right to an interview. The MPSC issued letters of reprimand for site survey results that remained below thresholds, organ refusals after acceptance that led to an organ's discard, failure to comply with data submission requirements, and repeated violation of policy 5.3. No member recommended for Probation or Member Not in Good Standing has ever waived its rights to an interview. Historically, when a member waived the right to an interview, it did not submit additional materials for MPSC consideration; therefore, the MPSC did not review additional evidence or reconsider its original decision. Standardizing this process for future MPSC recommendations would be consistent with historical practice; however, proceeding directly with the MPSC's proposed action offers no opportunity for the committee to reevaluate its decision.

If the MPSC decides to formally standardize this practice, the resolution to consider recommending an adverse action or issuing a Letter of Reprimand, combined with the member's waiver of its right to an interview, will result in the MPSC imposing its proposed action.

Operational Principles

Outcomes—applies to Large and Small Volume outcomes Is the program active? — Membership database.

Is the program already under review? — CMRS.

If program released in last 2 meeting cycles, no action required—CMRS.

Has program had a death or graft failure since the date of most recent release from review? — Transplant Log Access Database.

Rule	*Type*	*Approved By*	*Approved Date*	*Retired Date*	*Supporting Documentation*	*Active*	*Comments*
Process for member waiving interview. If a member waives an interview, we will take the issue back to the MPSC to determine what action they want to take.	Process	MPSC	7/23/2009		Memo	Yes	Changes to Appendix L 6/13/18 have made slight changes to this, but we would still go back to the committee and ask their opinions on it.
Large and Small volume outcome review principles: how the MPSC approaches outcomes reviews.	Outcomes	PAIS	Varying dates	7/1/2022	Guidance doc	Ending soon	Retiring with introduction of new performance metrics—may re-introduce something for recently released programs as time goes on.
Inactivity Review principles: how the MPSC approaches inactivity reviews.	Outcomes	PAIS	Varying dates		Guidance doc	Yes	
Review of Compliance cases on Committee Management.	Process	PCSC	3/27/2012		Slides	Yes	Documents refer to PCSC but subcommittee does not exist anymore, all cases go to Committee Management.
Allocation—reportable allocation events: provides a list of criteria for allocations that the MPSC does not need to review because members are acting to prevent organ wastage.	Policy	PCSC	4/1/2013		Documents	Yes	Even if the allocation meets these criteria, allocations can be referred if there are questions or something seems unusual. Updated 4/22/21.
LDAE—not reporting outside 2 years as FYI: previously all living donor events, even those that occurred longer than 2 years after donation, were reported to the MPSC as an FYI. Changed process to only refer those cases to the MPSC if the event appears that it could be donation-related.	Process	MPSC Chair	10/27/2015			Yes	
Vessel Storage—do not send members to the MPSC the first time they store prohibited vessels (HCV, HBV).	Policy	MPSC 1	0/27/2016		Summary	Yes	

For Submission to the U.S. Senate Committee on Finance (October 12, 2022) (Continued)

Rule	*Type*	*Approved By*	*Approved Date*	*Retired Date*	*Supporting Documentation*	*Active*	*Comments*
Site survey—support for changing sample sizes, creating a CAP template. NO OFFICIAL RULE CHANGE.	Policy	Internal	10/27/2016		Summary	Yes	Staff Summary
Two tiered review of SRTR 1-year post-transplant outcomes for kidney—if meets threshold for review with full cohort of transplants, remove higher risk kidney transplants and only send inquiry if meet threshold for review.	Outcomes	PAIS	10/27/2016	7/1/2022	Minutes	Ending soon	MPSC approved 37–0–0. Eliminated with change to metrics and reduction in number of programs identified.
Allocation—do not review extrarenal organs turned down in OR.	Policy	MPSC	7/13/2017		Staff summary	Yes	Approved 30, 0, 0 Updated 4/22/21.
Elimination of identification of programs for outcomes review based on small volume criteria.	Outcomes	PAIS	7/13/2017	7/1/2022	Minutes	Ending soon	MPSC approved 30–1–0 (Small volume no longer in bylaws after 7/2022).
NUV (now Notice of Noncompliance) for late key personnel reporting.	Application	MPSC	7/15/2017		Staff summary	Yes	Approved 30, 0, 0
Wait-list inactivity monitoring: the first instance of improperly notifying patients of wait-list inactivity will require a CAP, the second instance will be referred to the MPSC.	Process	MPSC	1/30/2018		Staff Summary	Yes	MPSC approved 19–0–0
Review of non-institutional member renewals: non-institutional renewal applications will be placed on a consent agenda if all requirements are met.	Application	MPSC	3/1/2018		Staff summary	Yes	MPSC approved 32–0–0
KPC Application Review Process Change: key personnel change applications will be placed on a consent agenda if the application clearly meets criteria.	Application	MPSC	7/18/2018		Staff summary	Yes	MPSC approved 34–0–0

Rule	*Type*	*Approved By*	*Approved Date*	*Retired Date*	*Supporting Documentation*	*Active*	*Comments*
Late Report to the OPTN of Potential Donor-Derived Disease Transmissions: if a member reports a potential disease transmission appropriately to other members, but does not report to the OPTN, the first instance will not be sent to the MPSC.	Policy	MPSC	7/18/2018		Staff summary	Yes	MPSC approved 34–0–0 with two changes: all members start with a clean slate, and FTNC time frame is 3 years, to be consistent with compliance history time frame when reviewing cases.
SET Tool introduction and implementation: approved use of Survey Evaluation Tool and for staff to close or review again without MPSC review.	Policy	MPSC	7/18/2018		Staff summary	Yes	MPSC approved 34–0–0
Revising Outcomes operational rule to no inquiry for 2 SRTR reporting cycles after release.	Outcomes	MPSC	2/27/2019	7/1/2022	Staff summary	Ending soon	MPSC approved 35–0–0 Eliminated with change to metrics, will likely reintroduce as metric review matures.
Determining that the minimum two year (2–5 yr) time in the Bylaws for physician/surgeon logs can be fulfilled by the person's employment at designated transplant programs, not just by the dates of the actual transplants.	Application	MPSC	2/27/2019		Minutes	Yes	Made a decision on interpretation, then approved an application with this issue to set precedent.
Add application rejections to Membership consent agenda: after an application has been rejected unanimously by the ad hoc subcommittee, the rejection will be placed on a consent agenda.	Application	MPSC	2/26/2020		Staff summary	Yes	Approved 37–0–0
Update older decision to close self- reported issues with no action to include placing self-reported issues directly on the consent agenda unless significant concerns with response or patient safety.	Process	MPSC	4/22/2021		Staff summary	Yes	Approved 26–0–0
Update use of Survey Evaluation tool to use SET to evaluate both routine and first desk review, place first desk review directly on consent.	Process	MPSC	4/22/2021		Staff summary	Yes	Approved 27–0–0
Made adjustments to allocation operational rules based on changes to policy.	Process	MPSC	4/22/2021		Staff summary	Yes	Approved 26–0–0
Review of lung donor COVID–19 testing.	Process	MPSC	5/24/2021		Staff summary	Yes	Approved 28-0-0

Small Volume Outcomes—all of the above and then #2 below.

1) SRTR data provided includes all programs with 9 or fewer transplants that had at least one event in the 2.5 year cohort.
2) Review to determine if the program has had a subsequent event in the year since the end of cohort. If not, no action required—Transplant log Access Database.

Additional Small Volume Guidance

To memorialize discussions regarding how to proceed with the several cases where programs that are currently under review have had a second component flagged (adult or pediatric) or are under review for inactivity.

- If a small volume program is flagged for outcomes that is already under review for inactivity, an outcomes case will be created, the inactivity case will be closed. No subsequent event is required.
- If a small volume component is flagged for outcomes when the program is already under review for the other component, the outcomes case will be combined into an all ages review without a subsequent event.
- In both situations, instead of automatically sending an initial outcomes survey, analyst should contact the reviewers for the existing case and determine if:
    - An initial outcomes survey should be sent.
    - If no initial outcomes survey, do the reviewers want to request:
        - Only synopses and activity information for the newly flagged component/ program.
        - Request additional information on the new flagged component/program.

Guidelines for Inactivity Review Transplant inactivity

Once receive Turndown Reports:

1) Is program currently active? If no, no action required—Membership database.
2) Is program currently under review—check Active PAIS Case report—CMRS.
3) Has program been in active status for one year? If not, no action required.
4) Has program been released in last 2 meeting cycles? If yes, no action required—CMRS.
5) No offers received/no candidates on wait list—get a pass for one cycle—review turndown report/wait list.

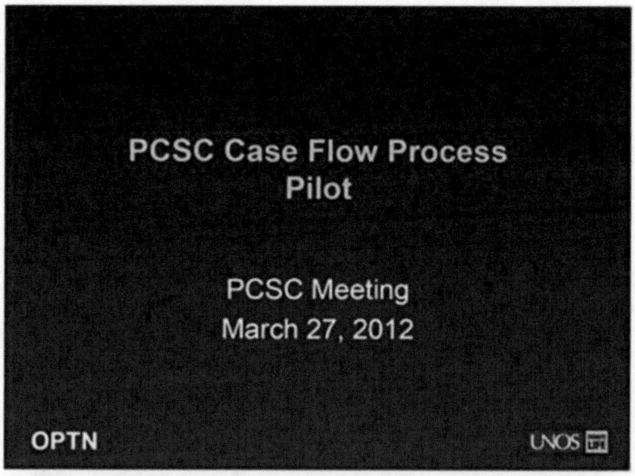
PCSC Case Flow Process
Pilot
PCSC Meeting
March 27, 2012
OPTN
UNOS

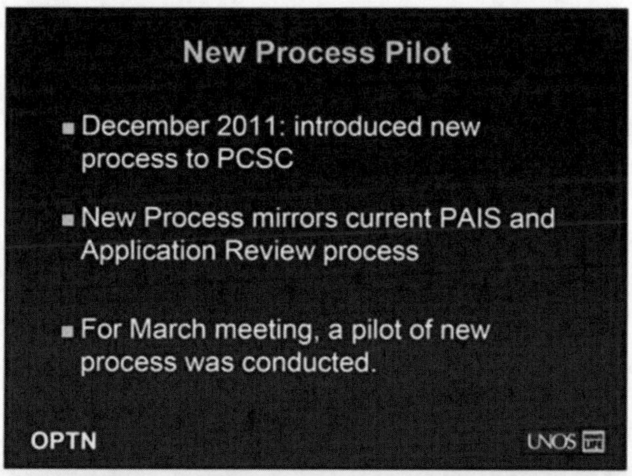
New Process Pilot
December 2011: introduced new process to PCSC
New Process mirrors current PAIS and Application Review process
For March meeting, a pilot of new process was conducted.
OPTN
UNOS

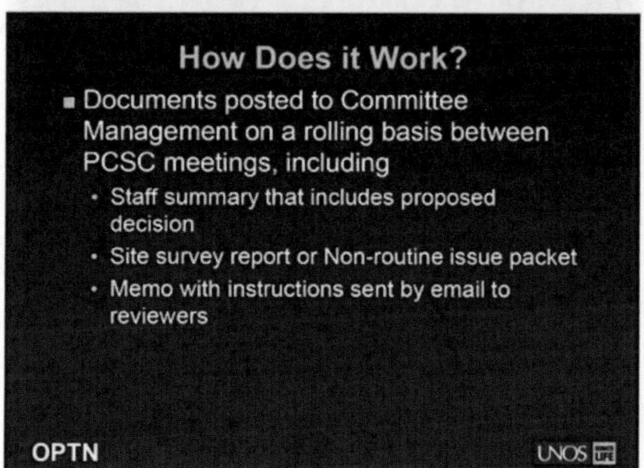
How Does it Work?
Documents posted to Committee Management on a rolling basis between PCSC meetings, including
Staff summary that includes proposed decision
Site survey report or Non-routine issue packet
Memo with instructions sent by email to reviewers
OPTN
UNOS

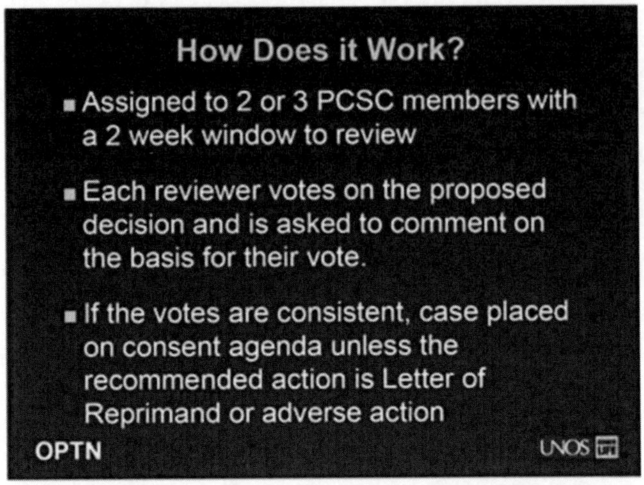
How Does it Work?
Assigned to 2 or 3 PCSC members with a 2 week window to review
Each reviewer votes on the proposed decision and is asked to comment on the basis for their vote.
If the votes are consistent, case placed on consent agenda unless the recommended action is Letter of Reprimand or adverse action
OPTN
UNOS

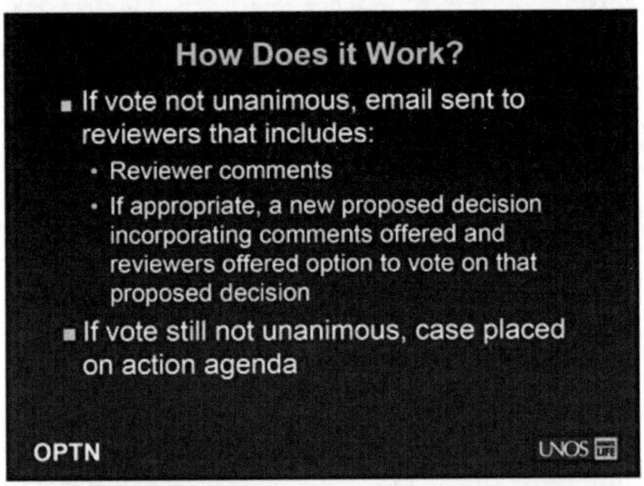
How Does it Work?
If vote not unanimous, email sent to reviewers that includes:
Reviewer comments
If appropriate, a new proposed decision incorporating comments offered and reviewers offered option to vote on that proposed decision
If vote still not unanimous, case placed on action agenda
OPTN
UNOS

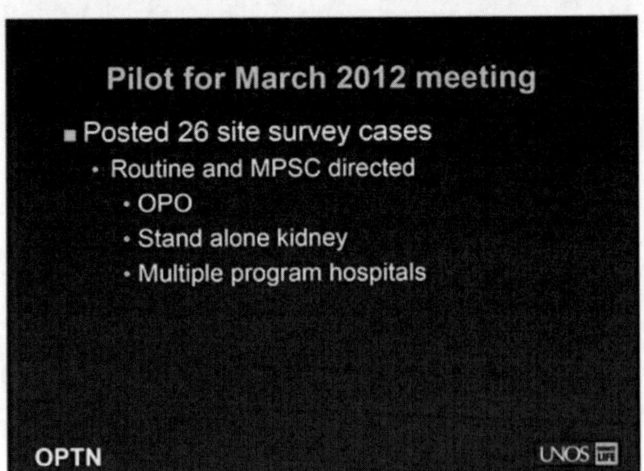
Pilot for March 2012 meeting
Posted 26 site survey cases
Routine and MPSC directed
OPO
Stand alone kidney
Multiple program hospitals
OPTN
UNOS

How Does it Work?

- If vote not unanimous, email sent to reviewers that includes:
  - Reviewer comments
  - If appropriate, a new proposed decision incorporating comments offered and reviewers offered option to vote on that proposed decision
- If vote still not unanimous, case placed on action agenda

OPTN UNOS

Site Survey Process

OPTN UNOS

Types of Site Surveys

DEQ's site surveyors detect potential policy violations nationwide across all organ groups through routine on-site, desk, and special reviews.

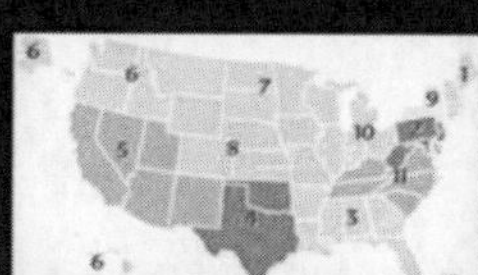

OPTN/UNOS Region Map

- 3-year reviews of all transplant centers and OPOs
  - Review medical records
  - Conduct staff interviews
  - Assess clinical and administrative compliance
- Patient safety reviews
- MPSC-directed reviews

OPTN UNOS

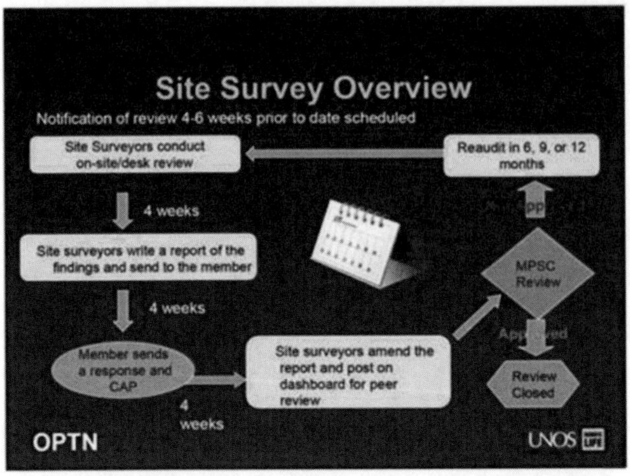
Site Survey Overview
Notification of review 4-6 weeks prior to date scheduled
Site Surveyors conduct on-site/desk review
4 weeks
Site surveyors write a report of the findings and send to the member
4 weeks
Member sends a response and CAP
4 weeks
Site surveyors amend the report and post on dashboard for peer review
MPSC Review
Review Closed
Reaudit in 6, 9, or 12 months
OPTN
UNOS

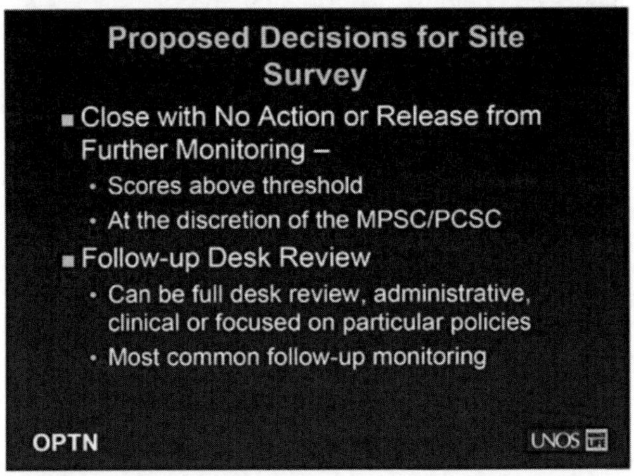
Proposed Decisions for Site Survey
Close with No Action or Release from Further Monitoring –
Scores above threshold
At the discretion of the MPSC/PCSC
Follow-up Desk Review
Can be full desk review, administrative, clinical or focused on particular policies
Most common follow-up monitoring
OPTN
UNOS

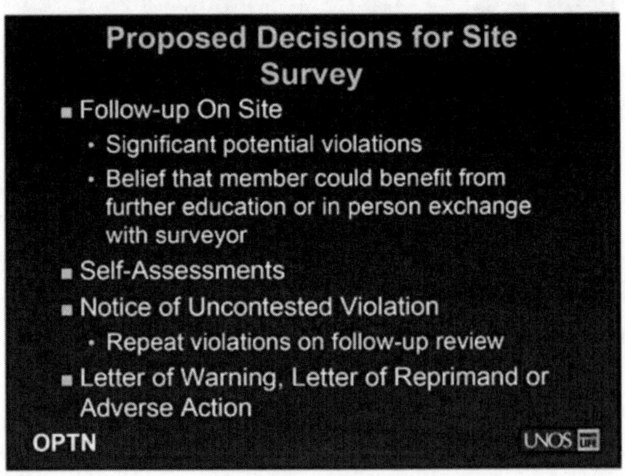
Proposed Decisions for Site Survey
Follow-up On Site
Significant potential violations
Belief that member could benefit from further education or in person exchange with surveyor
Self-Assessments
Notice of Uncontested Violation
Repeat violations on follow-up review
Letter of Warning, Letter of Reprimand or Adverse Action
OPTN
UNOS

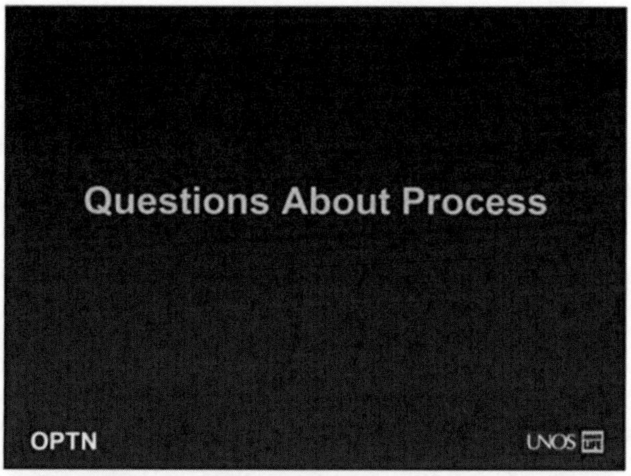
Questions About Process
OPTN
UNOS

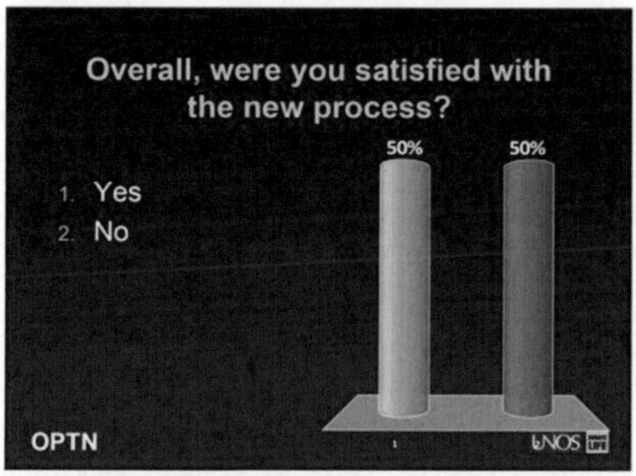
Overall, were you satisfied with the new process?
1. Yes
2. No
50%
50%
OPTN
UNOS

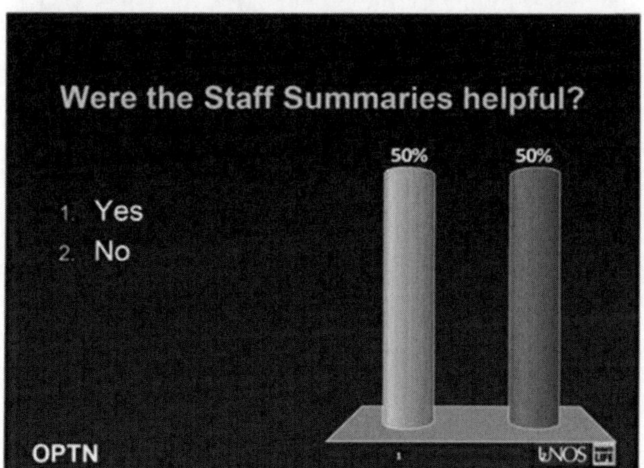
Were the Staff Summaries helpful?
1. Yes
2. No
50%
50%
OPTN
UNOS

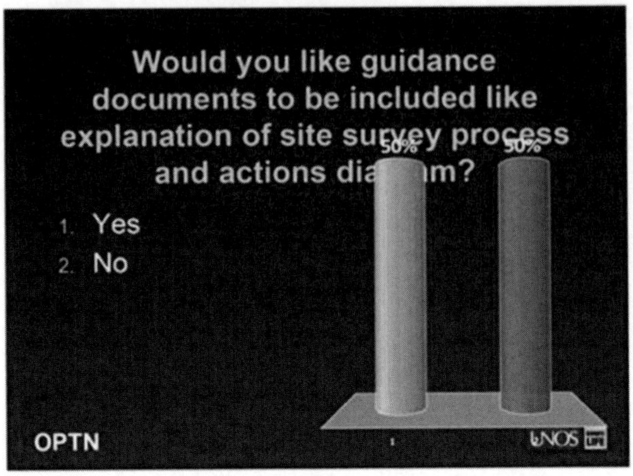

MPSC/PCSC Allocation Review

Exclusionary Criteria

The MPSC Allocation Analysis work group recommended that the UNOS staff not forward allocation cases involving the criteria listed below to the MPSC/PCSC for review.

1) Hep C positive donors.
2) Hep B Core positive donors.
3) Donors with age > 70.
4) DCD—for all organs EXCEPT kidney.
5) Local back up (Originally only in cases of actual vs. intended transplants associated with transplant center reviews. In October 2014 the MPSC work group expanded the scope to include OPOs that grant centers local back up to avoid organ wastage after late declines or try to and place organs that would otherwise be wasted).

For kidney allocations ONLY:

- ABO non-identical allocation not on a match run with appropriate documentation.
- Medical urgency with appropriate paperwork that local centers agreed.

The PCSC also discussed a number of possible improvements to PCSC/MPSC operational rules associated with site surveys and an educational referral to the OPTN Operations and Safety Committee. Specifically, the PCSC discussed potential changes to the process for requesting corrective action plans for each site survey violation, the timing and intent of follow-up focused desk reviews and the site survey sample size. The PCSC generally supported the following ideas, with the understanding that staff would continue to develop the ideas and bring them back to the PCSC for further discussion:

- The creation of a corrective action plan template for members.
- A tiered approach to which violations require a formal corrective action plan for MPSC review and which require another response such as self-audits, or potentially no response, if the member's policies and templates are updated at the time of the survey.
- A "check in" by UNOS staff after the routine survey to ensure the member has implemented its corrective actions and that the corrective actions are effective. This check in may delay the PCSC's review of the routine survey report, but would potentially provide enough information to allow the PCSC to close the review with no action instead of requesting a follow-up review.
- The creation of operational rules to identify which routine surveys automatically require follow-up reviews and which cases must go to the MPSC for the MPSC to determine whether a follow-up review, or more significant action is required.

The PCSC noted that smaller sample sizes, such as five records for small volume programs, would not provide statistically significant data. However, the PCSC supported the idea of considering other methods of identifying the appropriate sample size, such as a percentage of the program's total volume, and including the program's total volume as a reference point. The PCSC supported focusing reviews on the most recent and relevant data (by shortening the time frame of review) and focusing the review on identifying systematic issues.

The PCSC also reviewed the results of the UNOS staff analysis of prohibited vessel storage cases. Staff identified common root cause analyses and corrective action plans, and asked the PCSC to confirm whether their findings aligned with the PCSC members' review of these cases. The PCSC supported sharing the findings with the Patient Safety Advisory Group of the OPTN Operations and Safety Committee, to support the PSAG's development of educational resources for the transplant community. The PCSC generally supported the ongoing creation of such resources to share with the community.

In addition, based on its review of a number of prohibited vessel storage cases, the PCSC also approved a new operational rule to facilitate its review of these cases. Going forward, UNOS staff will automatically close with no action a member's first violation of the prohibited vessel storage policy. Staff will provide members with any educational materials available, will advise the member that the MPSC expects the member to implement a corrective action plan, and will advise the member that any additional instances of the member storing prohibited vessels will be forwarded to the MPSC for review. Staff will also inform the member that MPSC's review would include the initial violation.

UNOS Site Survey Discussion PCSC Meeting

October 25, 2016

Staff Summary

Item for Consideration

At the October 2016 PCSC/MPSC meeting, Member Quality staff would like the PCSC to provide feedback on:

- The need for corrective action plans/member responses to survey violations.
- A draft corrective action plan (CAP)/response template for members to use in response to their site surveys.
- The purpose and timing of follow-up desk reviews.
- Site survey sample sizes.

This feedback will help Member Quality staff as it continues to evaluate options and implement improved processes to promote value-adding monitoring and increasing efficiencies to reduce the burden on members, the MPSC and staff.

Site Survey Corrective Action Plans

Currently, Member Quality staff requires members to submit a CAP for each potential violation that will be forwarded to the MPSC for review. (Please note: we do not specify that the response must be a formal CAP with root cause analysis. Depending on the situation, a simple explanation may be sufficient, and we leave it up to the member to evaluate whether a RCA and CAP are appropriate. However, despite this guidance, we believe many members often feel obligated to provide a full RCA and CAP. In the rest of this document, we use the term CAP to mean any sort of formal response to the MPSC.)

During the site survey process, members receive an initial site survey report that details all potential policy violations identified during a site survey or focused desk review. Members are asked to either submit new documentation to verify compliance, or to submit a CAP to address the non-compliance. (We do not typically review or require a CAP for a policy that is no longer in effect at the time of the survey.) The final site survey report forwarded to the MPSC for review includes all potential violations and the member's corrective actions.

Staff are interested in the PCSC's feedback on what information it needs in order to decide on the appropriate action after a site survey? Does every identified violation need a CAP, or are there specific instances when the PCSC does need or want a formal response from members? Potential alternatives approaches include not requiring corrective actions for certain policies or issues such as data entry errors or not requiring corrective action plans for surveys that we know are going straight on the consent agenda.

Corrective Action Plan Template

Member Quality staff are also evaluating whether to create a CAP template that members can fill out to address the violations. The idea is similar to the template plan for quality improvement that members receive in response to MPSC-directed peer visits. Member Quality staff want to make sure that this tool is useful for members as they create their CAP and also useful for PCSC members in your review of site survey reports.

Please review the enclosed template and be prepared to provide feedback during the PCSC meeting. Are any fields missing that you think should be added? Are there any fields that you think can be removed? Is the formatting easy to read?

Please note that the attached version assumes that all policy violations require a response of some kind according to the current process, but the form could be adapted as needed to fit a revised process for requesting CAPs. We can also consider whether the MPSC wants to specify which policy violations require a CAP and which do not and update the template accordingly.

Follow-up Desk Reviews

Follow-up focused desk reviews are a key component of the site survey and MPSC monitoring process. Since July 2015, the MPSC has requested follow-up desk reviews in approximately 17.5% of transplant program and OPO site surveys and has requested follow-up desk reviews in approximately 38% of living donor surveys.

Historically, the MPSC has requested Member Quality staff conduct follow-up focused desk reviews when a member's site survey report shows non-compliance with one or more particular policies, and the MPSC continues to request follow up reviews until the member has demonstrated compliance and/or satisfactory improvement.

For example, if a member has errors in five of 10 records regarding informed consent, the MPSC will likely request a follow up focused desk review of compliance with the informed consent policy. If the follow up review finds errors in four or five records, the MPSC will likely request another follow-up desk review. This pattern would continue until the member shows improvement. On the other hand, if the follow up review finds no errors or just one error, it is likely that the MPSC would close the review. They key is that the member typically must have records available for review that show compliance before being released.

In another example, assume the member had errors in five records from 2015, but no errors in the other five records from 2016. The program explained that they self-identified and corrected the error in late 2015 by updating its informed consent template. Because the program has five records in their sample after they updated the template, the MPSC would consider the more recent records to be evidence of compliance and would typically not request a follow-up desk review. However, if the 10 records in the sample were all from 2015, prior to the template update, the member would have no records in the sample to show that its corrective action was working, and the MPSC would likely request a follow up review. Similarly, if the member updated the template immediately before the site survey and provided it to surveyors during the visit, the MPSC would likely request a follow up focused desk review to ensure the template is properly implemented and used.

Items to consider:

- Does the MPSC wish for the standard to remain that members must actively demonstrate compliance, or is having an appropriate template or policy in place by the conclusion of the survey sufficient to close a review with no action? Should the standard be different for administrative policies or policies with patient safety or allocation implications?
- If the MPSC wants to ensure members are showing improvement and compliance, would the MPSC consider having a "staff check in" in lieu of a formal follow up focused desk review in some cases? Example: the member with errors in five of 10 records submits an updated template during the site survey visit. Site surveyors check in with the member a certain amount of time after the site survey and review additional records to confirm the new process is working, and includes that information in the site survey report to send to members. This may delay the site survey report making it to the MPSC for review, but may give the MPSC sufficient information to close the review with no action rather than requesting a formal follow-up desk review. The MPSC may need to identify which situations are appropriate for such "check ins" to avoid following up on every potential policy violation.

- Are there any other factors or data the MPSC would like to consider when deciding whether a follow up survey is appropriate? Examples include any other information surveyors may already obtain or start obtaining during site visits, the member's compliance history, and/or the member's outcomes.

Site Survey Sample Sizes (for Transplant Program Surveys)

In addition to considering potential changes to the follow-up desk review process, staff are also considering ways in which the emphasis of site surveys can change from an intensive chart review to an evaluation of a member's practices from evaluation through to transplant, death or removal. The living donor surveys currently review a selected sample of donors throughout the evaluation process.

Current process:

- Routine on-site surveys are conducted approximately once every 3 years. The applicable timeframe from which records are identified for review is typically the two to three years prior to the survey.
- The number of records available for review varies by organ group and the type of policy being reviewed. Generally speaking, administrative policies such as notification of listing, removal, and the option to multiple list, as well as informed consent are limited to 10 records in the sample. Clinical policies such as verification of candidate status include up to 30–45 records in the sample depending on the organ group. This may include anywhere from 60 to more than 100 individual listings for review.

Proposed process:

In order to incorporate and focus on an overall process review rather than strict data review, to ensure surveyors are focusing on the most recent and relevant data, and to promote consistency across the number of records reviewed between organ groups and surveys, staff are evaluating whether to implement new and smaller sample sizes in their surveys.

- Centers will be categorized by size (based on the number of transplants performed the previous year and the nationwide percentile distribution of center volume per organ type).
- The program size category determines the number of records reviewed for all policies:
  - Small centers—5 records.
  - Medium programs—10 records.
  - Large programs—15 records.
    - Living donor kidney and liver programs would have 5 records for review.
    - Surveys would still be scheduled approximately every three years. Rather than reviewing 2 to 3 years' of data, surveyors would limit the review period to the most recent 12 month timeframe. This would promote the review of the most recent and relevant practices and policy requirements. (Less but more relevant records.).
    - Limiting the survey review period to the most recent year provides the most relevant data, but means we may never know if the program had significant issues in the other time between the surveys.

- A smaller sample may influence the effectiveness of current scorecards and thresholds. For example, intestine and pancreas programs do not currently have scorecards due to their low volumes, so we may need to discontinue using them in the smaller volume programs. We can of course revise the scorecards as needed, or develop an alternative method to identify surveys that can be placed on the consent agenda to close with no action.
- A smaller sample size may promote inconsistent review. If a survey shows errors in two of five records, will MPSC reviewers perceive that as only two errors, or as a 60 percent compliance rate? There is not a clear historical action in these cases.

Items to consider:

- Does the MPSC support the proposed sample sizes? If the site survey reports included fewer records, would the MPSC need any additional information to determine an appropriate action? If so, what information is needed? Examples include any other information surveyors may already obtain or start obtaining during site visits, the member's compliance history, and/or the member's outcomes.

Scientific Registry of Transplant Recipients (SRTR) Proposed Evaluation Plan for Transplant Program Performance Measures (Outcome Measures) Proposal

The proposal focuses on improving the utilization of high-KDPI kidneys through reduced oversight of "high-risk transplants," i.e., high-KDPI kidneys transplanted into high-EPTS candidates. The reduced oversight of high-risk transplants has raised concerns that unadjusted survival of high-risk transplants may worsen after the implementation of the proposal. It is therefore critical that the proposal has a detailed evaluation plan to ensure improved utilization of high-KDPI kidneys while maintaining adequate survival of high-risk transplants. The evaluation plan outlines the schedule and corresponding analysis to:

1) Estimate the impact of the proposal on the utilization of high-KDPI kidneys.
2) Estimate the impact of the proposal on the survival rate of high-risk transplants.

The proposal should impact the utilization of high-KDPI kidneys relatively quickly after implementation. Therefore, one year after the implementation of the operational rule, the discard rate of high-KDPI kidneys one-year pre-and post-implementation will be compared. Specifically, data for recovered kidneys with KDPI = 85% along with donor characteristics will be pulled from the SRTR database. An initial descriptive analysis will compare the unadjusted discard rates pre- and post-implementation. For the primary analysis, a generalized linear mixed model (GLMM) with a logit-link will estimate the effect of the proposal on the probability of discard with an indicator for recovery pre-or post-implementation. It is critical to account for differences in the donor pool as the proposal may lead to more aggressive OPO placement of high-KDRI kidneys. Thus, based in part on the June 2016 SRTR OPO yield model, the GLMM will account for potential differences in the donor pool pre-and post-implementation by including covariates for: age, KDRI, blood type, DCD donation, cause of death, cigarette use, circumstance of death, clinical infections (blood, lung, urine and other), cocaine use, gender, Hepatitis B serology, HCV serology, heavy alcohol use, CDC high infectious risk, history of cancer, history of diabetes, history of hypertension, insulin dependence, mechanism of death, organ recovery outside of contiguous 48 states and terminal serum creatinine. Penalized splines will estimate the effect of age, KDRI, and terminal serum creatinine. Finally, a random effect for donor will account for the potential correlation between kidneys from the same donor. The proposal will be determined to have a sig- nificant effect on discard rates of high-KDPI kidneys by having a one-sided p-value less than 0.05 on the indicator for recovery pre- or post-implementation. Missing data will be handled by indicators and continuous variables will additionally be set to the median of the non-missing values.

Due to the follow-up required for assessing post-transplant survival, the evaluation of the proposed operational rule on the survival rate of high-risk transplants will be completed two years after implementation. Specifically, data on high-risk transplants completed one-year pre- and post-implementation will be pulled from the SRTR database. Similar to the evaluation of post-transplant outcomes, recipients will be administratively censored after one year of survival. An initial descriptive analysis will compare the unadjusted one-year survival rates. For the primary analysis, a Cox proportional hazards model will estimate the effect of the proposal on post-transplant graft survival with an indicator for pre-or post-implementation transplant. Due to potential differences in recipient and donor characteristics, the Cox proportional hazards model will adjust for KDRI, EPTS, CDC high infectious risk and DCD donation. Penalized splines will estimate the effect of KDRI and EPTS. Every covariate in the SRTR post-transplant graft survival model cannot be used due to the relatively low number of expected events over two years within the subset of high-risk transplants. Missing data will be handled through multiple imputation as implemented in the most recent PSR cohort.

A non-inferiority test will determine whether post-implementation graft survival is appropriately maintained with the non-inferiority margin set to a hazard ratio of 1.75. That is, the proposal will be determined to have maintained appropriate graft survival if the indicator for pre-or post-implementation transplant has a one-sided p-value less than 0.05 for the null hypothesis that the hazard ratio is greater than 1.75. The non-inferiority margin was selected because the one-year graft survival rate for kidneys with KDPI = 85% was approximately 85% in the 2014 OPTN/SRTR Annual Data Report, and a hazard ratio of 1.75 would ensure that the one-year graft survival rate for kidneys with KDPI = 85% remains above 75%.

Sensitivity analyses will be completed for both objectives of the proposal. To assess the sensitivity to the assumptions made within GLMMs, the utilization of high- KDPI kidneys will include an analysis based on generalized estimating equations (GEE) with an exchangeable working correlation structure for donors. Post-transplant survival will include an analysis based on a frailty model accounting for potential correlation between kidneys from the same donor. Additional sensitivity analyses will be completed that consider covariates or interactions that were not included in the primary analyses, especially for covariates included in the SRTR post-transplant graft survival model. Finally, a sensitivity analysis will investigate the potential presence and impact of temporal trends on organ utilization and post- transplant survival.

The significant advantage of the evaluation plan is the primary analysis for both objectives is a priori specified including covariates for adjustment and their functional form. This improves the scientific validity by ensuring the false-positive rate of 5% is not adversely impacted by stepwise variable selection methods (e.g., backwards selection). Additionally, the analysis is not biased by post-hoc selection of sta tistical methods (e.g., the selection of GLMM versus generalized estimating equations) or the post-hoc selection of clinical outcomes (e.g., graft versus patient survival). A potential disadvantage is the omission of potentially important covariates or interactions in the primary analysis although appropriate sensitivity analyses should alleviate these concerns. Additionally, important risk factors may not be collected (e.g., cardiovascular risk factors) and could confound the analysis if the prevalence of the risk-factors in high-risk transplants increases post-implementation. Finally, the analysis may also be confounded by temporal trends in the organ utilization of high-KDPI kidneys or graft survival of high-risk transplants.

MPSC Staff Summary

Allocation Operational Rule Updates July 11, 2017
Item for Consideration:

At the July 2017 MPSC meeting, the MPSC will be asked to consider an update to its existing allocation operational rule. The proposed rule would automatically close cases with no action when an OPO expedites placement of an extra-renal organ if a transplant program declines the organ in the donor OR.

Background

Member Quality staff review the match run for all deceased donor organ allocations that result in a transplant. Each month, the Quality Assurance Analysts identify approximately 250-300 transplants with deviations from the match run. The analysts inquire with members and forward potential policy violations to the MPSC. Possible violations include instances when an OPO skips or bypasses patients on the wait list ("allocation out of sequence"), a transplant program accepts an organ offer for one patient but transplants another patient on the match run ("actual versus intended"), or a transplant program transplants a patient not on a match run ("not on the match run"). Analysts send the MPSC one summary per year for each member. The summary allows the MPSC to review any potentially concerning patterns of behavior over time.

The MPSC has closed almost all allocation deviations with no action; most members attempt to follow the match run as much as possible but deviate from the match run to avoid organ wastage. To streamline the review process, the MPSC developed operational rules to automatically close cases with no action when it is likely that allocation deviation was necessary to avoid organ wastage. The MPSC developed the current operational rules through 2012 and 2013, and the committee approved them in April 2013.

The MPSC does not review allocations when:

- An OPO expedites placement of any organ from a Hepatitis C positive donor.
- An OPO expedites placement of any organ from a Hepatitis B core positive donor.
- An OPO expedites placement of any organ from a donor more than 70 years old.
- A program transplants any organ into a patient other than the original intended recipient and the Host OPO granted the transplant program local back up.
- A program transplants a kidney patient out of sequence due to medical urgency as permitted by Policy 8.2.A.

- A program transplants a kidney recipient who does not appear on the match run as described in Policy 5.4.E.
- An OPO expedites placement of any organ except kidneys from a DCD donor.

Proposed Operational Rule

MPSC leadership asked Member Quality staff to review relevant data and suggest possible updates to the existing operational rules.

2016 MPSC Allocation Reviews:

- 270 total allocation reviews.
- 162 extra-renal organ allocations.
- 28 heart allocations, 3 declined in the donor OR.
- 36 lung allocations, 7 declined in the donor OR.
- 98 liver allocations, 66 declined in the donor OR.

The MPSC closed all 76 extra-renal allocations where a transplant program declined the organ in the donor OR with no action. While reviewing these cases, MPSC members often commented that the OPOs appropriately expedited placement to avoid organ wastage.

Does the MPSC wish to add instances where an OPO expedites placement of an extra-renal organ after a transplant program declines the organ in the donor OR to its list of exclusionary criteria? This could eliminate approximately 25 percent of the allocation cases the MPSC currently reviews. Staff can make details of any case automatically closed with no action available at any time. In addition, staff can provide data on organs declined in the OR as needed for any allocation review projects.

The Subcommittee also considered whether the current criteria for identification of small volume programs for lower than expected graft or patient survival be removed from the Transplant Program Performance bylaw. New criteria for identification of programs for review was implemented in January 2015. The bylaw included new Bayes criteria for identification of large volume programs and retained the previous criteria for small volume programs of one death or graft failure in a two and half year cohort. Programs that perform 9 or less transplants in two and a half years are considered small volume under the Transplant Program Performance bylaw. The MPSC uses operational rules to decrease the number of small volume programs that receive an initial inquiry.

The MPSC retained the small volume criteria in the proposal because of some concerns that the Bayes methodology may not adequately identify small volume programs that need improvement. However, the MPSC committed to evaluate whether this small volume criteria could be eliminated post-implementation. The Sub-committee reviewed data regarding small volume program reviews since implementation of the new bylaw. Based on this review, the Subcommittee recommended that the MPSC approve elimination of the small volume criteria from OPTN Bylaws, Appendix D.11.A. Transplant Program Performance. The Subcommittee further recommended that the MPSC approve implementation of an operational rule that would operationalize this change until the Bylaws can be revised. The operational rule would provide that only those small volume programs that are identified using the large volume Bayes criteria be sent an initial outcomes inquiry.

The Committee approved the following resolution by a vote of 30 For; 1 Against; 0 Abstentions:

RESOLVED, the MPSC approves the elimination of the separate small volume program criteria from OPTN/UNOS Bylaws, Appendix D.11.A. Transplant Program Performance; using the current Bayes criteria for identification of programs regardless of volume; and implementation of an operational effective immediately to operationalize this change until the OPTN/ UNOS bylaws can be revised.

MPSC Staff Summary

Late Notification of Key Personnel
Departure Proposed Operational Rule

Item for Consideration

At the July meeting, the MPSC will be asked to consider an operational rule to automatically place late notifications of key personnel departures on a MPSC consent agenda with a recommendation to issue a Notice of Uncontested Violation.

Summary

Transplant programs and histocompatibility laboratories must notify UNOS within 7 days of learning of a key personnel departure. These members must also submit a key personnel change application 30 days prior to the current key personnel's departure. (If the member receives less than 60 days notice of the key personnel's planned departure, the program must submit the key personnel change application within 30 days of the departure). These requirements are in place to allow the member to submit and the MPSC to review any key personnel change applications prior to the current key personnel's departure and to avoid periods where a program is without approved key personnel.

The following is a description of the current MPSC process for late notifications of key personnel changes:

- Staff identify a late notification and prepare a staff summary.
- Staff present each late notification as a discussion item at the in-person MPSC meeting.
- The MPSC issues an action, generally a Notice of Uncontested Violation.

The MPSC will discuss six late notification cases at the July 2017 meeting.

In an effort to reduce the MPSC's workload and to promote consistent MPSC actions, staff are constantly evaluating potential operational rules to place items on the MPSC's consent agenda. This minimizes the number of cases posted for MPSC reviewers and the meeting time spent discussing cases.

Based on the number of late notifications, the consistent MPSC action and limited discussion or debate typically associated with these cases at MPSC meetings, staff have developed the following operational rule for the MPSC's consideration:

- Staff identify a late notification.
- If the member notified UNOS more than 7 days after hospital learned of key personnel departure and submits a key personnel change application at least 30 days before the current key personnel departs, staff will document and close the late notification with no further action needed. Staff will educate the member on the late notification requirements.
- If the:
  - Member fails to notify UNOS within 7 days after the hospital learned of a key personnel departure; and
  - The failure to timely notify results in an inability to submit a key personnel change application at least 30 days before the current key personnel departs; and
  - This is the member's first late notification.
  - Staff will place the item on the Applications Consent agenda with a recommendation to issue a Notice of Uncontested Violation.
- If the:
  - Member fails to notify UNOS within 7 days after the hospital learned of a key personnel departure; and
  - The failure to timely notify results in an inability to submit a key personnel change application at least 30 days before the current key personnel departs; and
  - The member has at least one previous late notification in its compliance history or if there are any extenuating or unusual circumstances.
  - Staff will post a staff summary and case packet for reviewers.
  - If reviewers agree on a recommendation, staff will add the recommendation to the Applications Consent Agenda.
  - If reviewers disagree on a recommendation, the MPSC will discuss the issue at its next meeting.
- The MPSC will receive a copy of the consent agenda in advance of the meeting. An MPSC member may request to see the corresponding documentation and/ or move any consent agenda item to the discussion agenda.

Examples

- Notice of Uncontested Violation: Program notifies UNOS 2 days after primary surgeon departed. Upon inquiry, the member states that the surgeon notified the hospital of the departure date 6 months earlier.
- Notice of Uncontested Violation: Program notifies UNOS 15 days prior to primary surgeon departure and states that the surgeon had given notice of his departure to the hospital 6 months earlier. Application cannot be completed, processed and approved by MPSC prior to departure resulting in a period where the program is without an approved primary surgeon.

- Document and close with no action: Program notifies UNOS 2 months prior to primary surgeon departure and states that the surgeon had given notice of his departure to the hospital 6 months earlier. Application sent to member and received 30 days prior to departure date.
- No Bylaw Violation: Primary surgeon notifies hospital that he is departing effective that day. Hospital notifies UNOS and submits application within 30 days.

Relevant OPTN Bylaw or Policy

Appendix C.5 Changes in Key Laboratory Personnel

A. Change in Laboratory Director, Technical Supervisor, or Clinical Consultant
When the histocompatibility laboratory is informed that the laboratory director, technical supervisor, or clinical consultant plans to leave or otherwise ends active participation in the laboratory, the laboratory must:

1) Notify the OPTN contractor in writing within 7 business days of when the laboratory becomes aware of the change in key personnel.
2) Submit a completed Personnel Change Application to the OPTN contractor no less than 30 days before the end of the individual's active employment or change in status. The Personnel Change Application must document that the new or acting laboratory director, technical supervisor, and clinical consultant meet the requirements of these Bylaws.
3) Submit an updated Laboratory Coverage Plan no less than 30 days before the date of departure that specifies how continuous coverage will be provided at the laboratory by all key personnel during and after the transition period to a new or acting laboratory director, technical supervisor, or clinical consultant.
4) If the histocompatibility laboratory receives less than 60 days notice of the key personnel change, then the laboratory must submit a completed Personnel Change Application and updated Laboratory Coverage Plan to the OPTN contractor within 30 days of the date of departure.

Appendix D.7 Changes in Key Transplant Program Personnel

Designated transplant programs must have key personnel, specifically a primary surgeon and a primary physician, who meet the required minimum levels of commitment to and knowledge of organ procurement and transplantation as specified in these Bylaws. All transplant programs should develop a succession plan that addresses changes in these key personnel.

When a designated transplant program is informed of a change in key personnel, it must notify the OPTN contractor within 7 business days in writing and follow the procedures that are described below. A change in key personnel can be any of the following:

- Departure of the primary surgeon or primary physician.
- Change in position from primary surgeon or primary physician to an additional surgeon or physician.
- Temporary leave.
- Reinstatement of the previously designated primary surgeon or physician.

Transplant programs are also responsible for maintaining Program Coverage Plans as described in Section D.6.B. Surgeon and Physician Coverage (Program Coverage Plan) above during changes in key personnel. The Program Coverage Plan must address instances when key personnel are unavailable to perform their transplant duties for short periods of time.

A. Primary Surgeon or Primary Physician Departure

When the transplant hospital is informed that either the primary surgeon or primary physician plans to leave the hospital or otherwise end their active participation in the transplant program, the transplant hospital must:

1) Notify the OPTN contractor in writing within 7 business days.
2) Submit a completed Personnel Change Application to the OPTN contractor no less than 30 days before the end of the individual's active employment. The Personnel Change Application must document that the new primary surgeon or primary physician meets the requirements of these Bylaws.

If the transplant hospital receives less than 60 days advance notice of the key personnel change, then the transplant hospital must submit a completed Personnel Change Application to the OPTN contractor within 30 days from the date the OPTN contractor was notified.

If a program is unable to demonstrate through a completed Personnel Change Application that it has on site both a transplant surgeon and a transplant physician who meet the requirements for primary surgeon and primary physician, the transplant hospital must *either:*

- Inactivate the designated transplant program.
- Withdraw its designated transplant program status as described in Section K.4: Withdrawal or Termination of Designated Transplant Program Status of these Bylaws.

B. Primary Surgeon or Primary Physician Change in Role

When the transplant hospital plans to propose a new primary surgeon or primary physician and the currently designated primary surgeon or physician will remain on staff as an additional surgeon or physician, the transplant hospital must:

1) Notify the OPTN contractor in writing within 7 business days.
2) Submit a completed Personnel Change Application to the OPTN contractor no less than 30 days before the change will take effect. The Personnel Change Application must document that the new primary surgeon or physician meets the requirements of these Bylaws.

The transition to the new primary surgeon or primary physician is effective after the application has been reviewed and approved by the MPSC or an Ad hoc Sub-committee of the MPSC, as described in Appendix A: Membership Application and Review of these Bylaws.

C. Primary Surgeon or Primary Physician Temporary Leave

If the primary surgeon or physician must take a temporary leave of absence or otherwise temporarily cease their active participation with the transplant program, the transplant hospital must:

1) Notify the OPTN contractor in writing within 7 business days.
2) Submit a completed Personnel Change Application to the OPTN contractor no less than 30 days before the individual's leave begins. The Personnel Change Application must document that the replacement primary surgeon or physician meets the requirements of these Bylaws.

Temporary leave is defined in these Bylaws as greater than 30 days but less than one year. If the transplant hospital receives less than 60 days advance notice of the leave, then the transplant hospital must submit a complete Personnel Change Application to the OPTN contractor within 30 days from the date the OPTN contractor was notified.

If a program is unable to demonstrate through a completed Personnel Change Application that it has on site both a transplant surgeon and a transplant physician who meet the requirements for primary surgeon and physician, the transplant hospital must either:

- Inactivate the designated transplant program.
- Withdraw its designated transplant program status as described in Appendix K of these Bylaws.

D. Reinstatement of Previously Designated Primary Surgeon or Primary Physician

If the previously designated primary surgeon or primary physician returns to the same transplant program within one year of departure the individual can be considered for reinstatement as the primary surgeon or primary physician. The transplant hospital must submit a written reinstatement request to the OPTN contractor.

The written reinstatement request must include all of the following:

- A letter from the Transplant program director, department chair, or chief of the division, verifying the individual's current working knowledge and experience.
- A letter from the individual confirming the individual's on-site availability and commitment to the program.
- A current letter from the hospital credentialing committee verifying that the individual meets the requirements and is qualified and able to resume as primary surgeon or primary physician.

The MPSC or an Ad hoc Subcommittee of the MPSC will review requests for reinstatement, as described below. In cases where reinstatement of a surgeon or physician affects the transplant program's current status, the MPSC will recommend the appropriate new program status, along with any resulting special conditions.

E. Failure to Notify the OPTN Contractor of Key Personnel Changes

Any member who fails to inform the OPTN contractor of a change in the primary surgeon or primary physician or to submit the required Personnel Change Application within the periods specified above will be reviewed by the MPSC. The MPSC may impose a sanction, including any of the following:

- A Notice of Uncontested Violation.
- Letter of Warning.
- Letter of Reprimand.

Each of these sanctions and other adverse actions that may be taken by the MPSC are further described in Appendix L: Reviews, Actions, and Due Process of these By-laws.

Failure to inform the OPTN contractor of changes in primary surgeon or primary physician or to submit the required Personnel Change Application will result in a recommendation that the Board of Directors take appropriate adverse actions. Additionally, the Board of Directors may notify the Secretary of Health and Human Services (HHS) of the violation.

MPSC Staff Summary

Wait-List Inactivity Operational Rule Proposed Operational Rule
January 30, 2018

Item for Consideration

During the January 30, 2018 teleconference meeting, staff will present a proposed operational rule regarding member compliance with the requirements for patient notification in OPTN Bylaws Appendix D.11.B which require a member to notify all candidates on its wait list when a threshold of 15 consecutive days of inactivity and/ or 28 cumulative days of inactivity is met. The MPSC will be asked to vote to approve the rule.

Summary

Historically, compliance with this bylaw was reviewed at each PAIS meeting. Notification letters submitted to staff were posted to committee management for review, and the committee would often issue a Notice of Uncontested Violation for any instance of noncompliance identified.

The site survey team has assumed responsibility for reviewing member compliance with this bylaw and will perform member reviews on an annual basis. Site Survey would like to propose an operational rule, similar to the rules that Safety Analysts and Allocation Analysts use; a first event of noncompliance would be "closed" and not forwarded to the committee, and language would be communicated to the member that any subsequent instance would then be forwarded on for committee review (as well as the first event).

Proposed rule: "Site survey staff will request members to implement corrective actions for first event of identified noncompliance with the wait-list inactivity notifications bylaw and will not forward the matter to the MPSC for review. If staff identifies a second event of noncompliance in a subsequent annual review, staff will gather documentation from the member and provide all events' documentation to the MPSC for review."

If approved, the rule will be effective immediately.

Examples

Member ABCD's kidney transplant program met the 28 cumulative day inactivity threshold in 2016. UNOS's Research department provides to the site survey team a random sample of 10 candidates on member ABCD's kidney wait list. Site Survey mails an inquiry letter with the patient sample to Member ABCD and requests that the member submit all required patient notifications. Member ABCD responds that they failed to notify their candidates when they met the cumulative day inactivity threshold, although they had notified their candidates of their plan to inactivate their list per other bylaw requirements. Site Survey requests a Corrective Action Plan and provides education to Member ABCD about the requirements in Bylaws Appendix D.11.B. Site Survey mails a Closing Letter to Member ABCD notifying them that the review is closed, that the event will not be forwarded to the MPSC, and that if another event of noncompliance is identified on a future annual review, all events will be forwarded to the MPSC at that time.

Relevant OPTN Bylaw or Policy

OPTN Bylaws Appendix D.11.B Patient Notification Requirements for Waiting List Inactivation.

A transplant program must provide written notice to candidates if it does either or both of the following:

1) Inactivates its waiting list for 15 or more consecutive days.
2) Inactivates its waiting list for 28 or more cumulative days during any calendar year.

A transplant program must provide written notice each time it reaches either of the inactive waiting list thresholds listed above. Written notice must include all of the following:

1) The reason for the inactivity.
2) The expected length of time that the waiting list will be inactive.
3) The explanation that during the period of inactivity, organs cannot be accepted on the candidate's behalf at this transplant program.
4) The options available to the candidate during this period, including multiple listing or transferring of accrued waiting time to another Transplant Hospital.
5) How the candidates will be notified when the waiting list is reactivated or if the expected length of inactivation is extended.
6) A copy of the OPTN contractor's Patient Information Letter.

Note: If written notice is required because a transplant program exceeded the inactive waiting list threshold due to cumulative periods of inactivation, then the written notice must also include the dates of each instance of waiting list inactivation.

Written notice must be provided within the periods defined in the table below:

For . . .	Written Notice Must Be Provided . . .
Periods of waiting list inactivation scheduled at least 30 days in advance.	30 days before inactivity begins.
Periods of waiting list inactivation scheduled less than 30 days in advance.	No more than 7 days following the initial date of waiting list inactivation.
Any periods of waiting list inactivation related to a cumulative period of inactivation.	No more than 7 days following the last date of the inactive period that caused the transplant program to exceed the inactive waiting list threshold.

MPSC Staff Summary

MPSC Review of Non-Institutional Member Renewals
Proposed Operational Rule
March 1, 2018

Item for Consideration

During the Applications agenda review at the MPSC meeting on March 1, 2018, staff will present a proposed operational regarding MPSC review of non-institutional member renewals under OPTN Bylaws Article 1. Non-institutional members are required to renew their OPTN membership every 2 years. Staff are proposing that the MPSC adopt an operational rule that would place these renewal applications directly on an MPSC Consent Agenda if all requirements are met. The MPSC will be asked to vote to approve the operational rule.

Summary

Non-institutional members of the OPTN include:

- Medical/Scientific.
- Public Organization.
- Business.
- Individuals.

Non-institutional members must meet the fairly minimal requirements for membership contained in OPTN Bylaws, Article 1. For example, a medical/scientific member needs to be a non-profit organization whose members include medical or scientific professionals with an interest in organ donation or transplantation and that has either of the following:

- Been in operation for at least one year.
- Letters of recommendation from at least three OPTN transplant hospital, OPO, histocompatibility laboratory, public organization or medical/scientific Members.

The non-institutional members have two year terms and need to apply for renewal of their membership at the end of each term.

Currently, all of the applications, new members and renewals, are posted for review by an ad hoc subcommittee and then placed on the applications consent agenda for the full MPSC.

UNOS staff is proposing that renewals for non-institutional members be placed directly on the MPSC consent agenda to approve if all requirements under OPTN By- laws, Article 1 are met.

Below are the non-institutional member application numbers for 2016 and 2017:

	2017		*2016*	
Member type	*New*	*Renewals*	*New*	*Renewals*
Medical/Scientific	0	2	0	11
Public Organization	1	3	0	2
Business	1	2	0	1
Individual	0	6	0	2
Totals	*2*	*13*	*0*	*18*

Relevant OPTN Bylaw or Policy

OPTN Bylaws, Article 1

1.5. Medical/Scientific Members

A medical/scientific member is a non-profit organization whose members include medical or scientific professionals with an interest in organ donation or transplantation and that has either of the following:

1. Been in operation for at least one year.
2. Letters of recommendation from at least three OPTN transplant hospital, OPO, histocompatibility laboratory, public organization, or medical/scientific Members.

1.6. Public Organization Members

A public organization member is an organization with an interest in organ donation or transplantation and must have been in operation for at least one year. A public organization member must also be one of the following:

1. A hospital that refers at least one potential organ or tissue donor per year.

2. A non-profit organization that engages in organ donation activities, or represents or directly provides support and services to transplant candidates, recipients or their families.
3. A non-profit organization that has letters of recommendation from at least three OPTN transplant hospital, OPO, histocompatibility laboratory, public organization, or medical/scientific members.

1.7. Business Members

A business member must be an organization in operation for at least one year that engages in commercial activities with two or more active OPTN transplant hospital, OPO, or histocompatibility laboratory members.

1.8. Individual Members

An individual member must be a person who meets any of the following criteria:

1. Has served or is presently serving on the OPTN Board of Directors or an OPTN committee.
2. Is a transplant candidate, recipient, or organ or tissue donor.
3. Is the family member of a transplant candidate, recipient, or organ or tissue donor.
4. Is presently employed by or is an independent contractor to OPO, transplant hospital, or histocompatibility laboratory members.
5. Is formerly employed by or is formerly an independent contractor for OPO, transplant hospital, or histocompatibility laboratory members.
6. Is formerly employed by a Federal or State government agency involved in organ donation or transplantation, and who demonstrates continued interest and involvement in organ donation or transplantation.
7. Has an active interest and involvement in organ donation or transplantation demonstrated by at least three letters of recommendation for membership from three other OPTN individual members.

MPSC Staff Summary

Proposed Process Change Key Personnel Change Applications
July 18, 2018

Item for Consideration

During the July 18, 2018 meeting, staff will present a proposed process change regarding moving Transplant program Key Personnel Change applications directly to an MPSC consent agenda if staff review reveals the application clearly meets the OPTN bylaws membership criteria. The MPSC will be asked to vote to approve the rule at this meeting.

Summary

Ad hoc subcommittees of the MPSC review every key personnel change application for compliance with the membership requirements in the OPTN bylaws. In 2017, these subcommittees reviewed 175 transplant program key personnel change applications. The OPTN bylaw membership requirements are detailed and the membership applications request specific information designed to demonstrate whether a proposed primary surgeon or primary physician meet the requirements. Most proposed transplant program key personnel clearly meet the requirements of the OPTN bylaws. Therefore, MPSC ad hoc subcommittee review does not appear to be a value added activity and is not a productive use of MPSC members review time.

Proposed rule: Transplant program key personnel change applications that clearly meet the OPTN bylaw membership requirements will be placed directly on the MPSC consent agenda for the next scheduled meeting (conference call or in person). UNOS staff will post for MPSC ad hoc subcommittee review any application where expert judgment is needed to determine if the application should be approved.

If approved, the rule will be effective immediately.

Example(s)

UNOS staff have identified the following examples that would require posting of an application for MPSC ad hoc subcommittee review:

- The program is requesting conditional approval for key personnel or extensions of conditional approval.
- Coverage plans that require approval of exceptions provided for in the OPTN bylaws.
- Letters of recommendation that do not clearly contain all requirements.
- Situations where a letter of attestation must be used such as for procurements from a long time ago.

Relevant OPTN Bylaw or Policy

OPTN Bylaws, Appendix D, D.7 Changes in Key Transplant Program Personnel

Designated transplant programs must have key personnel, specifically a primary surgeon and a primary physician, who meet the required minimum levels of commitment to and knowledge of organ procurement and transplantation as specified in these Bylaws. . . .

A. Primary Surgeon or Primary Physician Departure

When the transplant hospital is informed that either the primary surgeon or primary physician plans to leave the hospital or otherwise end their active participation in the transplant program, the transplant hospital must:

Notify the OPTN contractor in writing within 7 business days.

1) Submit a completed Personnel Change Application to the OPTN contractor no less than 30 days before the end of the individual's active employment. The Personnel Change Application must document that the new primary surgeon or primary physician meets the requirements of these Bylaws.

If the transplant hospital receives less than 60 days advance notice of the key personnel change, then the transplant hospital must submit a completed Personnel Change Application to the OPTN contractor within 30 days from the date the OPTN contractor was notified.

If a program is unable to demonstrate through a completed Personnel Change Application that it has on site both a transplant surgeon and a transplant physician who meet the requirements for primary surgeon and primary physician, the transplant hospital must either:

- Inactivate the designated transplant program.
- Withdraw its designated transplant program status as described in Section K.4: Withdrawal or Termination of Designated Transplant Program Status of these Bylaws.

B. Primary Surgeon or Primary Physician Change in Role

When the transplant hospital plans to propose a new primary surgeon or primary physician and the currently designated primary surgeon or physician will remain on staff as an additional surgeon or physician, the transplant hospital must:

1. Notify the OPTN contractor in writing within 7 business days.
2. Submit a completed Personnel Change Application to the OPTN contractor no less than 30 days before the change will take effect. The Personnel Change Application must document that the new primary surgeon or physician meets the requirements of these Bylaws.
3. The transition to the new primary surgeon or primary physician is effective after the application has been reviewed and approved by the MPSC or an Ad hoc Subcommittee of the MPSC, as described in Appendix A: Membership Appplication and Review of these Bylaws.

C. Primary Surgeon or Primary Physician Temporary Leave

If the primary surgeon or physician must take a temporary leave of absence or otherwise temporarily cease their active participation with the transplant program, the transplant hospital must:

1. Notify the OPTN contractor in writing within 7 business days.
2. Submit a completed Personnel Change Application to the OPTN contractor no less than 30 days before the individual's leave begins. The Personnel Change Application must document that the replacement primary surgeon or physician meets the requirements of these Bylaws.

Temporary leave is defined in these Bylaws as greater than 30 days but less than one year.

If the transplant hospital receives less than 60 days advance notice of the leave, then the transplant hospital must submit a complete Personnel Change Application to the OPTN contractor within 30 days from the date the OPTN contractor was notified.

If a program is unable to demonstrate through a completed Personnel Change Application that it has on site both a transplant surgeon and a transplant physician who meet the requirements for primary surgeon and physician, the transplant hospital must either:

- Inactivate the designated transplant program.
- Withdraw its designated transplant program status as described in Appendix K of these Bylaws.

D. Reinstatement of Previously Designated Primary Surgeon or Primary Physician

If the previously designated primary surgeon or primary physician returns to the same transplant program within one year of departure the individual can be considered for reinstatement as the primary surgeon or primary physician. The transplant hospital must submit a written reinstatement request to the OPTN contractor.

The written reinstatement request must include all of the following:

1) A letter from the Transplant program director, department chair, or chief of the division, verifying the individual's current working knowledge and experience.
2) A letter from the individual confirming the individual's on-site availability and commitment to the program.
3) A current letter from the hospital credentialing committee verifying that the individual meets the requirements and is qualified and able to resume as primary surgeon or primary physician.
4) The MPSC or an Ad hoc Subcommittee of the MPSC will review requests for reinstatement, as described below. In cases where reinstatement of a surgeon or physician affects the transplant program's current status, the MPSC will recommend the appropriate new program status, along with any resulting special conditions.

Applicable membership requirements for organ specific primary transplant surgeons and physicians can be found in:

- *Appendix E: Membership and Personnel Requirements for Kidney Transplant Programs.*
- *Appendix F: Membership and Personnel Requirements for Liver Transplant Programs.*
- *Appendix G: Membership and Personnel Requirements for Pancreas and Pancreatic Islet Transplant Programs.*
- *Appendix H: Membership and Personnel Requirements for Heart Transplant Programs.*
- *Appendix I: Membership and Personnel Requirements for Lung Transplant Programs.*

MPSC Staff Summary

Proposed Process Change Late Reports of Potential
Disease Transmissions to the OPTN July 18, 2018

Item for Consideration

During the July 18, 2018 meeting, staff will present a proposed process change regarding late reports of potential disease transmission to the OPTN required in Policies 15.4, 15.5, and 15.6. The MPSC will be asked to vote to approve the rule.

Summary

Policies 15.4.A and 15.4.B require host OPOs to submit certain potential donor-derived disease transmissions to the OPTN Improving Patient Safety Portal as well as to the receiving transplant centers within 24 hours. Policy 15.5.B requires transplant centers to notify both the host OPO and the OPTN Improving Patient Safety Portal within 24 hours after learning of a potential donor-derived disease transmission. Policy 15.6.A requires recovery hospitals to notify the receiving transplant program and the OPTN Improving Patient Safety Portal within 7 days when new information is learned about a living donor that indicates a risk of potential disease transmission or malignancy within two years post-donation.

Currently, events that are appropriately reported to the applicable members within required time frames but submitted late to the OPTN are referred to the MPSC for review, even though the patient safety risk was appropriately mitigated.

In an effort to reduce MPSC and UNOS staff workload and promote process improvement, staff are proposing a First-Time Non-Compliance (FTNC) process change in certain late reports of potential disease transmission to the OPTN. If a case meets FTNC criteria, Safety Analysts would investigate the cause of the delayed report, request the results of any root cause analyses (RCA) performed, and request documentation of any corrective action plans (CAP) per the normal investigative process. Assuming the RCA and CAP appropriately address the gap that led to the late report, the new process change would allow Safety Analysts close the case instead of sending it to the MPSC for review. This allows the member to develop corrective actions without a MPSC referral and reduces the workload of MPSC members and UNOS staff.

FTNC Conditions

Member has no late report non-compliances since August 1, 2016, and meets one of the following three circumstances as appropriate:

1) A host OPO who did not report a Pathogen of Special Interest, malignancy or other finding highly suggestive of malignancy recognized after procurement, or discovery of recipient disease to the Improving Patient Safety Portal within 24 hours, but did make the required notifications to all recipient centers per OPTN Policy 15;
2) A transplant center who did not report to the Improving Patient Safety Portal within 24 hours when an organ recipient has, is suspected to have, or has died from a potentially donor-derived transmissible disease, infection or malignancy, but did notify the host OPO within 24 hours per OPTN Policy 15;

3) A living donor recovery hospital who notified the receiving transplant program of new information indicating a risk of potential disease or malignancy transmission during the first two years post-donation, but did not report it to the Improving Patient Safety Portal within 7 days per OPTN Policy 15.

The FTNC process change can only be applied to a member one time. Thus, if a member has a subsequent case of a late report to the OPTN, that case would be referred to the MPSC even if the other members were notified within time frames required. If a second case is identified and referred to the MPSC for review, the first case will also be included for MSPC review.

Since August 2014, Member Quality has investigated 26 cases of potential donor- derived disease transmissions and malignancies reported late to the OPTN and/or to the required members. Of these 26 cases, 14 (54%) were reported to the necessary members as required by policy and were reported late only to the OPTN. To date, none of those centers have reported a potential donor-derived disease transmission late a second time, which suggests the member implemented appropriate corrective actions in response to those events.

Proposed rule: Cases that meet FTNC conditions would be investigated, with RCAs and CAPs obtained and reviewed by Safety Analysts, but would be closed and would not be referred to the MPSC for review. Should subsequent non-compliances be identified, those cases would be sent to the MPSC for review and the first case initially closed would be included.

If approved, the rule will be effective August 1, 2018.

Example(s)

OPO ABCD received donor test results that resulted positive for Chagas in the left kidney recipient of a donor who also donated a right kidney, heart, and liver. OPO ABCD notified all other recipient centers immediately upon receiving the notification, but did not submit the information to the OPTN Improving Patient Safety Portal for five days. Investigation into the late reporting revealed that internal policy did not specify the need to report Pathogens of Special Interest to the OPTN Improving Patient Safety Portal within 24 hours so staff believed the timely reporting to the receiving centers was all that was required. Internal policy was updated and staff were re-educated on Policy 15.4. Because the appropriate notifications were made to protect patient safety and the OPO had no prior non-compliances with regard to reporting potential disease transmissions, this case would not be referred to the MPSC for review.

Hospital EFGH identified adenocarcinoma in the heart recipient and upon review of donor and recipient records, had substantial concern that the malignancy could be donor-derived. The Hospital immediately notified the OPO but did not submit a report to the OPTN Improving Patient Safety Portal. During the investigation, the hospital reported that they believed hospitals were only responsible for notifying the OPO and that the OPO was responsible for all notifications and reports thereafter. The Hospital updated all process checklists, internal policy, added a note in their EMR to remind staff to notify the OPO and the OPTN, and re-educated staff. The hospital notified the OPO within 24 hours and had not had a prior late report to the OPTN, so this case would not be referred to the MPSC for review.

A living kidney donor is diagnosed with breast cancer one year post-donation. The hospital documented the information in the donor's chart, but did not notify the receiving center until two months later when a new coordinator identified the error during chart review. The hospital had no prior non-compliances related to potential disease transmissions, but had not made the required notification to the receiving transplant program so this case would be referred to the MPSC for review.

Relevant OPTN By Law or Policy

15.4.A. Host OPO Requirements for Reporting Post-Procurement Donor Results and Discovery of Potential Disease Transmissions

The host OPO must report all positive test results and other relevant information received post-procurement for each donor as soon as possible but no later than 24 hours after receipt as follows:

1) All results indicating Pathogens of Special Interest must be reported to the receiving transplant program's patient safety contact and the OPTN Improving Patient Safety Portal. The OPTN contractor provides a list of Pathogens of Special Interest, including any results that can be excluded from reporting. The OPTN contractor reviews and updates this list at least annually.
2) All other positive test results and relevant information must be reported according to Table 15–1 below.

Table 15–1. Host OPO reporting requirements for positive post- procurement donor results and discovery of potential disease transmissions

The host OPO must report all of the following positive results:	To:
Samples relevant to all recipients	
Serologic, NAT, or antigen results indicating presence of parasites, virus, or fungi	The receiving transplant program's patient safety contact
Cultures from the following specimens: • Ascites • Blood • Cerebrospinal fluid (CSF) • Deep wound • Genital • Pericardial • Pleural fluid	The receiving transplant program's patient safety contact
Mycobacterial smears and cultures	The receiving transplant program's patient safety contact
Fungal smears and cultures with the exception of *Candida* species	The receiving transplant program's patient safety contact
Relevant information	

The host OPO must report all of the following positive results:	To:
Respiratory samples (bacterial or *Candida* species) *only* to transplant programs receiving lungs or head and neck VCAs	The receiving transplant program's patient safety contact
Urine cultures (bacterial or *Candida* species) *only* to transplant programs receiving kidneys or genitourinary VCAs	The receiving transplant program's patient safety contact
Malignancy or other findings highly suggestive of malignancy recognized after procurement	The receiving transplant program's patient safety contact The OPTN Improving Patient Safety Portal
Histopathology results reported post-procurement	The receiving transplant program's patient safety contact
Relevant information	
All final culture information for any culture results that were reported according to these requirements	The receiving transplant program's patient safety contact
Other psycho-social history, medical history, autopsy, testing, and laboratory findings identifying infectious conditions that may adversely affect a potential transplant recipient	The receiving transplant program's patient safety contact

15.4.B. Host OPO Requirements for Reporting Post-Procurement Discovery of Recipient Disease or Malignancy

If the host OPO is notified that an organ recipient is suspected to have, is confirmed positive for, or dies from a potential transmissible disease, infection, or malignancy and there is substantial concern that it could be from the transplanted organ, then the host OPO must do all the following:

1) Communicate the suspected donor's and affected organ recipient's test results and diagnosis that may be relevant to acute patient care, as soon as possible but no more than 24 hours after receipt, to any transplant program patient safety contacts and tissue banks that received organs, vessels, or tissue from the donor. This includes any test results that were not available at the time of procurement or that were performed after procurement. The host OPO must document that this information is shared with all receiving transplant programs and tissue banks.
2) Report the event to the OPTN Improving Patient Safety Portal as soon as possible but no more than 24 hours after notification or receipt of recipient test results or diagnosis.

15.5.B. Transplant Program Requirements for Reporting Post-Transplant Discovery of Recipient Disease or Malignancy

When an organ recipient is suspected to have, is confirmed positive for, or has died from a potential transmissible disease, infection, or malignancy and there is substantial concern that it could be from the transplanted organ, then the transplant program must do all of the following:

1) Notify host OPO or living donor recovery hospital that procured the organ without waiting for all medical documentation that may eventually become available. The transplant program must notify the host OPO or living donor recovery hospital by phone and provide documentation as soon as possible but no more than 24 hours after learning of the event.
2) Report the event through the OPTN Improving Patient Safety Portal as soon as possible but no more than 24 hours after learning of the event.
3) Provide additional related information or specimens if requested.

15.6.A Living Donor Recovery Hospital Requirements for Reporting Post- Donation Discovery of Living Donor Disease or Malignancy
If a living donor recovery hospital learns new information about a living donor during the first two years post donation that indicates risk of potential transmission of disease or malignancy, then the living donor recovery hospital must do all of the following:

1) Disclose to the living donor that the potential disease transmission or malignancy will be reported to the receiving transplant program and the OPTN Improving Patient Safety Portal.
2) Notify the receiving transplant program.
3) Report the potential transmission through the OPTN Improving Patient Safety Portal as soon as possible but no more than 7 days after receipt of the new information.

MPSC Determination

At its meeting on July 18, 2018, the MPSC accepted the proposal with two changes:

1) All members will begin with a "clean slate," i.e., any instances of late reports that have occurred prior to implementation of this process change are not counted towards the member's FTNC conditions considerations.
2) The FTNC condition will be maintained for three years. Because the MPSC reviews a member's compliance history going back three years, members thought a similar time frame should be applied here.

No other changes were recommended. With the above two changes added into the proposal, the MPSC voted 33–0–0 to accept and implement this change.

Member Quality Site Survey

Process Proposal MPSC Meeting July 18, 2018

Staff Summary

Item for Consideration

At the July 2018 MPSC meeting, the MPSC will consider changes to the process by which the MPSC reviews member site survey reports. The proposed process revisions will decrease the MPSC's case review workload and will better identify for the MPSC review members that have ongoing compliance issues. The process change will also reduce the amount of time members must wait to learn the outcome of their survey and the amount of time between the initial survey to and follow-up surveys.

Background

The site survey "scorecard" is a tool used to determine which site surveys can be placed straight on a MPSC consent agenda to close with no action and which site surveys must be posted for MPSC reviewers to determine an appropriate action. The chart below summarizes the current "scorecard" thresholds for different survey types:

HR KI LI LU Transplant Programs	95% Clinical Score Threshold 90% Administrative Score Threshold Posted for reviewers if member's score is below either threshold
IN PA Programs	No scorecard, posted for reviewers if survey has any errors
Living Donor Component of KI and LI Program	No scorecard, posted for reviewers if survey has any errors
OPOs	Clinical scorecard only; posted for reviewers if survey has any errors.

Problems with the current scorecard and MPSC site survey review process include the following:

- Members rely on their "score" as a determination of their overall effectiveness. For example, members under outcomes review may cite their "100% clinical compliance score."
- Changes to the scorecard are difficult to make. Because each policy is weighted within the scorecard, adding or changing a policy to the survey process requires re-evaluating the weight assigned to every other policy.
- Surveys without an established scorecard and threshold must be posted for MPSC review. This results in the MPSC reviewing surveys with a small number of errors that the member has already corrected.
- The MPSC reviewers typically must decide whether to close the review with no action or request a follow-up desk review of certain policies. Feedback received from MPSC reviewers in the past has suggested that they are often happy to defer to staff recommendations on whether to close the review or conduct a fol- low-up survey.

Proposed Process Change

The proposed process would completely eliminate the current scorecard approach for determining which cases are posted for MPSC review. Instead, Member Quality staff will use a Survey Evaluation Tool (SET) to determine whether a survey can be closed with no follow-up, whether a follow-up focused desk review of certain policies is needed, or whether the survey should be sent to MPSC reviewers to determine the appropriate action.

Survey Evaluation Tool

All policies reviewed will be placed into a category based on the potential risk to patient safety. OPOs will have four categories while transplant programs, including living donor, will have three categories based on assigned risk. Each category will have a threshold for compliance as described in the charts below.

Survey Evaluation Tool—OPO

	Examples of Policies in this Category	*Required Compliance Rate*
Tier I	Policy 2.6.B—A2 and A2B Requirements	100%
Tier II	Policy 2.4 requires documentation of communicating factors associated with an increased risk for disease transmission	90%
Tier III	Policy 2.8 requires OPOs to have a urinalysis within 24 hours of cross clamp	80%
Tier IV	Policy 18.1 requires accuracy of data submitted on DDRs	No follow-up

Survey Evaluation Tool—Transplant Programs (including Living Donor)

	Examples of Policies in this Category	*Required Compliance Rate*
Tier I	Policy 5.8.B—Pre-Transplant Verification Upon Organ Receipt Policy 14.4.A—Living Donor Medical Evaluation Requirements	90%
Tier II	Policy 3.9—Removing Candidates from the Waiting List Policy 14.3—LD Informed Consent Requirements	80%
Tier III	Policy 3.2—Notifying Patients of Their Options Policy 18.1—Data Submission Requirements Accuracy	No follow-up

Members continue to be asked to submit a corrective action plan for noncompliance with any policy in any tier.

If an OPO member does not meet the required compliance threshold for a policy in Tiers I, II and III, UNOS staff will automatically conduct a follow-up desk review of that policy. Transplant programs that do not meet the required compliance threshold for a policy in Tiers I and II will automatically have a follow-up desk review of that policy within six or twelve months, depending on the program's transplant volume. If a member meets all the required compliance thresholds, UNOS staff will automatically close the review with no action, without posting the case for MPSC review.

UNOS staff will post for MPSC review the results of any follow-up focused desk review where the member continued to not meet the required compliance threshold.

Benefits of the proposed process include:

- A reduction in cases posted for MPSC review. For example, staff anticipate the MPSC will review approximately 18 fewer heart program surveys and 20 fewer liver program surveys each year under this rule, which will free up time the MPSC can use for other purposes.
- Continued ability to post any unusual or concerning cases for MPSC review. Currently, staff will send a case for MPSC review based on concerns regarding patient safety or any unusual findings, regardless of whether the case meets the established scorecard threshold. Staff will continue to prioritize posting for MPSC review any such survey report, regardless of the program's compliance rate with given policies.
- Ability to easily adapt the survey evaluation tool to policies. For example, if site survey adds a newly implemented policy to the list of policies reviewed during a survey, site survey will only need to determine which tier to assign the policy; adding or removing a policy from the site survey process will not impact the assigned tier or compliance rate for any other policy.
- Emphasis on member's improvement rather than strict adherence to compliance. Members who have errors on their initial survey but demonstrate improvement in their follow-up survey will automatically be released from monitoring.

Data Modeling

Data modeling comparing review via the SET with prior MPSC review show the outcome is the same or slightly more conservative than the outcomes determined by MPSC reviewers, as shown in the chart below.

Survey Type	*Same outcome in current and proposed processes*	*More follow-up desk reviews in proposed process*	*Fewer follow-up desk reviews in proposed process*
HR KI LI LU IN PA	305 reviews	45 reviews	5 reviews
Living Donor KI and LI	33 reviews	17 reviews	3 reviews
OPO	19 reviews	9 reviews	3 reviews

Data modeling also indicates there will be a significant reduction in MPSC workload, as described in the table below.

Survey Type	Date Range	Surveys Performed	Number Reviewed by MPSC Under Current Process	Number Requiring MPSC Review Under New Process
Heart	March 2017–March 2018	74	22	4
Liver	March 2017—March 2018	53	22	2

Recommendation

The Policy Compliance Subcommittee (PCSC) of the MPSC heard a report from site survey staff on this proposed process change during the PCSC's June 25 conference call and unanimously recommended that the MPSC vote to support the proposed concept. The MPSC will be asked to vote on this concept as a part of the PCSC consent agenda during the MPSC meeting on July 18, 2018.

MPSC Staff Summary

Possible Revision to Operational Rule

No inquiry 2 meeting cycles from release in outcomes cases February 26, 2018

Item for Consideration: During the February 26, 2018 PAIS meeting, staff presented possible options for revision of the operational rule regarding postponement of new MPSC outcomes inquiry. The PAIS recommended that the operational rule be revised to make a program ineligible to receive a new inquiry for 2 SRTR reporting cycles which results in a time period of ineligibility which is more consistent regardless of when the program is released. The PAIS approved this recommendation by a vote of 15 for, 0 against and 1 abstention.

Summary: Under the current operational rule, the MPSC will not send an inquiry to a program for 2 meeting cycles following release from review for lower than expected post-transplant outcomes. In July 2017, the PAIS/MPSC endorsed the elimination of the data request for updated Spring SRTR reports for use at the October Subcommittee/MPSC meeting. UNOS staff have noticed that the elimination of this October report has resulted in an inconsistent result when applying the 2 meeting cycle operational rule:

Release date	2 meeting cycles	Inquiry if still flagged	Results
March 2018	July 2018, October 2018	March 2019	Skip if flagged in July 2018 SRTR report and send inquiry if flagged in January 2019 SRTR report—1 year from release
July 2018	October 2018, March 2019	July 2019	Skip if flagged in January 2019 SRTR report and send inquiry if flagged in July 2019 SRTR report—1 year from release
October 2018	March 2019, July 2019	March 2020 (3 meeting cycles)	Do not receive SRTR reports in October 2019 so skip January 2019 and July 2019 SRTR reports and receive inquiry if flagged in January 2020 SRTR reports—1 year and 5 months from release

The MPSC adopted this operational rule to accommodate the fact that there is a 1 year lag in the SRTR reporting of one-year post-transplant outcomes but the MPSC reviews current data and events when a program is under review. For example, the MPSC will have reviewed synopsis of events and improvement efforts through April 30, 2018 for a program that is released in July 2018. In addition to the 2 meeting cycle operational rule, the MPSC does not send an inquiry if there have been no new events at the program since the program's release from review.

If the MPSC was to change the operational rule to use the SRTR reporting periods as the deciding factor for when a new inquiry would be sent, the following would be the effect for skipping 1 reporting cycle or 2 reporting cycles: Two SRTR reporting cycles:

Release date	2 SRTR reporting cycles	Inquiry if still flagged	
March 2018	July 2018, January 2019	July 2019	Eligible for new inquiry 1 year, 4 months after release
July 2018	January 2019, July 2019	March 2020	Eligible for new inquiry 1 year, 8 months after release
October 2018	January 2019, July 2019	March 2020	Eligible for new inquiry 1 year, 5 months after release

One SRTR reporting cycle:

Release date	1 SRTR reporting cycle	Inquiry if still flagged	
March 2018	July 2018	March 2019	Eligible for new inquiry 1 year after release
July 2018	January 2019	July 2019	Eligible for new inquiry 1 year after release
October 2018	January 2019	July 2019	Eligible for new inquiry 9 months after release

Questions for PAIS/MPSC

1) Should the current operational rule postponing new inquiry for 2 meeting cycles be revised to be based on SRTR reporting cycles?
2) If answer to question 1 is yes, should the new inquiry be postponed for 1 SRTR reporting cycle or 2 SRTR reporting cycles?

If revisions to the rule are approved, the new rule will be effective immediately.

1) Following the decision on the operational rule, the PAIS/MPSC will need to vote on whether to send inquiries to the following programs that were released in March 2018, are flagged in the SRTR reports from January 2019 and have had additional events since release:
   - 03953N LU pediatric component; identified for lower than expected graft and patient survival
   - 21440N KI adult component, identified for lower than expected graft survival
   - 41540N KI pediatric component, identified for lower than expected patient survival

Relevant OPTN Bylaw or Policy:
OPTN Bylaws, Appendix D
Section D.11 Additional Transplant Program Requirements

A. Transplant Program Performance

Appendix D.12.A does not apply to VCA transplants

The MPSC will conduct reviews of transplant program performance to identify underperforming transplant programs and require the implementation of quality assessment and performance improvement measures. One measure of transplant program performance is triggered through a review of the one-year graft and patient survival rates. The MPSC utilizes performance metrics produced by the Scientific Registry of Transplant Recipients (SRTR) as the principal tool to identify transplant programs that have lower than expected outcomes.

For programs performing 10 or more transplants in a 2.5 year period, the MPSC will review a transplant program if it has a higher hazard ratio of mortality or graft failure than would be expected for that transplant program. The criteria used to identify programs with a hazard ratio that is higher than expected will include either of the following:

1) The probability is greater than 75% that the hazard ratio is greater than 1.2.
2) The probability is greater than 10% that the hazard ratio is greater than 2.5.

For programs performing 9 or fewer transplants in a 2.5-year period, the MPSC will review a transplant program if the program has one or more events in a 2.5-year cohort.

The MPSC review will be to determine if the higher hazard ratio or events can be explained by patient mix or some other unique clinical aspect of the transplant program. If a program's performance cannot be explained by patient mix or some other unique clinical aspect of the transplant program, the program, in cooperation with the MPSC, will adopt and promptly implement a plan for quality improvement. The member's failure to adopt and promptly implement a plan for quality improvement will be considered a noncompliance with OPTN Obligations and may result in an OPTN action according to Appendix L: Reviews and Actions.

As part of this process, the MPSC may conduct a peer visit to the program at the member's expense. The MPSC may also require, at its discretion, that the member participate in an informal discussion. The informal discussion will be conducted according to Appendix L: Reviews and Actions.

The MPSC may recommend that a member inactivate a program, or a component of a program, or withdraw its designated transplant program status based on patient safety concerns arising from review of the program's graft and patient survival. The MPSC must offer the member an informal discussion before recommending that the program inactivate or withdraw its designated transplant program status. A program's failure to inactivate or withdraw its designated transplant program status when the MPSC recommends it do so will be considered a non-compliance with OPTN Obligations and may result in an OPTN action according to *Appendix L: Reviews and Actions.*

Excerpt from 2/27/2019 MPSC Confidential Meeting Minutes

1) Clinical Experience Pathway—2- to 5-year requirement

Prior to review of the above described key personnel change application discussion, UNOS staff presented information about the requirement in the clinical experience pathways for all organs that the primary transplant surgeon perform a certain number of transplants or the primary transplant physician care for a certain number of transplant patients over a 2- to 5-year period. The language contained in the by-laws is vague and could lead to an inconsistent application or unintended application of the requirement. It is unclear whether the requisite number of surgeries or patient care must take place throughout the entire period. The Committee discussed various scenarios and two interpretation options under the bylaws. The

Committee expressed support for an interpretation that would require a proposed transplant surgeon or transplant physician demonstrate that they did the requisite number of transplants or cared for the requisite number of transplant patients over a 2-year period in which the surgeon or physician was employed and on-site at a designated transplant program(s). The transplants/patients used to satisfy the volume requirement do not have to span the entire two year period as long as the individual was employed and on-site at designated transplant programs for a consecutive 2-year period.

MPSC Staff Summary

Proposed Operational Rule
Adding Application Rejections to the Consent Agenda February 26, 2020

Item for Consideration

During the February 2020 meeting, staff will present a proposed operational rule regarding adding application rejections to the consent agenda. The MPSC will be asked to vote to approve the rule.

Summary

Currently, only applications where all subcommittee voters agree to approve are included on the Membership consent agenda. When the subcommittee votes to reject an application, the application is brought for discussion with the full committee. This has led to the MPSC having discussions to reject applications that do not meet the OPTN Bylaws, which the MPSC has no option to approve. To eliminate this discussion, which takes the MPSC's time but does not allow for the MPSC to take a different action than the subcommittee recommendation, staff propose that, when a subcommittee unanimously agrees on a rejection, that decision be placed on the Membership consent agenda. This change would be consistent with the way that Performance and Compliance create their agendas. For those cases, if the sub-committee agrees on an action, it goes on the consent agenda.

Staff will continue to review the application and prepare a staff summary. The summary will indicate whether the completed application meets the OPTN Bylaw requirements. The cases will still be posted for a subcommittee of reviewers so that they can confirm the staff assessment of the application.

Proposed Rule

If all reviewers agree to reject an application, the rejection will be placed on the consent agenda for the full MPSC to approve.

If approved, the rule will be effective immediately and used in creating the next consent agenda.

Example
A member submits an application for a Primary Surgeon who does not have logs for the appropriate number of procurements. The member provides a letter that states that he performed the procurements, but does not have the record information. Staff review the documentation and post it for reviewers, noting that the documentation submitted does not meet the OPTN Bylaw requirements. The sub-committee votes in Committee Management to reject the application, so staff puts the rejection on the consent agenda for the next full committee meeting.

MPSC Staff Summary

Proposed Process Change
Adding Self-Reported Cases to the Consent Agenda April 22, 2021

Item for Consideration

During the April 2021 meeting, staff will propose a change to the existing operational rule regarding closing issues that members self-report with no action. The change would allow self-reports to be added to the consent agenda for closure, rather than being posted for reviewers. The MPSC will be asked to vote to approve the rule.

Summary
During its December 2019 meeting, the MPSC approved an operational rule regarding closing issues that members self-report with no action. The MPSC changed the recommended action for self-reported compliance cases where there seems to be an appropriate response through a root cause analysis (RCA) and corrective action plan (CAP), no likelihood of recurrence, and no ongoing patient safety issues from a Notice of Noncompliance to closing the issue with no action. The MPSC intended this change to help support a plan to encourage self-reports and shift community perception of the committee from solely focused on compliance toward a focus on process improvement. Originally, reviewers still examined all of these cases to confirm that the proposed action was appropriate.

During the COVID–19 pandemic, staff and the MPSC agreed to a process change that allowed self-reports with an appropriate RCA and CAP, no concerns about recurrence, and no associated compliance history to be placed on the consent agenda.

Cases Reviewed

Issue	Total	Straight to Consent	Posted for Reviewers	Outcomes
Hemodilution	4	4	0	All closed
HLA errors	3	2	1	All closed
Packaging and Labeling, Laterality Errors	16	7	9	13 closed, 3 Notice of Noncompliance
Wait-list errors	4	3	1	All closed
Data entry errors	2	1	1	Both closed
Vessel errors	1	1	0	Closed
OPO Responsibilities	3	1	2	2 closed, 1 Notice of Noncompliance
Total	33 self- reported cases	19	14	29 closed, 3 Notice of Noncompliance

Reasons Posted for Reviewers

Issue	July 2020	October 2020	February 2021
Weak RCA/CAP	1 HLA error case	1 case—2 KI were accidentally discarded, went to discussion	
Patient safety issue/ member under review	1 KI program failed to place 35 KI candidates on wait list on time, 1 data entry error		1 case—HR surgeon left OR without allowing packaging
Recent Hx of similar event	3 packaging and labeling cases	1 KI laterality error case and 1 packaging and labeling case	1 hemodilution case, 4 packaging and labeling cases, one went to discussion because of history

As you can see, staff have posted 14 case for MPSC review. Of those 14, 10 were also closed with no action, and four received a Notice of Noncompliance. Based on this information, the MPSC is asked to officially approve that self-reported compliance cases where there seems to be an appropriate response through an RCA and CAP, no likelihood of recurrence, and no ongoing patient safety issues be added to the consent agenda with a recommendation to close the issue with no action.

All cases will still be reviewed for whether the RCA and CAP are appropriate, the member has a pattern of noncompliance, or the circumstances of the issue call for a stronger action. Any cases with concerns about these items will be posted for reviewers. As always, any cases with strong patient safety concerns will be posted for MPSC reviewers.

Proposed Rule

The MPSC will close self-reported policy issues with no action on a consent agenda, unless patient safety concerns, member history, inadequate response, or other circumstances indicate another action.

If approved, the rule will be effective immediately.

MPSC Staff Summary

Proposed Operational Rule
Use of Survey Evaluation Tool on Desk Reviews April 22, 2021

Item for Consideration

During the April 2021 meeting, staff will present a proposed operational rule regarding continuing to evaluate desk reviews with the Survey Evaluation Tool (SET) and adding them to the consent agenda. The MPSC will be asked to vote to approve the rule.

Summary

Since July 2018 Member Quality staff use a Survey Evaluation Tool (SET) to determine whether a survey can be closed with no follow-up, whether a focused desk review of certain policies is needed, or whether the survey should be sent to MPSC reviewers to determine the appropriate action. The tool separates policies reviewed into categories based on the potential risk to patient safety.

If a member does not meet the required compliance thresholds staff automatically conduct a desk review of that policy after six months. If a member meets all the required compliance thresholds, staff automatically close the review with no action, without posting the case for MPSC review. Prior to the COVID–19 pandemic, staff posted the results of any focused desk review where the member continued to not meet the required compliance threshold for MPSC review, as well as any surveys with concerns that the MPSC needs to address.

During the pandemic, staff began assessing both routine surveys and the resulting desk reviews with the SET, and adding the recommendation from the desk review to the MPSC consent agenda. The table below shows that site survey cases for the MPSC have decreased dramatically since the implementation of the SET (February 2019). It also shows that the number of surveys recommended for closing versus having a desk review has not changed drastically using the SET for 2020. For July 2019—February 2020, 80 surveys closed and 44 had a desk review. After the process change May 2020—February 2021, 57 surveys closed and 34 had a desk review.

	Closed	*Desk Review*
February 2019	150	53
July 2019	24	31
November 2019	28	4
February 2020	28	9
May 2020	14	4
July 2020	19	6
October 2020	6	4
February 2021	18	20

If the operational rules is approved, going forward the MPSC will review only a member's second desk review. In all cases, any surveys with serious concerns about patient safety, compliance, or corrective action plans can be sent to the MPSC for review despite the SET recommendation.

Proposed Rule

Staff will continue to evaluate routine site surveys with the SET and close or conduct a desk review as recommended by the tool. Staff will also evaluate the first desk review with the SET and add that recommendation to the MPSC consent agenda. The MPSC will review any second desk review results.

If approved, the rule will be effective immediately.

MPSC Staff Summary

Proposed Process Change Updates to Allocation Operational Rules
April 22, 2021

Item for Consideration

During the April 2021 meeting, staff will propose several changes to the existing operational rules for MPSC review of allocation deviations. The MPSC will be asked to vote to approve the changes to the rules.

Summary

Member Quality staff review the match runs for all deceased donor organ allocations that result in a transplant. Each month, the Allocation Analysts identify approximately 450–500 transplants with deviations from the match run. The analysts inquire with members and forward potential policy violations to the MPSC. Possible violations include instances when an OPO skips or bypasses patients on the wait list ("allocation out of sequence"), a transplant program accepts an organ offer for one patient but transplants another patient on the match run ("actual versus intended"), or a transplant program transplants a patient not on a match run. During the COVID pandemic, analysts have concentrated on making sure that they have adequate information about each allocation and have only referred the most egregious or clear policy violations to the Committee for review. As the analysts begin to return to a more normal review process, policy changes have led to the MPSC needing to review several of its current operational rules. After the MPSC moves back into normal monitoring of allocations, staff will continue to evaluate data for additional changes to these operational rules.

Analysts send the MPSC one summary per year for each member. The summary allows the MPSC to review any potentially concerning patterns of behavior over time. The MPSC has closed almost all allocation deviations with no action; most members attempt to follow the match run as much as possible but deviate from the match run to avoid organ wastage. To streamline the review process, the MPSC developed operational rules to automatically close cases with no action when it is likely that allocation deviation was necessary to avoid organ wastage.

Currently, the MPSC does not review allocations when:

- An OPO expedites placement of any organ from a Hepatitis C positive donor.
- An OPO expedites placement of any organ from a Hepatitis B core positive donor.
- An OPO expedites placement of any organ from a donor more than 70 years old.

- A program transplants any organ into a patient other than the original intended recipient and the Host OPO granted the transplant program local back up.
- A program transplants a kidney patient out of sequence due to medical urgency as permitted by Policy 8.
- A program transplants a kidney recipient who does not appear on the match run as described in Policy 5.4.E.
- An OPO expedites placement of any organ except kidneys from a DCD donor.

An OPO expedites placement of an extra-renal organ turned down in the Operating Room.

Kidney and Pancreas Allocation Changes

1) March 15, 2021 changes to kidney and pancreas allocation included a change to Policy 5.9 (Released Organs) which now states "The transplant program must transplant all accepted, deceased donor organs into the original intended recipient or release the deceased donor organs back to and immediately notify the host OPO or the OPTN for further distribution. If a transplant program released an organ, it must explain to the OPTN the reason for refusing the organ for that candidate. The host OPO or OPTN must then allocate the organ to other candidates according to the organ-specific policies. The host OPO may contact the OPTN for assistance allocating the organs. The host OPO may delegate the responsibility to the OPO serving the candidate transplant program's DSA, except in the cases of released kidneys, pancreata, and islets." (emphasis added)

Therefore, the idea of local backup involving the importing OPO running a match and reallocating organs is no longer permitted for kidneys and pancreata. While there may still be instances where the host OPO chooses to offer the organ to the same hospital for a different patient, it seems appropriate that the MPSC review these instances, especially while the policy is new. Therefore, the MPSC is asked to remove kidney and pancreas from the operational rule stating "a program transplants any organ into a patient other than the original intended recipient and the Host OPO granted the transplant program local back up."

2) Changes to Policy 8.5.A.i (Medically Urgent Status for Adult and Pediatric Candidates) have added medically urgent candidates as an allocation classification, and the offers for medical urgency are no longer dependent on each individual DSA approval. Therefore, the MPSC is asked to remove the operational rule "a program transplants a kidney patient out of sequence due to medical urgency as permitted by Policy 8.5.A.i (formerly 8.2.A)."

Liver Expedited Placement Policy Change

Policy 9.10 (Expedited Placement of Livers) recently went into effect, which provides OPOs with conditions under which they are permitted to make expedited liver offers and a process for those allocations. These conditions include the turndown of a liver offer after the donor has entered the operating room. Staff will confirm that the OPO allocates the liver appropriately using the new policy. Therefore, the MPSC is asked to remove liver from the operational rule "an OPO expedites placement of an extra-renal organ turned down in the Operating Room."

Conclusion

For any and all of these rules, staff can make details of any case automatically closed with no action available at any time. In addition, staff can provide aggregate data on reasons for closing cases for any allocation review projects. During their reviews, even with these rules, MPSC members often find that the OPOs appropriately expedited placement to avoid organ wastage.

Based on this analysis, the MPSC is asked to officially approve the rules as amended below.

Proposed Rules Summary

Rule	Applicable Organs
Hep C positive	All
Hep B Core positive	All
Over 70 years old	All
Transplanted a different recipient with local backup	Heart, Intestine, Liver, Lung
Kidney recipient not on match but follows 5.4.E	Kidney
DCD Donor	Heart, Intestine, Liver, Lung, Pancreas
Turndown in OR	Heart, Intestine, Lung, Pancreas

The MPSC will adjust the review of kidney, pancreas, and liver allocations based on the recent policy changes.

If approved, the rule changes will be effective immediately.

MPSC Staff Summary

Proposed Operational Rule
Lower Respiratory SARS–CoV–2 Testing for Lung Donors May 25, 2021
MPSC Meeting

Item for Consideration

During the May full MPSC meeting, staff will present a proposed operational rule regarding real-time monitoring of the emergency policy approved 4/26/21 that requires lower respiratory SARS–CoV–2 testing on all lung donors. The MPSC will be asked to vote to approve the rule.

Summary

This is a new policy that was proposed by the DTAC and it was taken to the Executive Committee for emergency approval, to be implemented within 30 days of approval. It will go through the summer Public Comment cycle, while in effect, and then ultimately to the BOD in December, pending with changes or as is. Site Survey will monitor OPOs' compliance with this policy in real-time, by use of a weekly report provided from the UNOS Research department. If it is found that an OPO has not reported the test results in DonorNet and/or not uploaded the results to the Attachments tab of DonorNet, then Site Survey will send an inquiry email to the OPO to investigate. If it is found that the member did not perform the test, Site Survey will ask the OPO to provide an explanation and a plan for future potential lung donors. Site Survey proposes to "close" the first identified event for each OPO (same process as the operational rule for Wait-list Inactivity notification letters), without forwarding to the MPSC for review, and will communicate language to the member that any subsequent event would then be forwarded on for committee review (as well as the first event).

Proposed rule: "Site Survey staff will request members to provide an explanation and develop a plan for future potential lung donors after the first event of identified noncompliance with the Lower Respiratory SARS–CoV–2 Testing requirement in Policy 2.9 and will not forward the matter to the MPSC for review. If staff identifies a second event of noncompliance in a subsequent weekly review, staff will ask the member to provide an explanation as well as a corrective action plan and then staff will provide all events' documentation to the MPSC for review."

If approved, the rule will be effective immediately upon implementation of the policy on May 27, 2021.

Of note: The weekly report from the Research department will provide a list of donors where lower respiratory specimen results were not reported in DonorNet prior to the lung recipient's removal from Wait list.

Example

OPO ABCD recovers lungs from donor A on 5/31/21. As of the run time of the weekly report from Research on Friday 6/4/21, OPO ABCD has not entered lower respiratory specimen test results in DonorNet. Site Survey views the Attachments tab of DonorNet on 6/4/21 and confirms that OPO ABCD has not uploaded a source document of the test. On the afternoon of 6/4/21, Site Survey sends an Inquiry email to OPO ABCD to ask if the test was completed and if so, for the OPO to provide the test results to Site Survey and upload the source document to DonorNet. Site Survey requests an answer by COB 6/7/21. OPO ABCD responds that the test was not completed. Site Survey then requests an explanation and a plan for future potential lung donors by COB Thursday 6/10/21. Site Survey sends by email a Closure Letter to OPO ABCD noting the noncompliance. Site Survey logs this first event of noncompliance into an Excel tracker. OPO ABCD recovers lungs from donor B on 6/30/21. As of the run time of the weekly report from Research on Friday 7/2/21, OPO ABCD did enter lower respiratory specimen test results in DonorNet, in compliance with Policy. OPO ABCD recovers lungs from donor C on 7/31/21. As of the run time of the weekly report from Research on Friday 8/6/21, OPO ABCD had not entered lower respiratory specimen test results in DonorNet. Site Survey views the Attachments tab of DonorNet on 8/6/21 and confirms that OPO ABCD has not uploaded a source document of the test. On the afternoon of 8/6/21, Site Survey sends an Inquiry email to OPO ABCD to ask if the test was completed and if so, for the OPO to provide the test results to Site Survey and upload the source document to DonorNet. Site Survey requests an answer by COB 8/9/21. OPO ABCD responds that the test was not completed. Site Survey then requests an explanation and corrective action plan by COB Thursday 8/12/21. Site Survey sends by email a formal Closure Letter to OPO ABCD noting the noncompliance and informing the member that the events of donors A and C will be forwarded to the MPSC. Site Survey logs this second event of noncompliance into an Excel tracker. Site Survey provides a case packet to the COAs prior to the next MPSC meeting, for presentation and review by the MPSC. The MPSC will provide a final resolution.

Relevant OPTN Bylaw or Policy

New requirement: OPTN Policy 2.9, "3. Infectious disease testing for all potential deceased lung donors using an FDA licensed, approved, cleared, or emergency use authorized lower respiratory specimen test for SARS–CoV–2 (COVID–19) by nucleic acid test (NAT)

Lower respiratory specimen test results for SARS–CoV–2 by nucleic acid test (NAT) must be available prior to transplant."

Also relevant (current policy, no change)—OPTN Policy 2.2 #14 "Ensuring that documentation for all of the following deceased donor information is submitted to the OPTN upon receipt: . . . c. Infectious disease results source documentation "

Supporting Documents

See proposal and policy notice on OPTN site.

MPSC Staff Summary

Proposed Operational Rule
Sending Performance Inquiries to Newly Identified Members

Item for Consideration

The Performance Monitoring Enhancement Subcommittee is asked to consider a proposed operational rule regarding the timing of sending inquiries to members newly identified for performance review. The Subcommittee will be asked to recommend that the MPSC approve the rule.

Summary

Currently, staff receive the SRTR performance data twice a year, prior to the MPSC's February and July meetings. When the data arrives, staff determine which members are newly identified for review. Staff automatically then add a row to the upcoming meeting's consent agenda with a proposed action of "Send Initial Inquiry." Members do not receive their initial inquiry letter until after the MPSC approves the consent agenda.

Proposed operational rule: The MPSC approves sending an initial inquiry for members newly identified for outcomes review when the data is available automatically, without a committee vote.

Benefits of this proposal are:

- Newly identified members will receive their inquiry earlier, which may allow both more time for their response and more time for MPSC review before the next meeting.
- The rule is consistent with the process used for inquiries in other MPSC case types.
- Shorter performance consent agendas and reduction of potential errors.

If questions arise about whether to send an inquiry to a particular program, staff will have the option to place the item on discussion for MPSC consideration and decision.

If approved, the rule will be effective with the release of the Spring 2022 PSR in July.

United Network for Organ Sharing (UNOS)

700 North 4th Street Richmond, VA 23219
tel: 804–782–4800
fax: 804–782–4816
https://unos.org/

August 17, 2022
The Honorable Ron Wyden, Chairman
The Honorable Charles Grassley
U.S. Senate Finance Committee Washington, DC 20150

Dear Chairman Wyden and Senator Grassley,

United Network for Organ Sharing (UNOS) offers the following additional information to the Senate Finance Committee following the testimony of Mr. Brian Shepard, CEO, on August 3, 2022, concerning the U.S. organ donation and transplantation system. UNOS shares the Committee's desire to see a successful transplant for every patient in need. We ask that the Committee please include this letter and the attached documents in the record.

As Mr. Shepard testified, UNOS is and has always been committed to improving the U.S. organ donation and transplantation system. We heard the concerns shared by members of the Committee and will work in collaboration with Congress, our federal partners, and community members, to further improve the national system and save more lives. We have a demonstrated record of continuous improvement, and in partnership with Health Resources and Services Administration (HRSA) and the broader transplant community, we have played a key role in nine consecutive years of increases in the number of deceased donor transplants. In 2021, we saw record breaking numbers of kidney, liver, and heart transplants.

This sustained record of growth, which continued throughout a global pandemic, shows that the system is dedicated to serving patients through unprecedented challenges. The best course for our nation's transplant system is to continue building on this momentum and to identify and execute on new opportunities for continued improvement.

We would like to take this opportunity to reiterate our commitment to continuous improvement in four key areas in particular:

- *State of the art technology:* UNOS has always provided reliable, effective, secure technology services to support the organ donation and transplant community. The system UNOS built and operates to support the OPTN has 99.99% up time, is regularly audited by HRSA, and exceeds performance and security standards established by the federal government. Just within the last two weeks, UNOS has achieved high scores on two separate government reviews, and HRSA is currently preparing for a full audit that will begin in a few weeks.
- As with all developing technology, we are never satisfied with the performance of the system, however, and we bring the leading technology providers in the country together to make the system stronger. UNOS partners with Nutanix to host the OPTN systems in the cloud. UNOS has engaged Accenture to help apply human-centered

design principles to modernize the user experience of the OPTN system. UNOS uses Apigee to support Application Program Interfaces (APIs) for electronic data sharing, and more than 200 hospitals and OPOs provide data to UNOS through APIs.

- Attached to this submission are a copy of the IT presentation made to committee staff earlier this year and a letter to the HRSA administrator reiterating our commitment to government review of OPTN IT systems.
- *Organ transportation:* UNOS agrees with the consensus at the hearing that any organ lost in transit, damaged or arriving otherwise unable to be transplanted is a tragedy—both for the generous donor and the patient waiting.
- UNOS heard a desire from the community to improve the visibility of tracking unaccompanied organs as an opportunity to improve efficiency. UNOS has and offers a tracking solution, one of several on the market. Just last week, the 5,000th organ carrying a UNOS-provided tracker was shipped and transplanted. As mentioned during the hearing, we are also currently piloting an organ travel mobile app that will enable OPOs to more quickly determine the very best travel plan for an organ in transit, based on a variety of factors.
- UNOS is engaged with major commercial airline providers to design improved organ handling processes that comply with TSA regulations while safely and reliably delivering the organ. UNOS would be pleased to work with the Committee in making improvements to federal restrictions on organ handling, such as returning organs to the passenger cabin or cockpit, where they once were allowed to travel.
- *Organ Discards:* The hearing included discussions of the decade-long rise in the number of kidney discards. UNOS agrees that there are organs recovered by OPOs that could be acceptable for transplant yet go unutilized. The OPTN has undertaken a number of initiatives designed to empower transplant programs with relevant and timely information, providing data, tools and analytics to help centers get to "yes" faster, as noted by the NASEM study.
- UNOS recently deployed data-driven predictive analytics to help clinicians decide whether to accept organ offers. A new offer filters tool built by UNOS helps target organ offers to the candidates most likely to accept them, improving system efficiency and ultimately increasing the number of transplants. Similarly, the Center Acceptance and Refusal Evaluation (CARE) tool allows centers to see all of the outcomes for offers they accept, as well as those they refuse. The OPTN Image Sharing project offers surgeons access to high resolution images of a donor organ, enabling teams to make more informed acceptance decisions up front, and reduce the likelihood of having to reallocate an organ last minute. Further, the OPTN's Membership and Professional Standards Committee (MPSC) has recently implemented additional transplant center metrics to include Organ Offer Acceptance Rate Ratios, a risk-adjusted calculation with an intent to both ensure organs suitable and safe for transplantation are allocated to the appropriate recipients on the waiting list based upon established policy and to improve transparency of the offer system to patients and providers.
- *OPTN member performance improvement and peer review:* At times, it seemed that questioners at the hearing conflated the two complementary but distinct roles that the OPTN and CMS play in oversight of the national transplant system. By statute,

regulation, and contract the OPTN, through its Membership and Professional Standards Committee (MPSC), is designed to provide a collaborative quality improvement process. In contrast, CMS has authority to impose sanctions, including payment and decertification.

- As Mr. Shepard testified, full and frank participation in our peer review process is what we believe leads to understanding and improvement following adverse events. Confidential peer review is a quality improvement practice implemented across healthcare disciplines following the Institute of Medicine's seminal report, *To Err Is Human* (2000). The IOM recommended a two-pronged system, one that included both confidential peer review for near misses and lesser events, and stricter sanctions for serious events. We are committed to working with the Committee and with HRSA and CMS at ensuring that the two-pronged system is working correctly and cooperatively, and that the types of events to be reviewed by each part of the system are properly defined. However, we strongly believe that abandoning confidential peer review entirely would have a detrimental effect on honest disclosure, and ultimately on patient safety.

UNOS has a long and successful record of facilitating transplants in the United States, and we are proud to be a part of the most successful organ donation and transplant community in the world. It is our daily mission to continue to improve the donation and transplant system.

We welcome the support of the Senate Finance Committee in implementing improvements to the system, and continuing to pursue our shared goal of saving lives through organ donation.

Sincerely
Jerry McCauley, M.D., MPH
President, UNOS Board of Directors Chief, Division of Nephrology
Medical Director, Transplantation Services
Vice Chairman, Health Equity, Diversity and Inclusion
Thomas Jefferson University Hospitals
Philadelphia, PA

United Network for Organ Sharing (UNOS)

700 North 4th Street Richmond, VA 23219
tel: 804–782–4800
fax: 804–782–4816
https://unos.org/

August 2, 2022

The Hon. Carole Johnson,
Administrator Health Resources and Services Administration
U.S. Department of Health and Human Services Rockville, MD 20857

Dear Administrator Johnson,

United Network for Organ Sharing (UNOS) is proud to have served as the Organ Procurement and Transplantation Network (OPTN) since 1984. In partnership with HRSA, we are nearing a decade of continued growth in the number of organ transplants and we are proud that our partnership with HRSA has yielded the highly equitable and efficient system we know today. We continue to make improvements every day for the benefit of the patients we serve.

UNOS has recently been provided with a document that has since been leaked to the media purporting to be a "draft" United States Digital Service (USDS) report on the OPTN IT system. We have never received an official copy of this draft report, despite a FOIA request to the U.S. Office of Management and Budget (OMB). Unfortunately, the report contains significant factual errors and demonstrably false misstatements about the OPTN IT infrastructure. We understand HRSA may have seen a copy of this report, and so we wanted to extend this invitation to you to discuss these claims to clarify and correct its numerous inaccuracies.

By way of background, the draft USDS report appears to be based entirely on a ninety-minute presentation by UNOS on December 10, 2020, pursuant to a request from HRSA during its 2019 Market Research for the Modernization National Resource Allocation System, as well as UNOS's responses to a set of follow-up questions submitted by HRSA. The USDS neither engaged with nor sought further information from UNOS during the development of this report, nor were we provided a chance to comment on the report or identify and correct any inaccurate information.

In contrast, the HRSA team has consistently reviewed the performance and security of the OPTN IT system in great detail throughout our performance of the OPTN contracts. HRSA reviews all OPTN contractual requirements for compliance annually, as well as on a periodic basis throughout each year, and UNOS consistently meets or exceeds its contractual obligations. Specifically, UNOS submits to HRSA results of the cybersecurity penetration testing conducted by a 3rd party on a semiannual basis. Further, HRSA security audits are conducted annually to ensure the quality and security of the OPTN system. Just today, UNOS received another 100% score on the HRSA Office of Information Technology's Capital Planning and Investment Control (CPIC) dashboard.

With that background, UNOS offers the following selected clarifications to the certain statements contained in the draft USDS report:

- UNOS utilizes an industry best practice, cloud-based approach incorporating both private and public cloud service providers. There are no components hosted on-premises.
- UNOS has maintained an IT system up time of 99.99% (outside of scheduled maintenance) for more than 10 years.
- More than 200 transplant hospitals and OPOs are leveraging UNet system APIs for reporting or querying data, and in the past year alone, the system processed nearly one million API transactions for members, with no additional manual data entry required.
- UNOS shares segments of real code with HRSA as part of both our ongoing application security program and the government's annual audit.
- UNOS has documented version control and the ability to replicate historical matches based on the policies in effect at the time.

We note that this represents only a selection of the statements in the draft report about which we have factual concerns.

Further, we are also concerned that the draft report mischaracterizes what we view as UNOS' productive, cooperative relationship with HRSA and ignores HRSA's above-referenced robust audit and oversight functions. As you know, the relationship described in the USDS report bears no resemblance to the working partnership we have with the HRSA team, a partnership that has produced positive results for patients since its inception.

You already have access to your team's routine annual audit information about the reliable, safe IT system that UNOS operates, but we stand ready to provide any additional briefings or information you request or to host you and/or your team for additional onsite meetings so that you can further understand our systems and processes.

We appreciate your consideration of our concerns about the inaccuracies in the leaked draft report. It is our sincere hope that these assurances, in combination with HRSA's own records, addresses any concerns the draft report may have raised for you. We look forward to continuing our work together on the critical mission of our Nation's transplant system.

Sincerely,

Jerry McCauley, M.D., MPH
President, UNOS Board of Directors

CC: Cheryl Dammons, Associate Administrator, HRSA
Adriane Burton, Chief Information Officer, HRSA

United Network for Organ Sharing (UNOS)

700 North 4th Street Richmond, VA 23219
tel: 804–782–4800
fax: 804–782–4816
https://unos.org

March 2, 2022

The Hon. Ron Wyden,
Chairman The Hon. Charles Grassley
U.S. Senate Committee on Finance Washington, DC 20510

Dear Chairman Wyden and Senator Grassley,

We appreciated the opportunity to brief your staff regarding the issues raised in your January 31, 2022, letter concerning UNOS' IT security and technology infrastructure and practices. We are pleased to provide the following additional information and actions taken since our February 17, 2022 meeting, in addition to the presentation materials and requested root cause analysis submitted to HRSA on February 26, 2021.

Penetration Testing

Senate staff inquired about the role of external entities in conducting penetration testing. Below are clarifications about our most recent tests.

- A third-party commercial company conducted the 2021 tests. Penetration test was a web application test with and without credentials. Testing was conducted in our "production equivalent" environment.
  - The HHS Office of Inspector General (OIG) and HRSA accepted this test in lieu of performing their own penetration test for the 2021 Audit
  - No vulnerabilities were identified allowing escalation of privilege or ability for lateral movement
  - As promised, we are providing the results and remediations from the 2021 penetration test:
    - 0 Critical
    - 3 High: All closed immediately
    - 6 Medium: 5 Closed, 1 pending software update available in June 2022
    - 3 Low: 1 Closed, 2 pending closure with code roll-out May 2022
- A HRSA-selected vendor, Synack, will conduct the 2022 test. It will be a crowd-sourced penetration test. The test will be in non-credentialed and credentialed format.

UNOS Relationship with Cybersecurity and Infrastructure Security Agency (CISA)

Senate staff recommended UNOS seek out free cybersecurity resources and services, such as the EINSTEIN sensor, offered by CISA to private sector organizations operating "critical infrastructure" for the nation. At this time, the OPTN system is categorized by HHS as a "high-value asset" and is ineligible for all services provided to infrastructures with this more elevated designation.

We appreciate, however, the suggestion to secure cybersecurity hygiene scans from CISA and have taken steps to request this important service.

UNOS established a relationship with CISA in 2015 and at that time registered for and participated in the Government Telecommunications Service (GETS), Wireless Priority Service (WPS), and Telecommunications Service Priority (TSP) programs. We have since sponsored numerous OPOs in support of their participation in the program.

Security Clearances and Classified Warnings

- In response to a staff suggestion for gaining Top Secret clearance for pertinent UNOS staff so that UNOS may receive classified briefings from the U.S. government on security threats, a formal request to HRSA has been made to determine the requirements for Secret or Top-Secret clearances and sponsorship and is under review within HHS. To date, Secret and Top-Secret designations have not been required nor sponsored by HHS for the OPTN. UNOS currently receives unclassified email alerts from the FBI, HRSA, and CISA.

- UNOS meets the contractual obligation as stated in the Position Sensitivity Designations requirements within the current OPTN contract, which states: "All contractor (and/or any subcontractor) employees must obtain a background investigation commensurate with their position sensitivity designation that complies with Parts 1400 and 731 of Title 5, Code of Federal Regulations (CFR)."

Code Scanning and Review

- UNOS scans code throughout the software development lifecycle using Veracode technology.
- Snippets of code have been and will continue to be made available to HRSA for verification and closure of findings as needed.
- Over the past several months, HRSA and UNOS have been working to establish a process for reviewing code. We estimate that HRSA will begin code reviews in Q2 of 2022.

Vulnerability Management

- Infrastructure vulnerability scanning is performed weekly using Tenable, and all results are provided to HRSA.
- HRSA is provided access upon request and on a regular schedule to perform web applications scanning, using NetSparker, against a production equivalent environment.

Offsite Backup Storage

- Offsite backup storage practices have been in place since the OPTN system's inception in 1999 and continue in the present.
- 2010 Modernization Project
- As a follow-up to your question regarding the 2010 system modernization project:
  - A project called Chrysalis was terminated in 2012 after concluding that it would not go far enough to modernize and evolve the OPTN technology.
  - Following that decision, UNOS determined that the path forward needs to be centered on digital transformation of the OPTN System, embracing and practicing the Agile methodology, test automation, open-source frameworks, Application Programming Interfaces (APIs), mobile capabilities, elevated security practices, and cloud computing. As a result of this direction and culture, we have been able to —
    - React faster to the needs of the transplant community.
    - Establish and maintain a consistent feedback loop with the users of OPTN system.
    - Integrate cloud-based data analytics and machine learning capabilities.
    - Implement a variety of open-source frameworks to deliver value.
    - Enable members to benefit from our seamless integration with EHRs and EMRs.

- Empower members with secure mobile capabilities to perform work whenever and wherever.
- Reduce the threat landscape by implementing zero trust principles in conjunction with a defense-in-depth strategy.
- Maintain high quality of software, leveraging 24x7 automated testing.
- Deliver on the OPTN Board of Directors commitments.
- Retain and attract engineering talent.

February 2021 Service Outage

- To clarify our response in our meeting, the February 2021 one-hour service outage occurred as the result of a failure within a high-availability redundant pair of internal firewalls, not a manual human error. The human error occurred during the service restoration effort. As requested during the meeting, the root cause analysis previously provided to HRSA is included as part of this response. Since this incident, further automation has been added to service restoration procedures to eliminate the need for human intervention.
- Please note the graphic depicted in the provided RCA reflects the OPTN system architecture as of February 2021, while we were in transition to the current state architecture. The OPTN system architecture today reflects what was presented to the staff during our call. It has additional built-in redundancies and security components, advanced use of public and private cloud, and automation.

Please do not hesitate to contact me if you have additional questions or require further clarifications.

Sincerely,
Brian Shepard, CEO

Attachments (2): UNOS IT Security Presentation for Senate Finance (17 February 2022); UNet Root Cause Analysis (6 February 2021)

OPTN Technology & Security
Briefing

United Network for Organ Sharing
U.S. Senate Finance Committee Staff
February 17, 2022

UNOS UNITED NETWORK FOR ORGAN SHARING

Areas of Focus

- System modernization and reliability
- Sufficient backup systems

- Cloud utilization
- Security of the system from cyberattacks
- Basic features and security systems
- Ensuring that security flaws do not lead to preventable deaths
- Prevention of service interruptions due to ransomware attack, technical failure or inefficiency causing delays

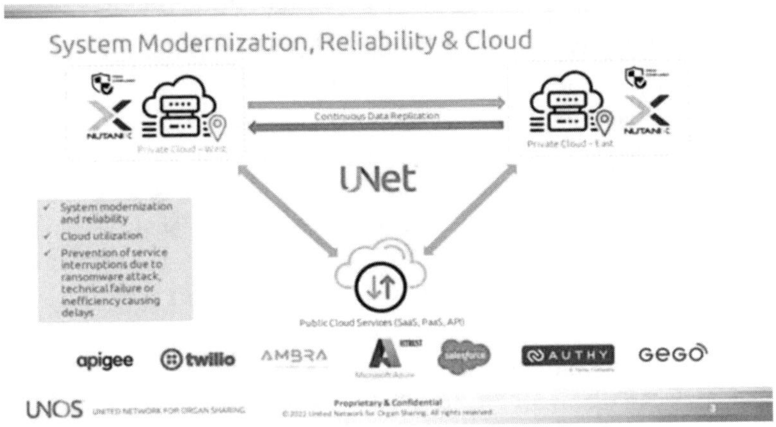

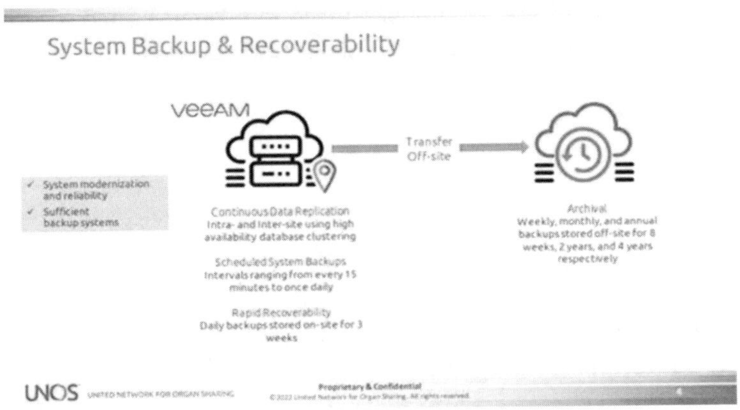

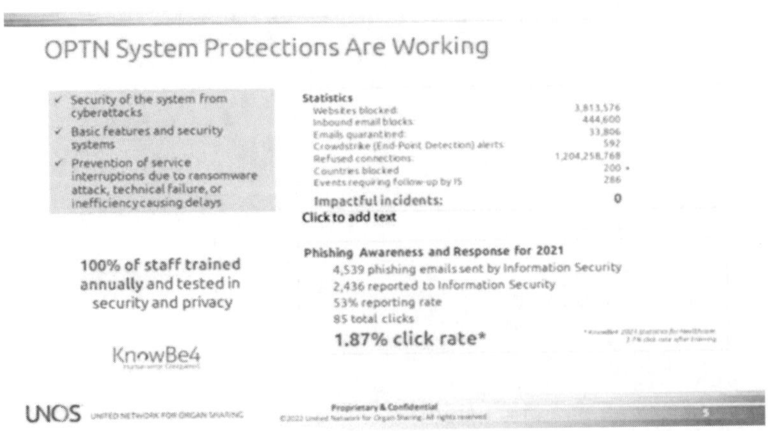

Access Management

Access to systems and data provided to the right individuals, at the right time, for the right reason

Areas of Focus	UNOS Capabilities
Basic features and security systems	✓ Role Based Access Control (RBAC) ✓ Multi factor authentication ✓ Encrypted data, channels and network drives
Ensuring that security flaws do not lead to preventable deaths	✓ Reduces risk of malware and ransomware propagation by preventing scope of administrator capabilities
Prevention of service interruptions due to ransomware attack, technical failure, or inefficiency causing delays	✓ Multi factor authentication ✓ Reduce risk of malware and ransomware propagation by preventing scope of administrator capabilities

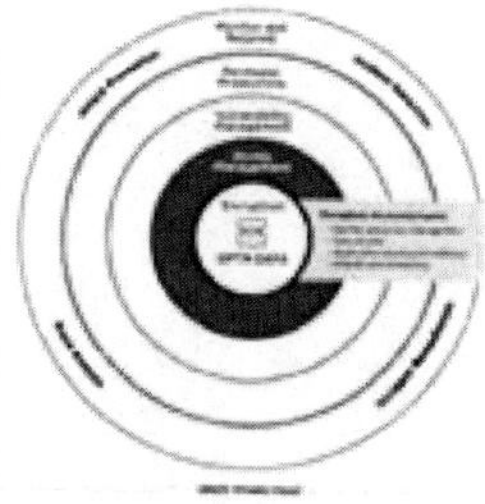

AUTHY Microsoft RSA NUTANIX

UNOS UNITED NETWORK FOR ORGAN SHARING

Proprietary & Confidential

7

Vulnerability Management

Ensures doors are shut

Areas of Focus	UNOS Capabilities
System modernization and reliability	✓ Automated software code analysis
Basic features and security systems	✓ Continuous vulnerability scanning ✓ Automated patching and remediation ✓ Scanning to detect code and on-line vulnerabilities in web applications (SAST and DAST)
Ensuring that security flaws do not lead to preventable deaths	✓ Continuous vulnerability scanning ✓ Automated patching and remediation ✓ Scanning to detect code and on-line vulnerabilities in web applications ✓ Penetration testing to simulate cyber attacks

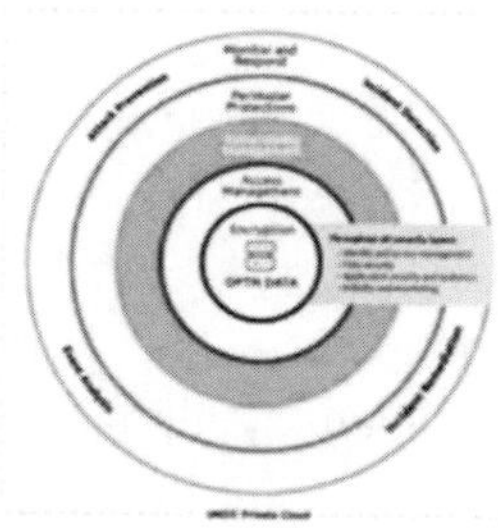

BURPSUITE WhiteSource Trustwave VERACODE tenable

UNOS UNITED NETWORK FOR ORGAN SHARING

Proprietary & Confidential

8

Perimeter Protections

Perimeter protections allow appropriate business activity

Areas of Focus	UNOS Capabilities
System modernization and reliability	✓ 5th generation firewalls ✓ End-point Detection and Response through Crowdstrike ✓ Canaries for early detection and alerting
Cloud utilization	✓ Crowdstrike cloud services to quickly update attack signatures, threat hunting and forensics ✓ 5th generation firewalls extended to Microsoft Azure
Security of the system from cyberattacks	✓ Intrusion detection and prevention to block attacks and suspicious traffic ✓ Attack identification and automated system containment to prevent spread of malware and ransomware
Prevention of service interruptions due to ransomware attack, technical failure, or inefficiency causing delays	✓ Intrusion detection and prevention to block attacks and suspicious traffic ✓ Attack identification and automated system containment to prevent spread of malware and ransomware ✓ Threat hunting to seek out signs of an intrusion

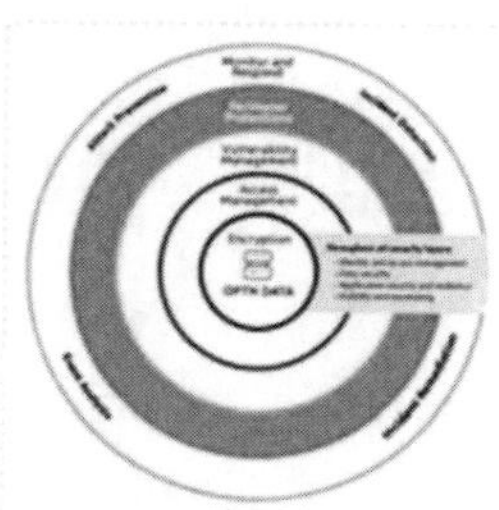

FORTINET CANARY

UNOS UNITED NETWORK FOR ORGAN SHARING

Proprietary & Confidential

9

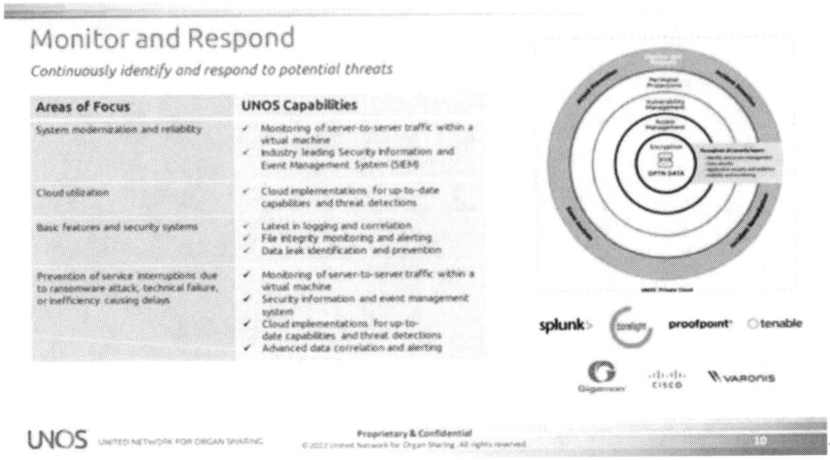

Appendix

UNOS Information Security Team

- More than 112 years of combined IT and Information Security Experience
- Holds 27 industry recognized certifications including:
  - Certified Ethical Hacker (CEH)
  - Certified Cloud Security Professional (CCSP)
  - Certified Detection Analyst (CDA)
  - Certified Incident Handler (CIH)
  - Certified Information Systems Security Professional (CISSP)
  - Certified Penetration Tester (GPEN)

<u>IT Operations RCA Report</u>

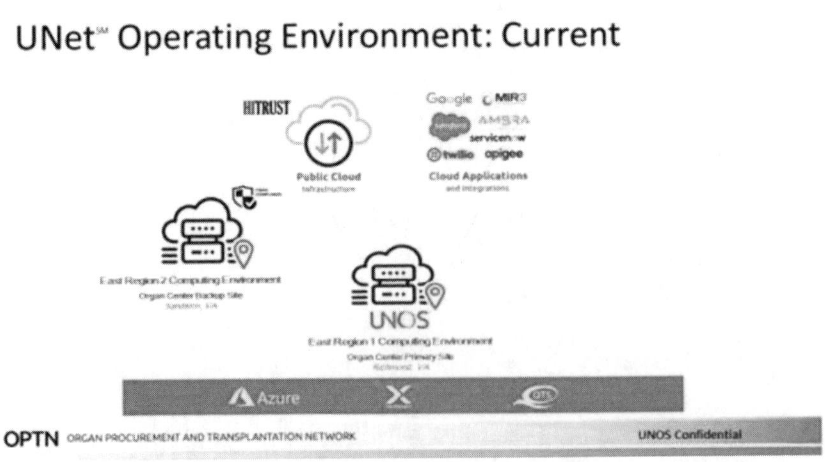

Incident: Periodic UNetSM Access Impact.
Date and Duration of Incident: 2021–02–06 8:10PM EST–11:00 PM EST.

Incident Summary

Starting around 2021–02–06 8:15PM EST, users began to experience periodic latency and errors in UNet functions.

Root Cause

East Region 1 (ER1) Computing Environment experienced a Network Equipment failure.

Detailed Description

UNet users experienced periodic latency or errors as a result of ER1 Networking Equipment failure.

Between 08:10pm and 08:15PM EST, one node of a clustered pair of internal Cisco firewalls experienced an interface failure which cascaded to the other firewall node, resulting in a total failure of the internal firewall cluster.

This failure, in turn, caused interruption to internal network traffic in ER1. Cisco technical support confirmed that the issue was caused by a defect in the Cisco firewall's firmware.

Issue resolution actions consisted of transitioning impacted workloads from ER1 to ER2 computing environment, as well as taking the ER1 internal firewall cluster offline and bypassing internal network traffic. Confirmed no impact to matching function or patients.

Additional Information

Throughout the incident some workloads running in ER1 remained there. Periodically, between 08:25 and 09:25PM EST, ER1 was not accessible to UNet users. Procedural errors made in the process of transitioning some workloads from ER1 to ER2 contributed to this incident. All other steps taken (manual and automated) during this incident were accomplished without any errors.

The equipment in question has not been put back in service.

Since the incident, ER1 has been and continues to be fully operational. All normal workloads/ activities have been and are functioning there.

Action Steps Taken During Incident

08:12PM EST	Initial *ThousandEyes.com* alerts received
08:25PM	Organ Center (OC) receiving Members Calls
	IT On-call responding engineer informs On-call manager and begins to evaluate the issue
08:33PM	Conference Bridge initiated
08:56PM	ER1 Networking Equipment failure identified as triggering event
	Systems Engineer enroute to ER1
09:10PM	Decision is made to move some UNet functions to ER2. Leverage external Transition Plan (TP) in *Attainium.net*
	Additional Systems Engineers are brought into the Conference Bridge to assist

09:23PM	TP procedures to ER2 are initiated
09:40PM	TP procedures to ER2 are completed Reviewing periodic *ThousandEyes.com* alerts reported in operational logs
09:45PM	UNet functions to add candidate or register donor are functional
10:01PM	Some functions transitioned from ER1 to ER2 generating periodic alerts
10:22PM	Issues in executing TP procedures to ER2 identified on the Conference Bridge: (1) External Plan not up to date; (2) Human data entry errors
10:30PM	Corrective Actions identified to address issues in TP procedures
10:58PM	UNet functions accessible both internally and externally

Corrective Action

We have completed our detailed investigation and compiled our corrective actions to prevent future incidents of this kind:

- All procedural documentation will be updated in Attainium.net first then synchronized with on premises copy. Attainium.net has no dependency to internal infrastructure. (Completed 2/8/21).
- Transition Plan (TP) procedures training will be updated to accommodate all scenarios. Staff retraining has commenced, and will be required for all new team members. Training will be ongoing as procedures are updated, and a quarterly review of all procedure documentation will be conducted.
- Continue with additional automation (scripting) to further reduce manual TP tasks, avoiding potential for human error and resulting in faster transitions. (2/28/21)
- Continue with West Region turn-on project (see below). Ensure Transition Plan is updated accordingly to incorporate Nutanix advanced management capabilities and staff are trained. (April 2021)

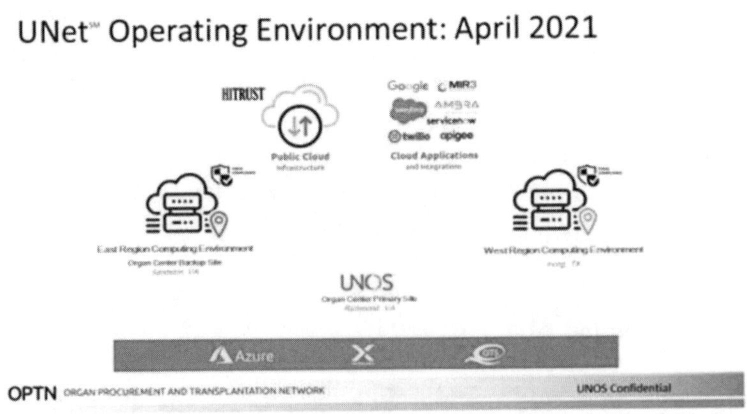

- Provide continuous updates to HRSA (2/9 and 2/11/21) and NOOC (2/19/21) on UNet availability to maintain confidence in the system.

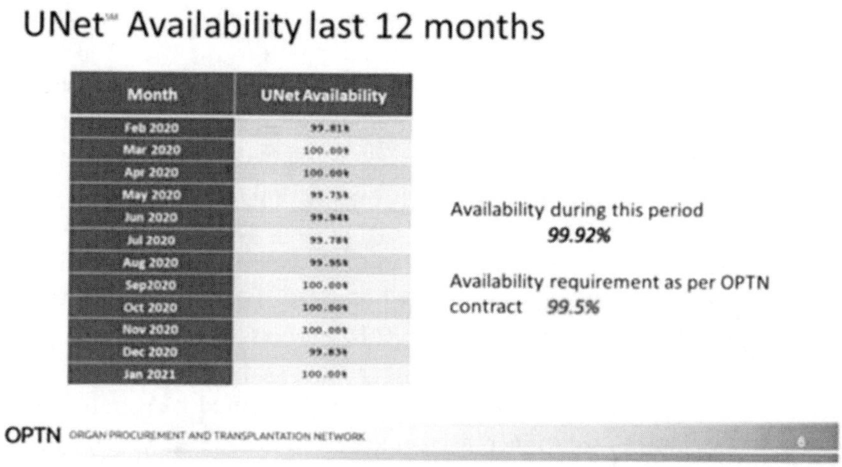

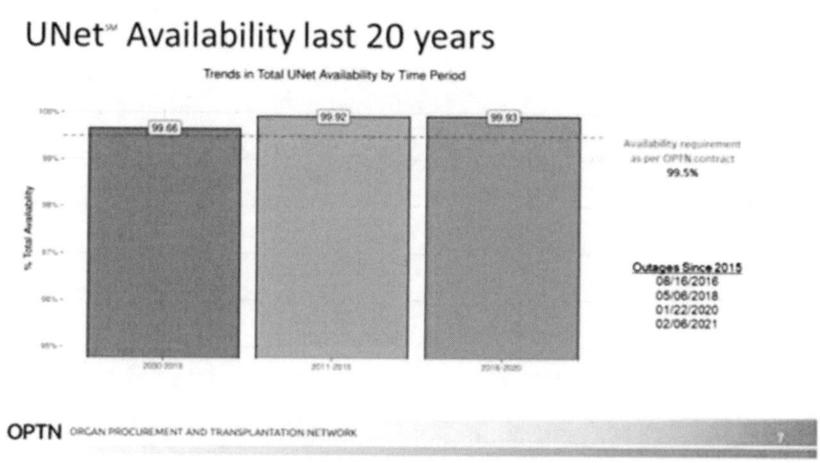

Questions Submitted for the Record to Brian Shepard Questions Submitted by Hon. Ron Wyden

Question. Black Americans are disproportionately impacted by the organ shortage. According to the 2022 OPTN kidney update, 28.5 percent of kidney registrations on the wait list are Black. This is essentially double their percentage in the population (2020 U.S. census data shows that 14.2 percent of the U.S. population is Black or identifies as Black). Additionally, minorities have much higher kidney disease burden than their Caucasian counterparts. The 1-year monitoring report for the new OPTN kidney allocation policy notes that transplant rates for minorities are approaching/similar to Caucasians. However, to be equitable, Black Americans would need to be transplanted at much higher rates than their Caucasian counterparts given this disproportionality of Black wait-list registrants.

Given the disproportionately large percentage of Black Americans on the waiting list, what kidney transplant rate for this community would the system need to achieve to reach equity for Black Americans? How has UNOS calculated this? How has this community's transplant rate changed over time?

Has UNOS calculated the equitable rates for other minorities? If so, please provide these rates, how each was calculated, and how they changed over time.

Answer. We agree that increasing equity in donation and transplant, especially among historically marginalized communities, is of paramount importance. Organ Procurement and Transplantation Network (OPTN) policies play a key role in addressing these inequities, and the data show that important gains in access for Black and other racial and ethnic minority wait-listed patients have accelerated since December 2014, when the OPTN Kidney Allocation System (KAS) was implemented. Following that policy change, we saw a dramatic expansion in the number of Black patients with long wait times on dialysis who were able to receive transplants. Six years later, despite the pandemic, 2020 deceased donor kidney transplant rates were similar for White and Black patients.

As the question notes, a new kidney policy was implemented in March 2021, and the 1-year monitoring report showed sharp increases in kidney transplant rates: 16- percent increase overall; 23-percent increase for Black patients; and 36-percent increase for patients with 3 or more years of dialysis time at listing.

Table 1: Comparison of Percent of Kidney Waiting List and Percent of Kidney Transplants by Ethnicity and Year, 2015-2021

	White, NH		Black, NH		Hispanic/Latino		Asian, NH		Other, NH	
Year	% Waiting List	% Transplants	% Waiting List	% Transplants	% Waiting List	% Transplants	% Waiting List	% Transplants	% Waiting List	% Transplants
2015	36.62%	46.01%	33.72%	28.05%	19.37%	17.61%	8.12%	6.99%	2.16%	1.94%
2016	36.64%	46.30%	33.27%	26.96%	19.52%	18.56%	8.38%	6.31%	2.20%	1.88%
2017	36.41%	46.54%	32.73%	26.58%	19.89%	18.19%	8.66%	6.80%	2.31%	1.89%
2018	35.96%	45.78%	32.32%	26.25%	20.34%	18.81%	8.96%	7.07%	2.43%	2.09%
2019	35.50%	45.22%	32.08%	26.81%	20.84%	18.97%	9.07%	6.96%	2.51%	2.05%
2020	35.33%	44.75%	31.83%	27.33%	21.11%	18.73%	9.19%	7.08%	2.53%	2.11%
2021	35.84%	42.08%	31.68%	28.67%	20.70%	20.06%	9.27%	7.16%	2.51%	2.02%

* Percent of waiting list is calculated based on a snapshot of the waiting list on December 31st of the stated year.

Since 2015, as shown in table 1, the discrepancy between the percentage of kidney transplants going to ethnic minorities in relation to the percentage of the kidney waiting list comprising ethnic minorities has been shrinking. This is seen most dramatically in the Black candidate population. As of December. 31, 2015, 34 percent of kidney waiting list registrations were Black, and 28 percent of 2015 deceased donor kidney transplants went to Black recipients. By December. 31, 2021, 32 percent of registrations on the kidney waiting list were Black, and 29 percent of 2021 deceased donor kidney transplants went to Black recipients.

The Hispanic candidate population has seen similar increases in equity; the percentage of candidates waiting for a transplant who are Hispanic and the percentage of transplants going to Hispanic candidates are now nearly on par, as of 2021. These improvements follow changes to OPTN policies relating to human leukocyte antigen (HLA) matching and typing as well as increased priority for highly sensitized patients. The percent of transplants going to Asian recipients has declined slightly relative to their waiting list presence, while the discrepancy between percent transplanted and percent waiting has remained stable over time for all other ethnic minorities.

While these gains are important, we agree that they are but one component of the effort to eliminate inequities in access to the transplant wait list. The community has long called for enhanced data collection to better understand the socio-economic factors that restrict access to the transplant wait list as well as to the care that is often required pre-listing, enabling the community to answer important questions like 1a above and many others. Further, while understanding the national disease burden is a key step toward addressing inequities in access to transplant, it is also crucially important to understand how many patients with end-stage organ failure are unable to seek transplant due to comorbidities or other clinical factors. Both factors are unknown.

While OPTN regulatory authority is limited to organ donors and wait-listed patients, the OPTN has still sought to contribute to understanding the barriers that exist to accessing the wait list. For example, in 2021, the OPTN Data Advisory Committee (DAC) proposed a project, currently under review with the Health Resources and Services Administration (HRSA), to collect prewait-list patient referral and evaluation data and to work with partners to study and improve equitable access to the wait list. The OPTN also requested and received additional funding from HRSA to study the feasibility and utility of linking existing external social determinants of health (SDOH) datasets with the OPTN dataset. That study led to the creation of two research studies that helped the OPTN understand the role of SDOH in determining waitlist outcomes among transplant candidates. As a result of these studies, the OPTN is currently working with committees to find ways to incorporate SDOH data into policy monitoring and evaluation. Finally, the OPTN recently supported an amendment by HRSA to the OPTN Systems of Records Notice, which added a new routine use to allow HRSA or its contractors to disclose OPTN records "to physicians or other health-care professionals providing clinical treatment to such individuals, for clinical purposes."[49]

This will allow the OPTN to share candidate information with physicians, such as nephrologists, and health-care professionals, such as dialysis providers, to assist in the evaluation and wait-listing process for their current patients who may be potential candidates for kidney transplant.

Question. According to UNOS 990s, in the year ending September 30, 2020, the organization brought in $4 million more in OPTN revenue than it spent on expenses. In the year ending September 30, 2019, the organization had $5.6 million more in OPTN revenue than expenses. Since at least FY 2019, UNOS has had a financial management policy that it could use revenues from OPTN contract fees that exceed reimbursable costs for its general expenditures, and as of the year ending September 30, 2021, UNOS total assets are reported to be $97.7 million not including property and equipment. What role did UNOS have in approving this policy and for how long has it been in place?

Please describe how the UNOS policy of using excess revenues from fees for general expenditures came about and how long it has been in place.

Who ultimately determined that UNOS could utilize OPTN fee revenues in this manner? UNOS management? The UNOS Board? HRSA?

Answer. UNOS has no such policy in place. While UNOS as a private corporation may have revenues exceeding its expenses, any excess OPTN Registration Fee revenue may *not* be used by UNOS for any purpose other than for allowable costs under the OPTN contract and only when such allowable costs are approved by the HRSA Contracting Officer. In order to support the committee's understanding of our financial processes and policies, however, we offer the below clarifying information.

The Form 990s referenced above are for UNOS, a private nonprofit Virginia membership corporation. The OPTN is not yet a distinct private nonprofit entity and accordingly, its

---

[49] OPTN Systems of Record Notice, 87 Fed. Reg. 46967 (August 1, 2022). *https:// www.federal register.gov/documents/2022/08/01/2022-16344/privacy-act-of-1974-system-of-records.*

financial position is presented in consolidated financial statements with UNOS. In audited financial statements, OPTN assets are listed as "restricted cash" and "restricted investments" within those consolidated financial statements. As detailed in financial records provided to the Senate Finance Committee and available online, OPTN Registration Fees may only be used for allowable OPTN contract expenses, and only when a monthly voucher is approved by the OPTN Contracting Officer's Representative at HRSA. At the end of each fiscal year, OPTN Registration Fee revenue in excess of allowable contract costs remains in the OPTN operating account, and the amount may be carried forward to the next OPTN fiscal year budget and included in the OPTN budget calculations. The annual OPTN budget is developed by the OPTN Finance Committee and approved by the OPTN Board of Directors with oversight by U.S. Department of Health and Human Services (HHS) staff and ultimate approval by the HHS Secretary. From time to time, OPTN operating account funds are invested in a separate restricted OPTN reserve fund account.

To illustrate the funds transfer process, for the month of June, UNOS would pay all of its expenses during the month from UNOS' operating account. On behalf of the OPTN, UNOS continuously invoices, collects, and holds in a separate OPTN operating account all OPTN registration fee revenue received from OPTN member transplant hospitals who add a candidate to the OPTN candidate waiting list. At the end of June, UNOS prepares a voucher and submits it to the HRSA Contracting Officer, accounting for all allowable OPTN contract expenses that UNOS incurred during the month of June. HRSA reviews the voucher, and once approved, UNOS transfers funds from the OPTN operating account to the UNOS operating account to reimburse UNOS for expenses that UNOS has already incurred and paid. This process occurs every month.

In pre-hearing interviews, Finance Committee staff specifically asked about Note 4 in UNOS's most recent financial audit, which is readily available online.[50] The American Association of International Certified Professional Accountants' (AICPA) Financial Accounting Standards Board established a requirement that nonprofit organizations must disclose publicly the amount of liquid resources available to cover 12 months of expenses, in order for readers of the financial statements to more accurately assess the organization's financial stability.[51] Note 4 of the UNOS financial audit details the amount of assets that are available to pay organizational expenses in the next 12-month period.

An auditor completing the type of information contained in Note 4 evaluates whether there are limitations or restrictions on a nonprofit organization's cash or cash equivalents that would make those assets unavailable for general expenditures that will arise in the next 12 months. General expenditures are not defined but are understood to mean those costs associated with the ordinary course of business. Cash or cash equivalents are restricted if, for example, a donor places limitations on the purpose for which a cash donation can be used, or the time period during which it must be used.

It is also important to read Note 4 in conjunction with the preceding Notes in the report. In particular, Note 1 describes that UNOS "functions as the sole national network whose mission is to improve the effectiveness of the United States organ procurement and transplantation

---

[50] 2021 UNOS Audited Financial Statement. https://unos.org/wp-content/uploads/2021-Audited-Financial-Statement.pdf.

[51] Accounting Standards Update (ASU) 2016–14, Not-for-Profit Entities (Topic 958): Presentation of Financial Statements of Not-for-Profit Entities, available at https://www.fasb.org/ page/PageContent? pageId=/projects/recentlycompleted/statements-notforprofit.html&isstaticpage=true (accessed October 11, 2022).

system and to provide for the fair and equitable distribution of all donated organs. To carry out this mission, the Organization maintains a computerized database to identify potential transplant recipients and to provide for the systematic matching of donated organs with such recipients."

Thus, in Note 4, "when collection of OPTN registration fees exceed the reimbursable costs incurred at a given point in time by the Organization," the Organization "has determined that the use of the restricted cash and investments amounts will be for mission-related activities within 1 year and, accordingly, these amounts are included in financial assets available to meet general expenditures within 1 year." The mission being those OPTN activities described in Note 1.

To reiterate, excess OPTN registration fee revenues are used only for allowable OPTN contract purposes and will remain in the OPTN operating account until authorized to pay allowable contract costs, or transferred to the OPTN reserve fund, as appropriate.

Question. One of the baseline requirements for Federal contracting, Medicare, and Medicaid costs is that they must be reasonable and necessary.

How does OPTN/UNOS define both "reasonable" and "necessary" for itself and other parties in the OPTN?

Answer. The OPTN and UNOS Board of Directors Finance Committees are composed of members of the donation and transplant community, along with non-voting advisors and, on the OPTN Finance Committee, representatives from HRSA. These Committees develop the annual OPTN and UNOS budgets and related fees before seeking approval from the Board of Directors.

The OPTN final rule requires the OPTN, annually, to establish the OPTN registration fee for patients registered on the wait list, and requires that the fee shall be determined by the OPTN and calculated to cover the "reasonable costs" of operating the OPTN, with approval from the Secretary:

> An OPTN member shall pay a registration fee to the OPTN for each transplant candidate it places on the waiting list. The amount of such fee shall be calculated to cover (together with contract funds awarded by the Secretary) the reasonable costs of operating the OPTN and shall be determined by the OPTN with the approval of the Secretary. No less often than annually, and whether or not a change is proposed, the OPTN shall submit to the Secretary a statement of its proposed registration fee, together with such supporting information as the Secretary finds necessary to determine the reasonableness or adequacy of the fee schedule and projected revenues. This submission is due at least 3 months before the beginning of the OPTN's fiscal year. The Secretary will approve, modify, or disapprove the amount of the fee.[52]

The budget development process applies these "reasonable cost" principles as is inherent in the budgeting process for public and private institutions. The OPTN Finance Committee considers multiple factors when determining what the "reasonable costs" of operating the OPTN will be for the upcoming fiscal year. With respect to the OPTN contract, revenue will consist of the estimated number of candidates added to the waiting list multiplied by the approved OPTN Registration Fee, and the contracted amount for the Federal appropriation. The expense portion of the budget includes a detailed analysis of several factors including but not limited to: the strategic and operational goals of the OPTN; the estimated personnel costs to

[52] 42 CFR Sec. § 121.5(c)

deliver the requirements of the OPTN contract; the technology roadmap; and the estimated number of policy projects the OPTN is anticipating and developing.

The OPTN Finance Committee propose a budget to address these goals, and the board of directors approves the proposed budget. Ultimately, the Secretary of HHS must approve the OPTN budget and associated OPTN Registration Fee.

Neither UNOS nor the OPTN bill Medicare, Medicaid, or any Federal or State public health insurance program for services.

Question. In the August 3rd hearing, you stated that UNOS lacks strong enforcement levers to hold OPOs accountable. Specifically, you stated that, "The statute does not give UNOS any authority to offer sanctions . . . the certification, decertification and payment authorities belong to entirely to CMS." However, the OPTN final rule gives UNOS the ability to refer an OPO to the Secretary of HHS for decertification. In the 40 plus years of holding the OPTN contract, UNOS has only referred an OPO to the Secretary once.

Why has UNOS only used this enforcement authority one time? Does UNOS feel this appropriate reflects the overall performance of OPOs during its tenure as the OPTN?

Answer. Oversight, rigorous performance measures, and continuous improvement are essential parts of the Nation's organ donation and transplantation system. The OPTN maintains a robust system for monitoring member compliance with "OPTN Obligations." OPTN Obligations are defined in the OPTN Bylaws as ". . . all the applicable provisions of the National Organ Transplant Act (NOTA), OPTN Final Rule, OPTN Charter, OPTN Bylaws, and OPTN Policies." Pursuant to 42 CFR§ 121.10(b), the OPTN conducts ongoing and periodic reviews of each member OPO for compliance with these obligations.[53]

The final rule defines the scope of the OPTN's role in monitoring members, and that role was specifically designed by HHS to focus on member support and quality improvement.

The OPTN board-approved charge for the Membership and Professional Standards Committee (MPSC) requires that the MPSC monitor OPTN member compliance with OPTN membership criteria, OPTN bylaws and policies, and the OPTN final rule. Through a robust peer and effective peer review process, the MPSC analyzes events that are identified as presenting a risk to patient safety, public health or the integrity of the OPTN. The MPSC also evaluates and supports OPTN members by providing feedback on and making recommendations to improve members' performance, compliance and quality systems. The MPSC also identifies opportunities to educate the community about improving patient safety through effective practices.

When the MPSC considers members under review, the committee's discussion centers primarily on how the member can improve its performance, if corrective action planning or quality improvement planning is necessary, and what benchmarks the member can provide the MPSC to ensure they are correcting and improving. The MPSC is made up of experienced donation and transplant professionals who are in the best position to identify programs who can benefit from coaching and help them improve. The MPSC takes action or makes recommendations for further action to the OPTN board of directors as needed.

Based on law, precedent, policy, and longstanding effective practices for quality improvement in health care, the OPTN's role is to support its members in driving their improvement. Both the final rule and the OPTN contract require the OPTN to employ a peer review process and provide and facilitate confidential coaching of effective practices, in

[53] OPTN Compliance and Evaluation. https://optn.transplant.hrsa.gov/policies-bylaws/compliance-and-evaluation/.

contrast to the regulatory and financial oversight rules that CMS provides. Sanctions are indeed a tool, but actions such as decertification reside outside of the OPTN's mandated purview. Only the Secretary of HHS is empowered to remove a member from the OPTN, and the Secretary is not bound by the OPTN's recommendation, even in those instances in which a member is referred to them. If a referred member is not decertified, they remain a member of the OPTN. In all cases, the OPTN's focus remains on member improvement. As noted in our response to Senator Wyden, the MPSC will discuss specific potential improvements to the process at its October 2022 meeting.

UNOS supports enhanced communications with CMS in particular, as well as a more formal communication process between CMS and the OPTN. In that process, UNOS believes communication must flow both ways. UNOS would also be pleased to discuss with Congress, CMS, HRSA and HHS any ongoing concerns about this process, to provide additional information about how the review and member improvement approach works. We understand the committee's interest in promoting the sharing of valuable incident data within the OPTN and with Federal regulators. We believe it is critical that any mechanisms for increased sharing continue to protect patient privacy and to promote candid self-disclosure when incidents do occur.

Question. During the August 3rd hearing you stated that the OPTN "peer review process has significant persuasive authority, but all the payment authority and all the certification/decertification authority [for OPOs] live at CMS."

Does UNOS routinely provide CMS with critical information on each OPO's history of performance, policy compliance, and safe practice or lack thereof, so that CMS may adequately enforce these payment and decertification authorities?

If yes, please describe the mechanisms in place for UNOS to share this information on a routine basis.

At the hearing, you alluded to HRSA's role in communicating this type of information to CMS. Does UNOS routinely provide HRSA with critical information on each OPO's history of performance, policy compliance, and safe practice or lack thereof, so that HRSA may report this information to CMS?

We understand from your testimony that HRSA participates in MPSC discussions, but how does UNOS ensure HRSA is fully informed when less than half of the OPO patient safety cases reported to UNOS in recent years were referred to the MPSC?

Are OPOs and transplant centers required to report safety events to UNOS? If so, please describe the requirements.

Is UNOS aware of failures to report safety events by any OPOs or transplant centers? If so, what were the consequences of these failures?

Answer. As the OPTN contractor, we have always welcomed a substantive conversation about how best to share information with the Federal Government in this process to ensure that all parties remain informed. While we routinely provide HRSA information on member performance, we do not routinely provide CMS with the same information. Whether HRSA shares information with CMS is beyond our knowledge, as we have traditionally been required to limit sharing of information only to HRSA. However, we will be pleased to provide CMS with information if directed and permitted by the OPTN Contracting Officer's Representative (COR).

Engagement with HRSA and CMS: The OPTN board and committee structure as required by NOTA, the final rule, and the OPTN contract is designed to ensure HRSA is engaged and included at all levels of governance. HRSA representatives serve as non-voting members of all OPTN committees, as well as on the OPTN board of directors. Additionally, HRSA representatives are present for all closed sessions of the MPSC. If HRSA requests information from the OPTN, even information protected by confidential medical peer review, the OPTN is obligated to provide that information. The OPTN does not have discretion over what HRSA does with any of this information after it is provided and does not have insight over what HRSA provides to CMS.

We believe it is important that both HRSA and CMS fully understand the issues the MPSC addresses in its peer review and monitoring processes. Expanding communication to include direct engagement between CMS and the OPTN is likely important to have more coordinated oversight of the system and of OPOs in particular.

As mentioned above, HRSA is intimately involved in the OPTN's compliance processes, and is informed of all cases sent to the MPSC. In addition to being a part of the MPSC and the OPTN board of directors, HRSA attends weekly MPSC leadership calls, during which HRSA and MPSC leadership are apprised of any ongoing issues. HRSA has access to all MPSC meeting agendas and materials, consistent with contract requirements. If staff are not clear about whether a case should be referred to the MPSC, staff will brief the MPSC leadership, including HRSA, so that MPSC leadership can make an informed determination. Staff also provide the MPSC with a retrospective report of the issues reported in the previous year and provide a similar report to HRSA as required in the OPTN contract. Even if a case is not reported to the MPSC, it may nevertheless be reported to HRSA if it meets certain agreed upon criteria, or other criteria agreed upon in the OPTN contract.

Additionally, pursuant to the OPTN contract, UNOS staff annually provide HRSA a monitoring report, which includes aggregate information about the monitoring activities of both the MPSC and UNOS Member Quality. The report provides data on efforts to monitor members and improve member performance and compliance.

Reporting Patient Safety Events: Promoting patient safety is central to the integrity of the donation and transplant system. OPTN members are both required and encouraged to report safety events, and a dedicated Patient Safety Portal is available for members to report issues. However, the OPTN has been intentional about not explicitly defining a "patient safety event" in OPTN policy in order to avoid the risk of members potentially not reporting concerning events that might fall outside a strict definition.

The OPTN contract requires UNOS to "encourage OPTN member self-reporting of potential patient safety issues" but does not provide an explicit definition for patient safety, save for a reference to types of patient safety events described in the August 5, 2011 letter from former HRSA Administrator Mary Wakefield ("the Wakefield letter") to then-OPTN board president Dr. John Lake.

As an example of the emphasis on patient safety, regardless of definition, UNOS exceeds what is required in terms of providing expedited notice to HRSA should any event meet the criteria outlined in the Wakefield letter list of events; UNOS routinely provides notice about other events that appear to be patient safety events despite not being included on this list. This ensures that the broadest possible scope of events reaches the MPSC for expert review and reasoned deliberation to determine if an incident poses a risk to patient health or public safety.

There are a number of OPTN policies that require submission regarding specific kinds of patient safety events. Those policies include, but are not limited to:[54]

- 15.5 Transplant Program Requirements for Communicating Post Transplant Discovery of Disease or Malignancy.
- 15.6 Living Donor Recovery Hospital Requirements for Reporting Post-Donation Discovery of Disease or Malignancy.
- 16.2 Packaging and Labeling Responsibilities.
- 18.5 Reporting of Living Donor Events.

Additionally, when OPTN members use the Patient Safety Portal to file a report, the portal itself outlines the types of events that OPTN members should report, including: "situations or activities that could have affected patient safety. These situations may be related to patient safety, organ placement/availability, communications, clinical information accuracy, or risk of disease transmission that was prevented. Situations that may not directly impact safety, availability, or utilization but cause concern from a transplantation, donation and/or quality perspective may also be reported."

The OPTN becomes aware of patient safety events when events are reported directly or otherwise discovered by the OPTN. If a member does not report a patient safety event to the OPTN as outlined in OPTN policies, that would qualify as a separate OPTN policy violation and would be addressed on a case-by-case basis by the MPSC. Any noncompliance is serious, and we are committed to engaging in substantive conversations to address additional concerns the committee may have about the MPSC's processes, and welcome opportunities to work collaboratively to strengthen the rigorous, widely-used, and regulation and contract-mandated confidential peer review process.

Question. Is UNOS able to calculate how many organs are matched with a waitlist patient but ultimately not transplanted? If so, please provide this number for each organ type in each of the last 5 years. To the extent possible, please provide the reason the organ was not ultimately transplanted.

Answer. Increasing the number of transplants by improving organ utilization is a key strategic goal of the OPTN. The OPTN classifies organ "discards," or organs recovered for transplant but not transplanted, as an organ that is recovered for the purpose of transplant and ultimately not transplanted. The reasons for an organ not being transplanted are provided to the OPTN by the recovering OPO, and are categorized below:

1) Each transplant team who received the organ offer declined the offer until there were no remaining wait-listed patients who matched with the available organ.
2) There were biopsy findings that would make transplant unsafe.
3) There were poor organ function or organ disease that would make transplant unsafe.
4) There were anatomic abnormalities that would make transplant unsafe.
5) There were other unspecified medical reasons.

In most cases it is only kidneys, pancreata, and organs which will be used for research purposes that travel without an accompanying team of physicians. Livers, hearts, and lungs are

[54] OPTN Policies. https://optn.transplant.hrsa.gov/policies-bylaws/policies.

generally not recovered until the offer has been accepted by the candidate's transplant team; the organ is then recovered by the candidate's transplant team who maintain physical possession of the organ until the transplant surgery.

The following 2 tables provide the rate of "discarded" organs by year/organ and the reasons for "discard."

Table 2: Count and Percent of Deceased Donor Organs Discarded by Recovery Year and Organ, 2017-2021

	Overall		Kidney		Pancreas		Liver		Intestine		Heart		Lung	
Year	Count	Percent	Count	Percent	Count	Percent	Count	Percent	Count	Percent	Count	Percent	Count	Percent
2017	4905	13.47%	3542	18.96%	311	23.63%	742	8.86%	4	3.57%	33	1%	273	5.89%
2018	5086	13.44%	3756	19.13%	278	21.19%	707	8.34%	3	2.75%	23	0.66%	319	6.56%
2019	6054	14.52%	4460	20.08%	346	25.18%	874	9.55%	5	5.81%	31	0.85%	338	6.44%
2020	6515	15.16%	5052	21.28%	294	23.24%	860	9.34%	3	3.19%	39	1.04%	267	5.43%
2021	8207	17.75%	6468	24.58%	343	26%	946	9.92%	1	1.03%	39	1%	410	8.1%

Table 3: Most Common Reasons for Deceased Organ Discard by Recovery Year and Organ, 2017-2021

		Overall		Kidney		Pancreas		Liver		Intestine		Heart		Lung	
Year	Reason for Discard	Count	Percent	Count	Percent	Count	Percent	Count	Percent	Count	Percent	Count	Percent	Count	Percent
2017	No recipient located - list exhausted	1450	34.28%	1376	44.13%	48	18.18%	25	3.77%	1	33.33%	0	0%	2	0.95%
	Biopsy findings	1141	26.97%	863	27.68%	0	0%	273	44.75%	0	0%	0	0%	5	2.38%
	Other, specify	749	17.71%	388	12.44%	103	39.02%	174	28.52%	1	33.33%	13	52%	70	33.33%
	Poor organ function	355	8.39%	194	6.22%	16	6.06%	35	5.74%	1	33.33%	7	28%	102	48.57%
	Anatomical abnormalities	317	7.49%	173	5.55%	71	26.89%	58	9.51%	0	0%	3	12%	12	5.71%
	Diseased organ	218	5.15%	124	3.98%	26	9.85%	47	7.7%	0	0%	2	8%	19	9.05%
2018	No recipient located - list exhausted	1511	33.86%	1446	42.87%	30	13.57%	29	4.87%	0	0%	0	0%	6	2.37%
	Biopsy findings	1234	27.66%	989	29.32%	2	0.9%	240	40.34%	0	0%	0	0%	3	1.19%
	Other, specify	830	18.6%	444	13.16%	89	40.27%	201	33.78%	2	66.67%	7	41.18%	87	34.39%
	Poor organ function	388	8.7%	216	6.4%	16	7.24%	28	4.71%	0	0%	8	47.06%	120	47.43%
	Anatomical abnormalities	316	7.08%	173	5.13%	68	30.77%	55	9.24%	1	33.33%	2	11.76%	17	6.72%
	Diseased organ	183	4.1%	105	3.11%	16	7.24%	42	7.06%	0	0%	0	0%	20	7.91%
2019	No recipient located - list exhausted	1969	37.29%	1681	46.92%	43	14.83%	39	5.26%	0	0%	0	0%	6	2.9%
	Biopsy findings	1484	28.11%	1163	29.01%	5	1.72%	309	41.64%	0	0%	2	6.67%	5	2.42%
	Other, specify	873	16.57%	439	10.95%	107	36.9%	226	30.46%	2	100%	17	56.67%	84	40.58%
	Poor organ function	387	7.33%	237	5.91%	26	8.97%	45	6.06%	0	0%	5	16.67%	74	35.75%
	Anatomical abnormalities	356	6.74%	181	4.51%	89	30.69%	62	8.36%	0	0%	3	10%	21	10.14%
	Diseased organ	209	3.96%	108	2.69%	20	6.9%	61	8.22%	0	0%	3	10%	17	8.21%
2020	No recipient located - list exhausted	2570	44.81%	2434	53.98%	50	20.16%	62	8.49%	0	0%	0	0%	4	2.26%
	Biopsy findings	1296	22.6%	1011	22.22%	1	0.4%	281	38.44%	0	0%	1	3.45%	2	1.13%
	Other, specify	1008	17.58%	579	12.73%	96	39.92%	246	33.63%	0	0%	15	51.72%	69	38.98%
	Poor organ function	360	6.28%	242	5.32%	17	6.85%	29	3.97%	0	0%	7	24.14%	65	36.72%
	Anatomical abnormalities	312	5.44%	169	3.71%	65	26.21%	62	8.48%	0	0%	2	6.9%	14	7.91%
	Diseased organ	189	3.3%	96	2.09%	16	6.45%	51	6.98%	0	0%	4	13.79%	23	12.99%
2021	No recipient located - list exhausted	3879	53.75%	3708	63.4%	54	18.95%	84	10.73%	1	50%	1	2.94%	30	11.45%
	Other, specify	1208	16.74%	648	11.08%	113	39.65%	311	39.72%	1	50%	19	55.88%	116	44.27%
	Biopsy findings	1198	16.6%	939	16.05%	0	0%	257	32.82%	0	0%	1	2.94%	1	0.38%
	Poor organ function	389	5.39%	255	4.36%	17	5.96%	32	4.09%	0	0%	9	26.47%	76	29.01%
	Anatomical abnormalities	368	5.1%	216	3.69%	81	28.42%	49	6.26%	0	0%	3	8.82%	19	7.25%
	Diseased organ	174	2.41%	83	1.42%	20	7.02%	50	6.39%	0	0%	1	2.94%	20	7.63%

Question. For over 40 years, UNOS has remained the only organization to manage the OPTN. As the sole operator, UNOS is accountable for the outcomes that have occurred during their management.

How does UNOS plan to address concerns raised by members during the committee's August 3rd hearing, as well as concerns raised in the committee's report?

What is UNOS doing, or planning to do, to improve its performance in its role as the OPTN? Please provide these plans for improvement, as well as when and how UNOS plans to accomplish them.

Answer. The strength of the U.S. donation and transplant system lies in the hundreds of volunteer committee members who are integral to the policy development process. This governance system includes two patient and donor affairs representatives on all policy development committees, and one quarter of the national board of directors is composed of such representatives. As a whole, OPTN committees are made up of experienced medical professionals, recipients, donors and donor family members, and all are focused on honoring the gift of life by increasing transplant. These stakeholders come together to create policies after extensive collaboration, which also involves incorporating input received during a rigorous public comment process. The OPTN contractor is tasked with facilitating this process.

We agree that the OPTN contractor and all parties involved in the organ donation and transplant system should be held to extremely high standards and be held accountable for their performance. UNOS is proud to be part of a system celebrating 9 consecutive years of growth in the number of deceased donor transplants, 11 consecutive years of growth in deceased donation, and record numbers of kidney, heart, and liver transplants in 2021—a year in which the U.S. exceeded 40,000 transplants for the first time.[55][7] In this system, tireless and dedicated donation and transplant professionals continued to go above and beyond to serve patients, despite a global pandemic. Of course, though these are remarkable achievements, they are only made possible thanks to the generosity of organ donors and their families nationwide.

It is incumbent upon us as the OPTN contractor to honor these gifts of life not only by fulfilling the obligations of NOTA and the OPTN contract to develop policies that ensure organs are allocated safely, equitably and efficiently to the Nation's sickest patients, but also to contribute to the growth and development of the system by proactively offering system-wide, evidence-based and patient-focused policy solutions at all levels of governance. Accordingly, the OPTN board of directors adopts a new strategic plan every 3 years to guide the work of the OPTN and its committees.[56] The strategic plan maintains a balance between setting high level community goals and allowing committees the flexibility to design specific policy projects. The plan for 2021–2024 is built around four primary goals. The most important is *Goal 1: Increasing the Number of Transplants,* to which one third of the OPTN's committee project resources are allocated. The other three goals are *Provide Equity in Access to Transplants, Promote Living Donor and Transplant Recipient Safety, and Improve Wait-listed Candidate, Living Donor, and Transplant Recipient Outcomes.* Each goal is accompanied by a suite of performance metrics, which is presented as an annual report to the Board by the OPTN Executive Director. HRSA also receives this report as a deliverable in the OPTN contract.

In addition, the OPTN maintains a publicly accessible OPTN metrics dashboard online, which displays key system performance indicators related to donation, transplantation, wait-list details, patient and graft survival, and transplant and mortality rates.[57] The OPTN also publishes the Equity in Access Dashboard, which shows how the OPTN monitors trends related to equitable access to deceased donor transplants among active waiting list candidates in the U.S. through an Access to Transplant (ATS) score. The ATS follows the National Institute on Minority Health and Health Disparities' Minority Health and Health Disparities Framework, which lays out potential conditions that can influence a person's health outcomes.[58][10]

---

[55] All-time records again set in 2021 for organ transplants, organ donation from deceased donors. Organ Procurement and Transplantation Network. *https://optn.transplant.hrsa.gov/news/all-time-records-again-set-in-2021-for-organ-transplants-organ-donation-from-deceased-do- nors/.* January 11, 2022.

[56] 2021–2024 OPTN Strategic Plan. https://optn.transplant.hrsa.gov/about/strategic-plan/.

[57] OPTN Metrics Dashboard. https://insights.unos.org/OPTN-metrics/.

[58] OPTN Equity in Access Dashboard. https://insights.unos.org/equity-in-access/.

As indicated in her inaugural message to the entire organ donation and transplant community, interim CEO Maureen McBride, Ph.D., said UNOS will remain responsive to feedback received from the public, the Federal Government, Congress, and other stakeholders.[59] Dr. McBride will seek engagement and support from the board of directors and community as a whole in developing responsive improvements that continue to accelerate system growth, increase patient and public engagement, and seek to address challenges that face the system within and outside the scope of the OPTN contract. Dr. McBride has identified key areas of focus, including:

1. Engage patients, donors and their families to reimagine public engagement, information and resources: In partnership with an external vendor, Accenture Federal Services, a consulting firm and expert in human-centered design, UNOS launched a research project to better understand what specific information, tools and resources patients need the most to support them in their jour ney. To date, UNOS and Accenture have conducted more than 50 interviews with a broad spectrum of patients, caregivers, living donors and transplant coordinators to better understand their perspectives. The results of these interviews, which will include members of the OPTN Patient Affairs Committee, will serve as a foundation for operational, policymaking, and strategic changes to UNOS and the OPTN in service of a more patient-focused organization.
2. Organ tracking and transportation: We share your concern about organ transportation and agree that one organ lost is one too many. Both UNOS and the OPTN have supported system-wide improvements in this area, from the launch of UNOS's own organ tracking service to the recently board-approved enhancements to OPTN data collection related to organ logistics and allocation.[60] Pending OMB approval, the data collection is expected to begin in May 2023. OPTN committees are currently building upon this work, exploring the development of common, community-wide guidance outlining the importance of organ tracking data and effective practices, as well as possible pathways within the authority of the OPTN for enhancing organ tracking system-wide. UNOS is also developing a technology product to help OPOs identify the most expeditious transportation options for organs given the dynamic challenges in the allocation system.
3. Enhancements to the MPSC peer review process: At its October 2022 meeting, the MPSC plans to review and reaffirm its operational rules and discuss the current construct of peer review as a mechanism for its reviews. The committee also plans to assess potential improvements to the way it shares information with the broader community, as well as other OPTN committees, for the benefit of the system and, ultimately, patients. Several recent system enhancements focused on increasing patient safety were a direct result of the MPSC peer review process. The MPSC is also driven to connect community members with peer mentors in order to improve the system and disseminate effective practices. Continuing to broadly disseminate MPSC learnings and improvement structures may inform future OPTN policymaking, lead to additional technology enhancements and spur future collaborative improvement initiatives. The

---

[59] UNOS names interim CEO. https://unos.org/news/unos-names-new-interim-ceo/. October 1, 2022.

[60] "Notice of OPTN data collection changes: Data collection to evaluate organ logistics and allocation." *https://optn.transplant.hrsa.gov/media/5accb1s3/policy-notice_osc_data-collection. pdf.*

OPTN Board will review and discuss the MPSC's recommendations at its December 2022 meeting.

4. Seek support from HHS to expand data collection throughout the transplant journey: Referral to a transplant program for a medical eligibility evaluation is the initial step to receiving a transplant, but patient referral information is siloed and not available in a systematic fashion. The barriers in these initial steps in the transplant process may be exacerbated by a number of social determinants of health. The OPTN will seek support from the Secretary to expand data collection of patient referral information as a next step to evaluating and enhancing equity in access to the transplant wait list.
5. Changes to UNOS senior leadership: On October 1st, Dr. McBride announced a restructured senior leadership team. Her new team includes key positions that renew a focus on streamlining operations to ensure UNOS is providing an equitable and inclusive environment for the volunteer workforce, the donation and transplant community, and the patients it serves; ensuring UNOS is the best possible steward of the resources it manages, promoting excellence and efficiency; and taking a holistic, databased approach to how it drives strategy across the organization.
6. Separating the OPTN and UNOS boards: UNOS board leadership finalized a work plan to formally separate the OPTN and UNOS boards in September 2022, developed after ongoing discussions that began in 2021. UNOS will work with HRSA to take the necessary legal, contractual and operational steps to implement the plan.
7. Serve as a "convener" for system-wide initiatives and improvements: UNOS will continue to partner with other key stakeholder groups and leaders in the fields of medicine, technology and data on strategic initiatives that contribute to the advancement of the field of organ donation and transplant. For example, UNOS hosts an annual conference for transplant administrators annually, sponsors a professional education forum, and hosts meetings with key stakeholders in the community. To this end, UNOS also will seek to expand relation ships with patient advocacy groups and other public health organizations. Together, UNOS and its partners will identify and advocate for evidence-based, patient-centered, systems improvement policy solutions.

Questions Submitted by Hon. Chuck Grassley

Question. The U.S. Digital Service (USDS) found UNOS's information technology (IT) systems outdated and voiced concerns that it operates on local data centers, rather than the cloud, and relies on manual data entry, resulting in user error and unacceptable downtime. USDS recommended that the Federal government take action to create a better organ transplant system including that the Organ Procurement and Transplantation Network (OPTN) IT contract be bid separately because UNOS has "denied nearly 100 Federal requests to audit source code."

Why has UNOS denied Federal requests to audit its source code?

How can Congress—or patients—trust UNOS to oversee its IT systems when reports show that it is fragile and antiquated?

Has UNOS provided a demonstration of its IT system for the Health Resources and Services Administration (HRSA) or discussed its IT modernization efforts with them? If not, why not?

Will you commit that UNOS will have this discussion with HRSA or other Federal agencies?

If the technology component of the OPTN contract is awarded to a different vendor, will UNOS commit to working with the Federal government to ensure a smooth transition for transplant patients?

Answer. UNOS appreciates the opportunity to address this concern and clarify any lingering misconceptions. The entirety of the report, as provided by a member of the media earlier this year, appears to be based on a 90-minute presentation by UNOS on December 10, 2020, pursuant to a request from HRSA during its 2019 Market Research for the Modernization National Resource Allocation System, as well as UNOS's responses to a set of follow-up questions submitted by HRSA.

The USDS has never conducted a review of our systems, and to date, they have not reached out to UNOS directly regarding the results of their report. UNOS continues to welcome the opportunity to review our systems with the USDS and discuss our architecture, code base and infrastructure. In an August 2, 2022, letter to the HRSA Administrator, UNOS reiterated our willingness to undergo any additional review deemed necessary. UNOS was and continues to be eager to engage directly with USDS in the interest of continually improving our technology systems and infrastructure.[61]

HRSA conducts an annual audit of our entire IT infrastructure, and consistently reviews the performance and security of the OPTN system in detail, as required by the OPTN contract. Their 2022 audit of our systems is currently underway. HRSA also reviews all OPTN contractual requirements for compliance annually, as well as on a periodic basis throughout each year. UNOS consistently meets or exceeds all contractual obligations. Semiannual tests are also conducted on OPTN IT systems by a verified third party. UNOS has also just shared with HRSA the results of the most recent cybersecurity penetration testing conducted by a third party in August.

The topics discussed have included the IT 3-year strategic plans, API strategy and updates, new concepts requested by the transplant community, information security, business continuity and disaster recovery, cloud transformation, test automation, establishment, and updates on the organ allocation assurance program, collaboration/ innovation events at various transplant conferences and numerous others. Multiple times every year, and outside of annual audits, UNOS has discussed a modernization strategy and updates on efforts for the IT system with HRSA and the OPTN board of directors. Since 2016, this has been a standing agenda item at every technology committee meeting and annually at the OPTN board meeting. These discussions are memorialized in OPTN Network Operations and Oversight Committee (NOOC) meeting summaries published on the OPTN website.[62]

On February 9, 2017, HRSA staff (including the program office, information technology and procurement) conducted an onsite, all-day visit where various UNet functions were demonstrated, and where an IT modernization strategy and progress were presented. More recently, our IT system was demonstrated to HRSA at the December 2020 HRSA Market Day presentation and again in September 2022, during the kickoff of the annual HRSA audit.

---

[61] Letter to HRSA Administrator. https://unos.org/wp-content/uploads/20220802_UNOS-McCauley-Letter-to-HRSA-Administrator.pdf.

[62] OPTN Network Operations and Oversight Committee (NOOC) meeting summaries. https://optn.transplant.hrsa.gov/about/committees/network-operations-oversight-committee-board-of-di-rectors/.

Since April 2019, the start of the current OPTN contract, and at every subsequent contract year kickoff meeting with HRSA, UNOS IT has presented technology modernization accomplishments for the prior year, as well as plans for the current contract year. These meetings are with the HRSA OPTN Contracting Officer's Representative (COR) and other HRSA staff.

UNOS's technology systems are uniquely designed to support complex allocation policies; they are flexible, modular and integrated within the policy development framework, so as policies and clinical requirements evolve, our systems can quickly evolve and change with them. Additionally, our technology experts have deep experience and understanding of transplant allocation algorithms, business rules and logic, making for a seamless transition from policy to technology. A dedicated IT liaison is assigned to each policy-making committee and regularly attends committee and leadership meetings to ensure the committee understands how the system works, and how intended changes to policies might impact data collection and workflows. As part of the interdepartmental team supporting committees, the IT liaison participates in policy development from the idea stage, through public comment, and board approval, refining business requirements and ensuring that the policies can be supported with scalable technology solutions that meet policy intent. IT's engagement with the solution development allows a variety of technology options to be shared with the committee as new policies are developed. Weekly meetings among support staff and with committee leadership ensure alignment between policy and system implementation at each stage.

However, UNOS is never satisfied with the status quo. That is why we remain committed to constantly improving our IT systems and responding to shifts in the technology and cybersecurity landscape to make our systems as safe, secure, efficient, and responsive to our members' needs as possible.

Since 2019, UNOS has maintained a cross-departmental team that is focused on creating public cloud patterns that can scale our ideas and core infrastructure for the capabilities found in the public cloud. While building this expertise, we have partnered with the Microsoft Tech for Social Impact team to align our vision with a reality we can bring to the transplant community.

In 2021, UNOS completed a transformation to a multi-regional hybrid cloud environment built using Nutanix cloud infrastructure and Microsoft Azure public cloud. In line with a cloud-first approach for all new functionality, UNOS has implemented new cloud-native real-time capabilities in Predictive Analytics decision support for organ offer acceptance, while actively executing a roadmap to move existing core infrastructure to the public cloud. Building microservices is critical to driving a seamless experience for a scalable solution that is built both by UNOS teams and vendors in the community. As of January 2022, UNOS has built hundreds of microservices as well as APIs with key integrations with vendors through our developer portal that is supported by Google Cloud's API management platform, Apigee.

One of the greatest challenges remains community adoption. Building and providing members with APIs does not guarantee that transplant hospitals, organ procurement organizations and histocompatibility laboratories will use them. Decisions to adopt APIs are at times driven by cost considerations between OPTN members and their Electronic Health Records (EHRs, such as Epic, CareDX, Transplant-Connect, etc.) who integrate with our APIs. There are also cases when the OPTN members decide not to leverage APIs because of previously implemented automation, where the information they submit to OPTN is created automatically within their EHR versus being entered manually. This automation was built years ago in collaboration between UNOS and the EHRs servicing OPTN members.

UNOS believes that APIs are still the path forward for seamless data exchange between systems and have staff who work directly with OPTN members and their software vendors (EHRs) to promote awareness and adoption of our APIs. To build on that investment, UNOS is partnering with Accenture Federal, a consulting firm and tech leader, to expand and extend our API strategy to increase API adoption. This strategy is focused on working with OPTN Member organizations to help them understand what APIs they have access to but are not yet leveraging, assisting them with implementation and testing, and driving process improvements to further streamline future adoption.

There are opportunities to continue to improve the usability of UNet applications to save users time and streamline customer experience. To accomplish this, we also are working with our strategic partner Accenture Federal, given their expertise in digital transformation for Federal agencies using human-centered design, to redesign the user interface and workflows within UNet applications. Our goal is to make it more convenient, easier and faster for transplant coordinators to manage patients in the national transplant system.

UNOS welcomes the opportunity to have focused and open discussions about how we can continue to improve the information technology systems that support the national transplant system. It bears repeating that we invite the USDS and HRSA to participate in meaningful conversations about our systems and improvements, and UNOS welcomes any additional feedback they can provide.

Based on the data, annual HRSA audits, demonstrations, third-party reviews and the fact that the system has remained safe for 36 years despite over 3 million hacking attempts each day, Congress and patients can trust the technology that powers the Nation's transplant system, which remains safe, secure and efficient.

Question. During the committee's August 3, 2020 hearing, you testified that UNOS's IT system was "paid for in part by taxpayers."

How much of UNOS's IT system was paid for by taxpayers?

How much of UNOS's IT system was paid for by OPTN members?

Answer. The National Organ Transplant Act (NOTA), 42 U.S.C. 273 et. seq. requires that the OPTN operate a national system to allocate organs using computer systems, and thus the costs of operating the OPTN include the costs of operating a national system using computer technology to allocate organs, including updates to reflect changes in organ allocation policies, data collection, security, privacy, reliability, improvements and architecture. The OPTN contract requires the OPTN contractor to provide computer systems and software to meet the statutory obligations of the OPTN, as well as meet extensive Federal requirements for security, operability, privacy, and reliability.

Within the UNOS budget, which is separate and distinct from the OPTN budget, approximately 8–10 percent of UNOS revenues come from Federal appropriations. Because UNOS does not directly bill Medicare, Medicaid, or any other public insurance program or system, UNOS cannot provide insight into the reimbursements hospitals and transplant centers receive from public or private insurance. UNOS bills the hospital directly and in turn is reimbursed by the hospital directly.

Approximately 85–90 percent of the OPTN budget is from a one-time fee transplant hospitals pay per patient registered on the wait list.

Question. During the committee's August 3, 2022 hearing, you acknowledged that over 3,000,000 attempts are made each day to hack into UNOS's IT system. Does UNOS report these hacking attempts to the Cybersecurity and Infrastructure Security Agency (CISA)? If so, what types of information does UNOS share with CISA, and how often?

Answer. CISA conducts cyber hygiene scans of our external-facing network weekly for vulnerabilities. Our scanning efforts with CISA began this year, resulting in one "low" priority finding to date. We subscribe to their alert program and are provided alerts for active attacks and vulnerabilities. We also receive Indicators of Compromise (IOCs) from them. We would report any impactful cybersecurity incidents to CISA.

Question. On April 27, 2022, UNOS acknowledged that it failed to report 35,000 deaths among patients on the waiting list. According to UNOS, "process improvement and automation" allowed it to verify this figure. This is deeply concerning and illustrates how the quality of information provided by UNOS complicates policy-makers' understanding of how to improve outcomes for patients.

Please explain what new "process improvement and automation" have allowed UNOS to report 35,000 additional deaths on the waiting list.

What caused the failure to identify to and report the additional deaths? Is the failure attributed to UNOS technology, and/or other factors?

Can UNOS provide a breakdown of the 35,000 additional deaths based on patient attributes such as race, religion, age, sex, veteran status, rural status, or physical or mental disability? If not, why not?

How many new or amended OPTN policies have relied on UNOS's faulty data?

How many times did UNOS cite incorrect patient death data in communications with policymakers and administrators in the executive or legislative branches?

Answer. We appreciate the opportunity to clarify this issue for the committee.

Prior to 2013, UNOS, as the OPTN contractor, had routine access to the full and publicly available Social Security Death Master File. That information supplemented the deaths reported to the OPTN by member institutions. As of 2013, however, that file has not been publicly available.

A new agreement between HRSA and CMS was established that allowed the OPTN to continue having access to death data, on the condition that the OPTN must verify each of the deaths with an external source prior to release in the publicly available OPTN dataset. As part of this workflow between 2013 and 2022, a multi-tiered process was used for this verification, which included a manual review of obituaries online. This process consumed significant resources each month, and the OPTN, in collaboration with HRSA, limited the process to verifying those deaths most likely to impact data analyses used for policy development and monitoring of member performance.

As part of our continuous improvement efforts, UNOS evaluated several technology and software solutions to automate the manual searching of obituaries. UNOS partnered with a vendor in 2021 whose technology was able to scan vastly more obituaries and match those deaths to become part of the publicly available OPTN dataset.

The first complete scan with this new software verified 35,087 deaths that had been previously unreported to the OPTN, and that dated back several decades. Following the data use agreement between HRSA and CMS, those data were then incorporated into the publicly available OPTN data set in the spring of 2022.

It is important to note that of these 35,087 deaths, roughly 23,000 were of transplanted patients who died at some point after their transplant (which in many instances could be years later). Fewer than 100 were of patients who were active on the waiting list at the time of their death, and roughly 12,000 were patients who died at some point after they had been removed from the wait list. Transplant programs remove patients from the wait list for a variety of reasons including the patient being too sick to transplant, their condition improves, they refuse a transplant, transplant programs are unable to contact them, or other reasons. In this verification process used by the OPTN, the reasons for death are unknown or unreported and could be for reasons unrelated to transplantation.

Religion and/or physical or mental disability are not part of OPTN policies and are not collected by the OPTN. Data regarding veteran status is not specifically collected; however, the primary source of payment is reported by transplant programs, and the Department of Veterans Affairs is one of the possible selections.

Below is a breakdown of the recently verified 35,087 patient deaths by race/ ethnicity, age (at listing or transplant), education status at time of listing, primary source of payment (at listing or transplant).

	Number of Patient Deaths	Percent of Patient Deaths
Total Individuals	35,087	100.0%
Race/Ethnicity		
White, Non-Hispanic	20,282	57.8%
Black, Non-Hispanic	8,425	24.0%
Hispanic/Latino	4,590	13.1%
Asian, Non-Hispanic	1,209	3.4%
American Indian/Alaska Native, Non-Hispanic	349	1.0%
Native Hawaiian/other Pacific Islander, Non- Hispanic	131	0.4%
Multiracial, Non-Hispanic	96	0.3%
Unknown	5	0.0%
Age at Transplant/Listing *		
< 1	1	0.0%
1–5	35	0.1%
6–10	74	0.2%
11–17	249	0.7%
18–34	3,097	8.8%
35–49	9,424	26.89%
50–64	15,860	45.2%
65+	6,347	18.1%
Education Level at Listing **		
Not Reported	2,948	8.4%
None	138	0.4%
Grade School (0–8)	1,821	5.2%
High School (9–12) or GED	13,284	37.9%
Attended College/Technical School	6,804	19.4%
Associate/Bachelor Degree	3,984	11.4%
Post-College Graduate Degree	1,700	4.8%
N/A (< 5 years old)	32	0.1%
Unknown	4,376	12.5%
Primary Source of Payment at Transplant/ Listing*, **		
Not Reported	2,418	6.9%
Private Insurance	13,704	39.1%
Public Insurance—Medicaid	1,780	5.1%
Public Insurance—Medicare FFS (Fee for Service)	8,236	23.5%

	Number of Patient Deaths	Percent of Patient Deaths
Public Insurance—Medicare & Choice	3,925	11.2%
Public Insurance—CHIP (Children's Health Insurance Program)	3	0.0%
Public Insurance—Department of VA	334	1.0%
Public Insurance—Other government	145	0.4%
Self	62	0.2%
Donation	3	0.0%
Free Care	35	0.1%
Pending	57	0.2%
Foreign Government	2	0.0%
Public Insurance—Medicare (further detail not collected)	4,169	11.9%
U.S./State Government Agency	214	0.6%

* For recipients with a transplant, age at transplant and source of payment at transplant were used. Age at listing and source of payment reported at listing were used for all other patients.

** Education at listing and primary source of payment were not collected throughout the entire period of OPTN data collection and therefore are not available for all patients.

Question. In 2018, UNOS made significant changes to heart transplant selection criteria in order to reduce wait-list times, among other reasons. I understand that some in the heart transplant community are beginning to raise questions about the impact these changes have had on physician practice patterns.

Is UNOS monitoring long-term changes in both clinical outcomes and quality of life for these post-transplant? If not, does UNOS intend to study the impact on these patients? If not, why not?

Is UNOS open to making any appropriate adjustments to the system to help improve patient outcomes and quality of life while maintaining shorter wait times? If not, why not?

Answer. Policy development does not end with implementation. A key aspect of the community-driven OPTN policy process is how it monitors both the short- and long-term outcomes and impacts of policy changes on patients and the system. Following the implementation of any policy, the OPTN begins monitoring the impact, looking for opportunities to potentially improve the policy, for any unintended consequences, and results that may require additional actions by OPTN committees and the board. The review process for any policy is agreed upon beforehand by committee leadership and is documented in the proposal that is ultimately reviewed and approved by the OPTN board of directors. Staff, committees and the board continue to analyze whether the policy is meeting stated goals. Additionally, UNOS researchers present their ongoing analysis to the sponsoring committee and interested external stakeholders. The committees' reviews of this analysis may result in new ideas to improve the policy and by extension, the overall transplant system. In this way, the policy development process comes full circle, resulting in continued innovations and improvements.

As it specifically relates to the 2018 heart policy change, the OPTN Heart Committee has reviewed monitoring reports gauging the ongoing impact of this policy at 1 year, 18 months, 2 years and 3 years post-implementation of the heart allocation policy changes. As noted in each report, a number of key metrics are monitored, including patients added to the heart wait list by medical urgency, patients waiting for a heart transplant by medical urgency, deaths on the wait list, post-transplant survival, the total number of transplants, the time it takes for a transplant hospital to accept offers, distance the heart travels between the donor and the recipient, uti lization rates, and many other metrics.[63] Where relevant, these metrics are then stratified by age, region, and urgency status to arrive at a fuller, more accurate picture of the policy's ongoing impact.

The 3-year report reviewed by the committee on October 10, 2022 is responsive to specific questions raised by the Heart Committee based on its review of past data, as well as the collective clinical experiences of its members who have been practicing under the new policy.[64] For example, based on previous findings and recent scholarly analyses, the Heart Committee has since emphasized the need to better understand wait-list mortalities associated with the individual criteria found in the adult heart medical urgency statuses 2, 3 and 4. The Heart Committee believes these data will provide a better idea of the medical urgency of patients who are being transplanted at each status and help to identify additional opportunities to assist any populations in need of improved access under the revised policy.

Consistent, rigorous, data-driven monitoring and responsive policy changes are essential to continuously improving the national system and ensuring the best outcomes for patients.

Question. In 2018, HRSA issued a request for proposal (RFP) for the operation of the OPTN. The RFP included conditions that required the contractor to submit a plan to ensure that the OPTN board of directors be separate from the contractor's board of directors. UNOS filed a protest with the Government Accountability Office, arguing that HRSA "does not have the authority under NOTA to direct the OPTN to have a board of directors that is separate from the entity that is awarded a contract to operate the OPTN." GAO rejected UNOS's argument and found "nothing in [the National Organ Transplant Act] prohibits the agency from issuing a solicitation that treats the UNOS and the OPTN as separate entities."

Has UNOS taken steps to separate the UNOS and OPTN board of directors? If not, why not?

How does the current board structure prevent conflicts of interest?

Answer. Yes, UNOS has taken these steps, and began the effort to separate the UNOS board and OPTN board in earnest in Spring 2021.

More recently, the UNOS board of directors leadership affirmed this plan, passing a resolution in August 2022 charging staff "to explore the separation of the boards to develop a viable framework for separate boards that provides clarity on roles and responsibilities, fiscal matters, and operational interactions between the OPTN board, HRSA, and UNOS. Staff are authorized to retain such experts as appropriate and will provide a report to the committee for its review within 30 days."

Currently, the existing OPTN contract with HRSA requires that the UNOS board of directors also serve as the OPTN board of directors. Thus, separation of the boards will require approval by HRSA, as it would require a significant modification to the OPTN contract.

Regarding conflicts of interest, the OPTN bylaws include specific provisions to address and avoid conflicts of interest for both board and committee membership. Additionally, the OPTN board has approved a plan to augment its current policies regarding potential conflicts of interest. Activities of the OPTN are clearly described and separate from UNOS's. The OPTN board of directors receives an annual orientation regarding its obligations to the OPTN, which

---

[63] OPTN Heart and Lung Resources: Heart Monitoring Reports. https://optn.transplant.hrsa. gov/professionals/by-organ/heart-lung/.

[64] Schellinger, E.; Bradbrook, K.; Lindblad, K. "Three-Year Monitoring of the Heart Allocation Proposal to Modify the Heart Allocation System Prepared for the OPTN Heart Committee." October 11, 2022. https://optn.transplant.hrsa.gov/professionals/by-organ/heart-lung/.

includes a presentation from HRSA staff. In addition, members of the OPTN board sign an attestation document acknowledging their obligation to the OPTN separate from any obligations to any other organization, including to UNOS.

As previously stated, efforts are currently underway to officially establish two separate boards, a process UNOS began over a year ago and which we believe will help address concerns about conflicts of interest and will provide another layer of transparency and accountability.

Question. Please identify the OPTN policy that prohibits organ procurement organizations (OPO) from discriminating against donor patients or their families based on attributes such as race, religion, age, sex, veteran status, rural status, or physical or mental disability?

Answer. OPTN policies do not allow for the segregation of patients or donors by distinguishing characteristics such as disability, race, religion, sex, age, veteran status or rural location.

OPTN Policy 2.2: OPO Responsibilities, includes the following provision:

- "The host OPO is responsible for all of the following 6. Establishing and then implementing a plan to address organ donation for diverse cultures and ethnic populations."
- *OPTN Policy 5.4.A: Nondiscrimination in Organ Allocation,* states the following:
- "A candidate's citizenship or residency status in the United States must not be considered when allocating deceased donor organs to candidates for transplantation. Allocation of deceased donor organs must not be influenced positively or negatively by political influence, national origin, ethnicity, sex, religion, or financial status."

Question. In May 2012, the former director of the Alabama Organ Center was sentenced to 13 months in prison in his role in a scheme to take kickbacks from a funeral home that did business with the organ center. Has UNOS ever addressed Medicare fraud and misuse of Medicare dollars among OPOs by implementing OPTN policies and procedures? If so, please identify the OPTN policy that addresses Medicare fraud among OPOs. How does UNOS monitor and enforce compliance?

Answer. Because Federal law does not provide the OPTN with the authority to investigate Medicare fraud or misuse of public monies, this issue is not within the scope of the OPTN's authority. CMS has direct access to OPO cost reporting and information relating to the OPO's business practices. Under the current regulatory and oversight construct, the OPTN would not have this information. Federal law and regulation for the OPTN primarily directs the OPTN to assist OPOs in organ placement and develop organ allocation and clinical data collection policies.

In this particular case from Alabama, we understand that the scheme related to tissue recovery from deceased donors, which is regulated by the Food and Drug Administration (FDA), and not the OPTN or HRSA. Because of this separation of oversight responsibilities, the OPTN does not collect data on payment or tissue recovery/ allocation.

Question. Studies show that, on average, kidney transplant candidates receive 16 organ offers while on the transplant wait list. However, studies also show that a large number of these offers are declined on their behalf by transplant hospitals, contributing to the shortage of available organs in the United States. It's critical that the OPTN be transparent with patients and their families when these decisions are made so that we improve trust in the OPTN.

Does UNOS have a system to alert patients when organ offers are rejected by transplant centers on their behalf? If not, why not?

Members of UNOS's Patient Affairs Committee (PAC) told committee staff that they discussed this issue with UNOS, but that UNOS did not listen to their concerns. If UNOS's PAC raised this issue, why hasn't it been addressed?

How will you alleviate concerns raised by PAC members that UNOS does not listen to their advice or counsel?

Answer. UNOS agrees that the continued rise in the number of organs recovered for transplant that are ultimately not transplanted requires a multi-pronged, systemic approach to address this issue, as noted in a February 2022 report from the National Academies of Science, Engineering, and Medicine (NASEM).[65] In this report recommendation, "Key Area for Improvement for Transplant Centers: Organ Offer Acceptance," the authors review in detail many of the factors that may contribute to this trend. The NASEM report also notes two OPTN tools, enhanced "refusal codes" and "offer filters" as having the potential to increase system efficiency and contribute to a hospital's understanding of its own acceptance practices with im proved data. UNOS agrees that patients, not just hospitals, need more information in key areas.

Shared Decision-Making

UNOS does not currently have a mechanism to alert patients when organ offers are declined on their behalf by their transplant teams. UNOS, however, supports and encourages clear communication between transplant teams and the patients they serve, and is in the discovery phase of developing a tool that members could use to help patients understand why they have refused organ offers.

UNOS is also currently conducting a research study with Accenture Federal Services, a consulting firm and expert in human centered design, to understand patient information needs throughout the transplant journey. More than 50 patients, caregivers, living donors and transplant professionals representing pre- and post-transplant, representing all organ types and geographic areas, along with members of the PAC, are being interviewed as part of the study. Findings will inform actions the OPTN can take to better meet patient's information needs and ensure equity in access to transplant.

UNOS agrees with recommendations in the NASEM report that empowering patients with information about their care leads to more positive transplant outcomes and is committed to pursuing tools and technology that will facilitate greater shared decision-making.

Patient Engagement

As of October 1st, UNOS has an interim CEO who is prioritizing listening to and determining how to better engage with patients. The patient, donor and family perspective are an essential component of both OPTN and UNOS governance and the interim CEO attended the in-person

[65] National Academies of Sciences, Engineering, and Medicine. 2022. "Realizing the promise of equity in the organ transplantation system." Washington, DC: The National Academies Press. *https://doi.org/10.17226/26364.*

Public Affairs Committee (PAC) meeting in September. In the coming months, UNOS will seek new ways to ensure the patient voice is heard and acted upon. The UNOS leadership team will engage the board of directors, the PAC and members of the donation and transplant community in identifying concrete solutions for addressing this concern.

UNOS has evolved support of the PAC over the past several years and made multiple operational changes to improve patient engagement both within our volunteer network and beyond, including:

- During the development of the current strategic plan, the PAC provided numerous and specific comments intended to improve patient engagement. Almost all of those comments were adopted and included in the plan. Following adoption of the strategic plan, several changes have occurred to follow up on that commitment:
  - An increase in the number of patient and donor affairs representatives to ensure a minimum of two on all policy development committees (the OPTN final rule at 42 CFR § 121.3(a)(4)(i) requires at least one transplant candidate, transplant recipient, organ donor or family member), with staggered terms so that new patient representatives will have the support of another representative that has experience on the committee moving forward.
  - Creation of a standard to include a patient representative on each of the regional nominating committees that nominate regional representatives to serve on the OPTN board of directors.
- Strengthened the patient voice by recruiting experienced PAC alumni to serve on other committees and the board of directors.
- Developed a two-step process for soliciting patient feedback on OPTN policy proposals, so that PAC members receive education and background on a topic first, and are asked for more detailed feedback on subsequent meeting, building on previous efforts to ensure and empower patients to provide informed, actionable feedback.
- Created focused, plain language prompts and a glossary of terms for proposals out for public comment, so patients and the general public are more empowered to influence policy development.
- Released new, patient-specific on-demand education modules on UNOS- Connect, UNOS's learning management system, designed to inform patient volunteers on the donation and transplantation system.[66]
- Promoted attendance and participation by patient representatives at OPTN Regional Meetings:
  - Highlighted and welcomed PAC regional representative at the beginning of each meeting (Winter cycle 2022).
  - Held prep sessions for PAC representatives prior to Summer 2022 regional meetings and provided opportunity for them to introduce themselves and their connection to transplant at the meetings.
  - Offered and committed to maintaining virtual attendance options for regional meetings to allow for increased patient accessibility.

[66] UNOSConnect. https://unos.org/resources/education/.

- Created and distributed a customized "what to expect" meeting guide to all registered patient and donor family attendees in advance of the meeting with contact information for questions/suggestions.
- Noted an increase in almost all regions with patients providing their feedback during the regional meeting, providing valuable perspectives to the transplant community in attendance.

Building on these accomplishments will require taking a holistic look at what information UNOS and the OPTN can provide to support patient empowerment. From their time on the wait list to their life post-transplant, treating patients as informed partners in their own care is a critical, system-wide goal.

Question. Section 5.4.A of OPTN policy mandates that "[a]llocation of deceased donor organs must not be influenced positively or negatively by political influence, national origin, ethnicity, sex, religion, or financial status." However, recent research demonstrates that some transplant centers factor in financial resources in wait-list determinations, causing otherwise eligible transplant candidates to be determined ineligible for transplantation based on socioeconomic status.

Is this behavior a violation of section 5.4.A of OPTN policy?

How does UNOS ensure that its members do not consider political influence, national origin, ethnicity, religion or financial status when making the initial wait-list decision?

Answer. It is important to distinguish between the allocation of deceased donors to transplant candidates who are on the waiting list, and access of potential transplant candidates to be placed on the waiting list. OPTN policies, including organ allocation algorithms, are programmed into the computer systems that allocate organs. The OPTN monitors every organ transplant to ensure that the organ allocation "match run" is followed, or that deviations from the "match run" are adequately explained by objective criteria. The question cites research that some transplant hospitals may deny patients access to the waiting list based on the financial resources of the patient, which is not addressed by OPTN Policy 5.4.A. Decisions on whether to add a patient to the OPTN waiting list are complex medical and social decisions made by a team of health-care providers at each transplant hospital.

To ensure that every transplant has the best chance for success and to prevent futile transplants, NOTA requires that patients demonstrate critical success factors for transplant, including availability of a full-time caregiver, transportation to the transplant center during the recovery period, and financially related matters among other things. Transplant teams conduct full psycho-social evaluations of every potential transplant patient as part of their decision to add them to the waiting list.

Question. UNOS's new organ allocation policy appears to have added significant chaos to the transplantation system. What is the OPTN doing to alleviate this chaos that is adversely impacting patients before making additional changes that require even greater travel distances—and more cold ischemic time—for organs? How can Congress—or patients—trust UNOS to effectively quarterback this system when investigative reports show it fails at even the basics of organ transportation, regularly losing track of organs in transit?

Answer. The data does not support the above assertions. In fact, similar arguments have been raised by certain plaintiffs in litigation in an attempt to block implementation of the national liver and kidney allocation policies. However, the GAO found no fault in their development, and the courts have upheld the OPTN's adoption of these policies.[67]

Since the implementation of new allocation policies in recent years, we have seen national increases in transplants for all major organs. In fact, the three organ types most commonly transplanted (kidneys, livers and hearts) all set records in 2021, despite a global pandemic. Liver transplant totals have set annual records for the past 9 years, and heart transplants have set a new record each of the past 10 years.

Specifically for kidney and liver, OPTN monitoring reports for recent changes to allocation policies for both organs have shown that these policies are fulfilling the obligations of NOTA by ensuring donated organs are shared as broadly as possible to reach the sickest patients first, regardless of where a patient is listed. These community- and data-driven allocation policies and ongoing efforts to further improve the system have resulted in more transplants and more lives saved; policies that have increased equity, expanded access and met the dual goals of ensuring that changes to cold ischemic time have no impact on the health of the organ (minimal increases were shown to be clinically insignificant) while also prioritizing the sickest patients first. Looking at this data and the policies that helped drive these outcomes, Congress as well as patients and their families can trust the Nation's organ donation and transplant system.

All organ allocation policy monitoring reports are available on the OPTN website for the public's review at https://optn.transplant.hrsa.gov/professionals/by-organ/

Questions Submitted by Hon. John Barrasso

Question. This committee has obviously been hard at work trying to identify shortcomings in the organ procurement and transplantation system over the past couple years. Also, within the past couple years, the Trump administration proposed and the Biden administration finalized the OPO final rule. This rule established new performance metrics for OPOs as well as helped promote more frequent oversight and competition among OPOs.

Are there other regulatory or legislative actions Congress or the administration should take to ensure the OPTN is performing to its maximum potential for patients and providers?

Answer. UNOS is pleased to offer the following items for your consideration:

1. Invest in innovations that may offer improved OPO regulatory oversight and increase organ donation: In order to improve regulatory oversight and identify underperforming OPOs, UNOS recommends automating donor referrals to collect data that will accurately measure true donor potential.[68] At least six OPOs with service areas across 15 States have partnered with donor hospitals to replace current manual data entry with automated donor referral, leveraging existing technology on the market to

---

[67] "Organ Transplants: Changes in Allocation Policies for Donated Livers and Lungs." U.S. Government Accountability Office. October 16, 2020. *https://www.gao.gov/products/gao-21-70.*

[68] "5 ways to improve the U.S. organ donation and transplant system: Automate real-time donor referral." Accessed October 10, 2022. *https://unos.org/news/media-resources/5-ways/automate-real-time-donor-referral/.*

automatically alert an OPO of a potential donor in a hospital ICU.[69,70,71] One study's analysis on three pilot hospitals in Texas found that electronic referral was associated with a 45-percent increase in referrals, an 83-percent increase in ap- proaches for donor family authorization, a 73-percent increase in donor family authorizations, and a 92-percent increase in organ donors.[72] A national investment into this innovation could not only save more lives by increasing the number of donor referrals, but also provide a more granular, independently reported and clinically accurate data set that would enable the OPTN and CMS to best assess performance.

2. Encourage HHS to enable the OPTN to collect data on inequities in access to pre-wait-list care and referral: Substantial research has documented inequities in access to the national wait list, and substantial variation across transplant programs with respect to transplant access.[73,74] However, what is unknown is the extent to which these inequities in access to transplantation are due to patient characteristics or to transplant program characteristics. OPTN data collection begins at the time a patient is wait-listed for transplantation. The transplant community, including clinicians,[75] community members,[76] and researchers,[77] has repeatedly called for pre-wait-list data collection to address this important problem, but no national data exist to identify patients who have end-stage organ failure and are appropriate candidates for transplantation. Authorizing the OPTN to collect this data would allow for better system evaluation and performance improvements. The OPTN Data Advisory Committee (DAC)'s request to HRSA to collect and study these elements is currently pending.
3. Support information sharing between the OPTN and CMS: As previously mentioned, CMS and the OPTN can mutually benefit from increased information sharing to aid in their respective roles in the system. UNOS continues to support the development of

---

[69] Niles, Patricia; Hewlett, Jonathan; Piano, John; Liu, Wade. "Automated Electronic Referrals Are Changing Donation." *Transplantation:* September 2020—Volume 104—Issue S3—p. S259 doi: 10.1097/ 01.tp.0000699788.52410.58.

[70] Glazier, A.; Moss, M.; Martin, L. (2021). "Electronic Health Records Can Improve the Organ Donation Process." Retrieved January 20, 2022, from *https://hbr.org/2021/12/electronic-health-records-can-improve-the-organ-donation-process.*

[71] "Cleveland Clinic, Lifebanc and Transplant Connect Develop Automated Donor Referral Process." April 30, 2021. *https://newsroom.clevelandclinic.org/2021/04/30/cleveland-clinic- lifebanc-and-transplant-connect-develop-automated-donor-referral-process/.* Accessed January 20, 2021.

[72] Levan, Macey L.; Trahan, Chad; Klitenic, Samantha B.; Hewlett, Jonathan; Strout, Tyler; Levan, Michael A.; Vanterpool, Karen B., Ph.D., MPH; Segev, Dorry L., M.D., Ph.D.; Adams, Bradley L.; Massie, Allan B., Ph.D.; Niles, Patricia, BS, RN. "Short Report: Evaluating the Ef- fects of Automated Donor Referral Technology on Deceased Donor Referrals." *Transplantation Direct:* August 2022—Volume 8—Issue 8.

[73] Ashby, V.B., J.D.; Kalbfleisch, R.A.; Wolfe, M.J. Lin; F.K. Port; A.B. Leichtman. "Geographic Variability in Access to Primary Kidney Transplantation in the United States, 1996–2005." *American Journal of Transplantation* 7, no. s1 (2007): 1412–23. *https://doi.org/10.1111/j.1600- 6143.2007.01785.x.*

[74] King, Kristen L.; Syed Ali Husain; Zhezhen Jin; Corey Brennan; Sumit Mohan. "Trends in Disparities in Preemptive Kidney Transplantation in the United States." *Clinical Journal of the American Society of Nephrology* 14, no. 10 (2019): 1500–1511. *https://doi.org/10.2215/ cjn.03140319.*

[75] Sehgal, Ashwini R. "Should Transplant Referral Be a Clinical Performance Measure?" *Jour- nal of the American Society of Nephrology* 28, no. 3 (2016): 721–23. *https://doi.org/10.1681/ asn.2016111169.*

[76] Fowler, Kevin John. "Accountability of Dialysis Facilities in Transplant Referral." *Clinical Journal of the American Society of Nephrology* 13, no. 2 (2018): 193–94. *https://doi.org/10.2215/cjn.13741217.* 2018;13(2):193–194.

[77] Patzer, Rachel E.; Laura McPherson. "Variation in Kidney Transplant Referral: How Much More Evidence Do We Need To Justify Data Collection on Early Transplant Steps?" *Journal of the American Society of Nephrology* 30, no. 9 (2019): 1554–56. *https://doi.org/10.1681/ asn.2019070674.*

such a process in a way that enhances and improves holistic oversight and improvement for the system.

Questions Submitted by Hon. Benjamin L. Cardin

Organ Transportation

Question. Since 2010, what penalties have OPOs or transportation companies received when an organ has been lost or damaged in transit such that it has to be subsequently discarded?

What is the exact number of organs lost, delayed, and/or damaged? Of those, what is the exact number of the resulting loss of prospective transplants, and how many patients died waiting for a new organ? Please provide a methodology to support your answer in a manner that is reproducible.

Does UNOS collect or have access to data regarding the number and percentage of organs that are transported with real time tracking (i.e., GPS) and organs transported with temperature tracking? If so, please provide that information you have from the last 5 years.

Given the overrepresentation of Black Americans waiting on a kidney, do transportation problems that seem to disproportionately impact kidneys impact the disparity we observe?

Answer. Any transplant opportunity lost due to transportation errors is one too many. As the committee is aware, organs are currently tracked by the OPTN's TransNetSM system, made mandatory by OPTN Board action in 2017, requiring the use of color-coded external, internal and vessel labels when shipping or transporting organs outside the donor hospital.[78]

Nonetheless, UNOS agrees that improving data collection and transportation tracking would benefit the system and supports an increase in data collection in this area to identify any appropriate, data-driven interventions that would support any improvements needed.

Should Congress wish to establish a central authority to track all organs unaccompanied by a transplant team (primarily kidneys) in transit across all transportation and logistics vendors, we submit the following for your consideration to support the development of potential policy solutions.

- At present, the only authority the OPTN has under both Federal law and regulation relates to its member institutions. The OPTN cannot make requirements or lodge penalties of transportation companies because they are not OPTN members and would not qualify as one per the OPTN final rule (42 CFR Sec. 121.3(b)(1)).
- Additional Federal appropriation may be required to develop and implement the technology required to track organs in transit across multiple commercial, non-clinical vendors and airlines, depending on the level of granularity of data and whether "real time" tracking is desired.
- Any policy solutions should clearly define a "reportable" transportation-related delay or damage, including how to determine if a specific incident played a role in the non-use of an organ or a transplant failure, or what individuals, organizations, private entities, businesses, etc. to hold ultimately accountable and under what authority.

---

[78] OPTN organ transport. https://optn.transplant.hrsa.gov/professionals/by-topic/organ-transport/.

We strongly believe the donation and transplant community, and especially patient and donor affairs representatives, should be engaged to develop requirements for such a solution, in addition to all other key stakeholders, to ensure all necessary considerations are identified. The OPTN would be pleased to provide a review of the previous Operations and Safety Committee, OPO Committee and MPSC's discussions on this topic to date should the committee desire.

As mentioned during the hearing, UNOS is taking action to address some of these challenges. In 2019, UNOS began developing an organ tracking solution to offer to OPOs. Since the product launched in June 2021, and as of September 22, 2022, 5,628 shipments have been tracked, accounting for roughly 8 percent of all packaged organs during that time period. Clients on average track 30 percent of all their packaged organs. Some OPOs don't track organs such as hearts, lungs and livers because they are traditionally accompanied by the procuring surgeon. Other OPOs only track kidneys and/or livers that use commercial air and/or are exported from their service area.

Based on currently available data, it is difficult to assess the impact that transportation might have on transplant disparities.

Please see additional transportation information in the responses to Senator Wyden's seventh question and Senator Young's first question.

Technology

Question. You testified that UNOS's IT system has a 99.99-percent uptime, and according to a report from the USDS entitled "Lives Are At Stake," UNOS told the Federal Government that it had "experienced 99.79 percent uptime since 1999." Since January 1, 2022, UNOS began reporting uptime excluding scheduled maintenance.

Please provide documentation of UNOS uptime including scheduled maintenance time.

Why is UNOS now excluding planned maintenance from its uptime calculation? Are there any contract requirements for downtime related to planned maintenance?

Is there a definition of planned maintenance in the service-level agreement?

Answer. Both during the oral testimony and in the written testimony, we have affirmed the fact that UNOS has consistently met or exceeded OPTN contract requirements across the board, including for system uptime.

The new uptime requirement, as referenced in your question, was adopted following a study requested by HRSA and conducted by the OPTN's Network Operations Oversight Committee (NOOC) to determine a "clinically acceptable" level of availability of the OPTN matching function. As detailed in a June 2022 report to the board, based on the committee's findings and supported by Gartner research into health-care applications on a national scale, the NOOC recommended that the OPTN maintain a 99.9-percent matching function uptime, not including planned maintenance.[79] The committee noted that any potential delay in organ matching as a result of downtime is managed at the donor level so that patient safety is protected, and organ offers are not missed.

---

[79] "Clinically acceptable availability of the OPTN matching function." OPTN Network Operations Oversight Committee report to the board. June 26, 2022.

As shown in the UNet Availability Summary below, the early years (2000–2005) of our systems' existence were challenging as new features and functions were being added. During 2005, core stability and scalability improvements were made and since 2006, the system has been consistently reliable and available. Additional high-availability improvements have been implemented between 2016 and 2022, including migration to multi-regional hybrid cloud.

Nonetheless, as shown below, UNOS has consistently exceeded 99.9 percent availability.

Planned maintenance is defined in the SLA as time when UNet is purposefully taken offline to perform regular system maintenance or to deploy organ allocation policy changes. To minimize impact to users, UNOS performs planned maintenance at low-usage times and with advance communication to users.

UNet Availability Summary

Year	Uptime/ Availability %	Planned (Maintenance) Availability %	Total Availability (Planned + Unplanned) %
2000	99.09%	98.90%	97.99%
2001	99.68%	99.51%	99.19%
2002	99.89%	99.90%	99.79%
2003	99.96%	99.95%	99.90%
2004	99.98%	99.89%	99.87%
2005	99.93%	99.95%	99.88%
TOTAL 2000–2005	99.76%	99.68%	99.44%
Significant scalability improvements made after 2005			
2006	100.00%	99.93%	99.92%
2007	99.98%	99.94%	99.92%
2008	99.99%	99.98%	99.97%
2009	99.98%	99.95%	99.94%
2010	99.97%	99.95%	99.92%
2011	99.99%	99.97%	99.96%
2012	99.92%	99.98%	99.90%
2013	100.00%	99.93%	99.93%
2014	100.00%	99.91%	99.91%
2015	100.00%	99.95%	99.95%
2016	99.99%	99.97%	99.96%
2017	100.00%	99.95%	99.95%
2018	99.98%	99.96%	99.94%
2019	100.00%	99.94%	99.94%
2020	99.99%	99.92%	99.91%
2021	99.99%	99.93%	99.92%
2022 (thru August)	99.99%	99.90%	99.89%
TOTAL since 2006	*99.99%*	*99.95%*	*99.93%*

In January 2022, after the recommendation by the NOOC, HRSA agreed to increase the Matching Function Service Level Agreement (SLA) from 99.5 percent uptime to 99.9 percent, excluding planned maintenance. This new SLA provides a more accurate picture of system stability by removing planned events from the measure, while also decreasing the contractually permitted amount of unplanned downtime from 0.5 percent to 0.1 percent. Further, it was determined that where practical, planned maintenance periods should not exceed 30 minutes per event.

Question. You testified that UNOS is "subject to 3 million attempts a day to hack the patient database."

How many hack attempts is UNOS receiving if you exclude attacks that are just routinely defended against using standard, commodity anti-virus, firewall software?

How many of those are targeted specifically and uniquely at UNOS, rather than just being the result of broad vulnerability scans of the Internet by attackers?

Answer. UNOS takes the position that all attacks have the potential to be targeted and we have implemented automation capabilities to block or respond to the wide threat landscape. Based on extensive and continuous system monitoring and alerting, there are attacks that are raised to levels of greater concern and are investigated by UNOS's Information Security team. Over the last year, almost 300 events were elevated for additional investigation, with zero impactful incidents.

The sources of these attacks are as follows:

Threat or vulnerability (CY 2021)	Quantity
Websites blocked for malicious or inappropriate content	3,813,576
Inbound email blocks for inappropriate content or spam	444,600
Emails quarantined based on confirmed security concerns	33,806
Crowdstrike—End-Point Detection	592
Refused connections	1,204,258,768
Events requiring follow-up by Information Security	286
Impactful incidents	0

Question. Given testimony during the hearing that UNOS has retaliated by withholding data access from researchers it disfavors, will UNOS commit to transparently sharing with all qualified researchers a full and complete reporting of the number of patients referred by hospitals to each OPO by month since 2010?

Answer. NOTA, the OPTN final rule, and the OPTN contract outline the criteria that members of the general public and researchers must meet to receive different types of data (i.e., identifiable data, limited datasets, etc.). The more identifiable the data, the more rigorous are the criteria for receiving access to such data.

UNOS, as the OPTN contractor, has always fulfilled all requests in compliance with these requirements. Further, Task 3.7 in the OPTN contract, quoted below, requires the OPTN contractor to report to HRSA when certain requests cannot be fulfilled.

Task 3.7: The contractor agrees to meet the following data disclosure standards (except sub-task 3.7.2, when it concerns requests from the Secretary of HHS): some data requests involve data that may be withheld under the terms of the Privacy Act of 1974 (5 U.S.C. 552a), the Trade Secrets Act (18 U.S.C. 1905), the Freedom of Information Act (FOIA) (5 U.S.C. 552), or other applicable laws. For example, any personally-identified or personally identifiable data will be maintained according to the OPTN/SRTR/HRSA Data System of Records, HHS/HRSA/ HSB/DoT, No. 09–15–0055, including data maintained electronically, must be disclosed consistent with the Privacy Act and the Systems Routine Uses, outlined in the applicable System of Records Notice (73 Fed. Reg. 19519, as amended). The contractor will provide a log of these requests and releases with level of effort for each request to the COR in the quarterly report.

The contractor shall notify the COR in the quarterly report if, in its view:

1) the data are not collected and/or verified;
2) release of the data violates the Privacy Act or applicable laws; or
3) the data and information are otherwise exempted from disclosure under the FOIA, when applicable.

The OPTN collects aggregate-level data on the number of referrals by hospital to each OPO by month. That data is submitted by the OPOs and is part of the OPTN dataset that we would provide to any researcher requesting it. UNOS, as the OPTN contractor, does not withhold data access from researchers for OPTN data. We don't know the specifics around the context that generated this question, but UNOS would be happy to talk with any researchers to get them the OPTN data they seek.

Question. In April 2022, UNOS acknowledged that it failed to report 35,000 deaths among patients on the waiting list. In 2019 alone, nearly one in four pre-transplant patient deaths were missed or mislabeled in UNOS data. Low-quality data provided by UNOS impedes researchers and Congress from understanding how to improve patient care.

How many new or amended OPTN policies have relied on UNOS's faulty data?

How many times did UNOS cite incorrect patient death data in communications with the Senate Finance Committee or its members?

Answer. Please see response to Senator Grassley's fourth question.

Question. Given one of your emails, which was included in the record at the Senate Finance Committee hearing, described UNOS's peer-review process as "Like putting your kids' artwork up at home. You value it because of how it was created rather than whether it's well done."

When and in how many instances has UNOS communicated to the Federal governing that UNOS's peer-review process was deficient?

If UNOS made such communications, please provide any supporting written communications from UNOS to the Federal Government.

Answer. The segment of the email as cited was a personal ad hoc reaction to a discussion taking place in the moment. It does not reflect an evidence-based conclusion that the OPTN peer review process is substantially flawed, nor was it intended as a specific, action-oriented recommendation for a change to the process.

Confidential medical peer review is critical to achieve improvements to the entire transplantation network and even more broadly, foundational to quality assessment throughout the health-care system and beyond.

Question. In 2022, UNOS approved the implementation of "bypass filters," allowing transplant centers to preemptively indicate donor characteristics that they are unwilling to consider for patients on their wait list. Currently, these filters are not shared with patients, who may be unaware if they are listed at a transplant center where they will not meet criteria to receive an organ. Bypassed organ offers are not currently included in the denominator of SRTR reported organ offer acceptance rates, further obfuscating choices for patients.

Did UNOS consult with the data advisory committee or SRTR review committee before implementing these bypass filters?

How is information regarding the use of bypass filters being shared with patients? Is UNOS monitoring how the use of these filters will adversely impact the probability of transplantation for patients at a given transplant center?

Has UNOS done any analysis to determine how bypass filters may impact organ discards, organ offer acceptance rates, or disparities by age, race/ethnicity, and geography in patients receiving a transplant?

Will UNOS commit to providing transparency to the public, especially to patients, regarding which bypass filters are being used by which transplant programs, and how these filters may impact the ability of wait-listed patients to obtain a transplant?

Answer. The OPTN implemented the Offer Filters tool as a system enhancement based on the organ donation and transplant community's feedback and collaboration. The goal of Offer Filters is to increase kidney utilization by helping transplant hospitals automate "refusal" of organ offers that they know they will not accept in accordance with their existing acceptance criteria, allowing the OPO to find an accepting center more quickly, especially for hard to place organs. In other words, Offer Filters screens offers that centers were already manually declining for their patients. Offer Filters significantly reduces the delays that could occur as a result of the former manual process.

By analyzing hospitals' kidney acceptance trends, Offer Filters reduces the time between offer and acceptance, bringing kidneys to patients faster and reducing non-utilization of organs ("discards").

The Transplant Coordinators Committee formed a work group to give feedback on the development of the Offer Filters project. In 2019, 29 kidney programs participated in the Offer Filters pilot. In 2020, UNOS conducted a second pilot with 34 more kidney programs. The results of these two pilots were used to refine the requirements for the national rollout of Offer Filters in 2022.

UNOS is committed to providing transparency to the public and to patients about all facets of its operations. UNOS recognizes the potential benefit to patients of using the Offer Filters tool for shared decision-making and will explore options for doing so.

Increasing the use of Offer Filters by transplant hospitals is currently under consideration by the OPTN Operations and Safety Committee (OSC). This summer, the committee released a concept paper to seek community and public feedback. The committee is considering proposing a policy change in this area, which could come with additions to the monitoring plan.[80] The current monitoring plan tracks 15 metrics at a national and program level. Changes in transplant volume are among these metrics tracked, as well as national and program-level rates of non-utilized organs.

Question Submitted by Hon. Robert P. Casey, Jr.

Question. The Finance Committee's investigation and witness testimony documented repeated instances of transportation errors leading to organs being damaged beyond use. However, the investigation found that transportation errors are rarely referred to the MPSC—of 53 transportation-related complaints, just 6 percent went to the MPSC for review. Accordingly,

---

[80] "Optimizing Usage of Kidney Offer Filters." OPTN Operations and Safety Committee. De- cember 20, 2021. *https://optn.transplant.hrsa.gov/policies-bylaws/public-comment/optimizing- usage-of-kidney-offer-filters.*

the Finance Committee recommended (1) increasing transparency and accountability for chain of custody and transportation of organs procured for transplant by providing for public reporting, as appropriate, on the status of organs in transport; and (2) increasing accountability for organs lost, damaged, or delayed in transport by requiring oversight and corrective action for such incidents.

What actions will UNOS take to implement these recommendations?

Answer. As shared in answer to question 7 of Senator Wyden, the OPTN agrees with the committee that increasing transparency and accountability for the transportation of organs would be an important system-wide improvement. The majority of organs that travel unaccompanied by surgical teams are kidneys, which are the most transplanted organ and thus impact the greatest number of patients on the waiting list.

The actions UNOS is taking to implement the committee's recommendations include discussions underway among the members of the OSC about ways to increase our understanding of the breadth and depth of transportation errors in the system. Discussion within both the OPO and OSC committees has acknowledged the complexity of implementing nationwide organ tracking and begun to review possible pathways to address the issue within the scope of the OPTN's authority.

UNOS provided data to the committee in a July 11, 2022, letter that offers some insight into the scale of transportation issues reported to the MPSC. The letter provided a more detailed accounting of data discussed in a UNOS Member Quality staff interview.

Over a 5-year period, there were 37 transportation-related cases out of 1,479 total OPO-related cases, or 2.5 percent of cases. Of those 37 unique cases over the same 5-year period, 14 were classified as involving commercial air transportation, 7 were classified as involving private or chartered air transportation, and 16 were classified as involving ground transportation. Of these 37 cases, 13 organs (or 0.88 percent of cases) over 5 years were ultimately unable to be transplanted for reasons that may or may not be related to the transportation error. During this same time period, 151,531 organs were transplanted.

While the OPTN is required to admit designated OPOs as members of the OPTN, not all organizations involved in the chain of custody for transporting organs are members of the OPTN. For example, commercial airlines, other common carriers, commercial shippers, and courier companies are not members of the OPTN, yet OPOs rely on these organizations to ship organs thousands of times a year. Please see question 20 of Senator Cardin for more detail on this issue.

Question Submitted by Hon. Tim Scott

Care Disparities

Question. Your unsealed emails reveal your belief that, in the transplant system which you have managed for a decade, "Only people who have means can get transplants."

Why, despite this awful care disparity which you yourself acknowledge, has UNOS spent its considerable resources lobbying against reforms, like the previous administration's Executive Order on Advancing American Kidney Health, that have been universally championed by patient groups?

Answer. This quote from a personal email of former UNOS CEO Brian Shepard has been routinely mischaracterized by plaintiffs in an ongoing lawsuit seeking to prevent more equitable distribution of livers. In the email, Mr. Shepard acknowledges the challenges of achieving equity in the U.S. health-care system, where access to insurance coverage or personal resources are so critical to accessing treatment. The transplant system is impacted by the flaws and challenges of the greater health-care system. UNOS would be pleased to work with the committee or individual Senators on initiatives that would expand access to health care, including organ transplantation.

UNOS routinely offered its support for important reforms, like the Executive Order on Advancing American Kidney Health, which issued ambitious and laudable goals for all actors in the system. In addition, while UNOS also strongly and routinely agreed with the need for improvements to OPO regulation, we were joined by many members of the community in cautioning against some of the technical aspects of the now-implemented rule that will harm patients if not addressed, such as mass decertification of OPOs without a transition plan in place.[81] UNOS and its partners also offered evidence-based, collaborative alternative solutions to achieve these goals.

Questions Submitted by Hon. Elizabeth Warren

Question. You testified that "the system has been paid for in part by taxpayers; approximately 10 percent of the budget of this contract is taxpayer funded, the rest of that is paid by hospitals when they list patients." Your answer spoke only to contract funding from HRSA, and entirely ignored Medicare dollars that have funded the system, as well as taxpayer dollars from Medicaid, Children's Health Insurance Program (CHIP), and the Department of Veterans Affairs (VA).

What percentage of the OPTN patient registration fees are ultimately reimbursed by all taxpayer funded sources? Please breakdown by source including Medicare, Medicaid, CHIP, and the VA.

What percentage of UNOS fees are ultimately reimbursed by all public sources, despite the fact that the UNOS fees are voluntary and not required to add a patient to the waiting list? Please breakdown by source including Medicare, Medicaid, CHIP, and the VA.

Answer. The OPTN final rule, 42 CFR 121.5(c) requires OPTN members to pay a registration fee to the OPTN for each transplant candidate it places on the waiting list. UNOS bills hospitals directly whenever a transplant center places a patient on the national transplant waiting list and requires the OPTN registration fee established by the OPTN board of directors, and approved by the Secretary, to cover the reasonable costs of operating the OPTN. Reimbursement is received from hospitals directly. Therefore, UNOS has no visibility to how public or private insurance programs are billed by the hospital. UNOS does not have information concerning hospitals' financial models, costs of care, or payor reimbursements.

Question. In October 2020, the Senate Finance Committee wrote to the Secretary of HHS with a concern about "double billing" from OPTN/UNOS.

---

[81] AST, ASTS and UNOS letter to CMS Acting Administrator Richter. https://unos.org/wp-content/uploads/UNOSGR-202210304-AST-ASTS-UNOS-Joint-Comment-CMS-3380-F2-OPO-Medicare-Conditions-for-Coverage-March2021.pdf. March 4, 2021.

Currently, to list the exact same patient on the organ waiting list, how much in fees does OPTN/UNOS charge to Medicare?

Answer. Federal regulation requires transplant hospitals to pay a fee to the OPTN to add a candidate to the organ transplant waiting list.[82] Neither the OPTN nor UNOS bill Medicare, Medicaid, or any other insurance provider for costs it incurs.

Authorized by Federal regulation and approved annually by the OPTN board of directors and the Secretary of HHS, the OPTN assesses a one-time registration fee (currently $868), billable to a transplant hospital at the time it registers a candidate for a transplant. Pursuant to section 121.5(c) of the final rule, the OPTN establishes the fee based on the reasonable costs of operating the OPTN, and HRSA approves that fee. The OPTN does not know the source of funding that OPTN members use to pay the OPTN registration fee. UNOS is a Virginia nonprofit membership corporation founded by the transplant community in 1984. UNOS members also pay a fee to UNOS, $100 per patient added to the waiting list in FY23, to fund UNOS operations and for the services that UNOS provides to the donation and transplant community and to its members. It is important to note that these are separate fees for different services to transplant hospitals; payment of the UNOS fee is not required for a transplant hospital to add a patient to the OPTN waiting list.

UNOS has no visibility to how public or private insurance programs are billed by the hospital. UNOS does not have information concerning hospitals' financial models, costs of care, or payor reimbursements. To supplement this response, please see our response to your first question.

Question. How much in fees does OPTN/UNOS charge to other public sources including Medicaid, CHIP, and the VA, including via hospital fees for which government payers reimburse?

Answer. See above answer.

Question. For each of the last 10 years (2012 to present):

What have been (a) per patient and (b) total OPTN fees received by UNOS as the OPTN?

What percentage of that total has been paid by Medicare?

What percentage of that total has been paid by other public sources including Medicaid, CHIP, and the VA, including via hospital fees for which government payers reimburse?

OPTN Fees

Fiscal Year	OPTN Fees Per Candidate	Fees Collected
2012	$603	$41,259,959
2013	$651	$43,682,960
2014	$810	$55,946,345
2015	$793	$57,081,282
2016	$812	$57,125,866
2017	$834	$59,310,720
2018	$834	$61,812,887
2019	$794	$65,479,021
2020	$748	$59,082,927
2021	$748	$60,461,138
2022 (August YTD)	$868	$66,270,399

[82] 42 CFR Sec. 121.5(c). "An OPTN member shall pay a registration fee to the OPTN for each transplant candidate it places on the waiting list. The amount of such fee shall be calculated to cover (together with contract funds awarded by the Secretary) the reasonable costs of operating the OPTN and shall be determined by the OPTN with the approval of the Secretary."

The OPTN final rule, 42 CFR 121.5(c) requires OPTN members to pay a registration fee to the OPTN for each transplant candidate it places on the waiting list. UNOS, serving as the OPTN contractor, bills hospitals whenever a transplant center places a patient on the national transplant waiting list. As such, UNOS does not have visibility into hospitals' financial models, costs of care, or payor reimbursements, and does not know the source of funding that OPTN members use to pay the OPTN Registration fee.

Question. For each of the last 10 years (2012 to present):

What have been (a) per patient and (b) total UNOS fees received by UNOS as the OPTN?

What percentage of that total has been paid by Medicare?

What percentage of that total has been paid by other public sources including Medicaid, CHIP, and the VA, including via hospital fees for which government payers reimburse?

Answer. The OPTN Registration Fee and the UNOS fee are for distinct and separate services. The OPTN Registration Fees, as outlined above, are required to be paid by OPTN members for the reasonable costs of operating the OPTN, outlined in the OPTN contract and below. The UNOS fee is collected from UNOS members and pays for services outlined below.

UNOS Fees

Fiscal Year	UNOS Fees	Fees Collected
2012	$122	$4,788,048
2013	$125	$5,131,425
2014	$147	$5,454,592
2015	$164	$6,410,040
2016	$145	$6,763,625
2017	$145	$7,980,220
2018	$145	$8,414,851
2019	$158	$9,657,618
2020	$178	$8,909,304
2021	$178	$10,845,896
2022 (YTD August)	$122	$7,063,800

UNOS does not have visibility into hospitals' financial models, costs of care, or payor reimbursements, and does not know the source of funding that UNOS members use to pay the UNOS Fee.

Question. On what activities are OPTN fees spent?

Answer. The OPTN registration fees and budget must be calculated to meet the "reasonable costs of operating the OPTN" and are approved annually by the HHS Secretary pursuant to 42 CFR § 121.5(c). Those costs will include sufficient resources to perform the following OPTN contract tasks:

1) Administering the OPTN contract through a project management plan; providing daily, weekly, quarterly, and annual updates to HRSA and other external audience; proposing the annual OPTN registration fee schedule and associated annual budget; providing HRSA monthly reports tracking revenue and expenditures associated with the OPTN contract; and maintaining various secure web-based platforms, including a platform for submitting contract deliverables to HRSA, and a document management platform to allow OPTN governance group members to share documents.

2) Supporting the OPTN board of directors (BOD) and executive committee, and OPTN BOD operating committees by: supporting an annual OPTN BOD composition review and recruiting plan; reviewing the OPTN charter; supporting the appointment of the OPTN executive director; supporting the operating committees and policy development committees; strategic planning to guide OPTN activity; providing ongoing education on OPTN legal and regulatory requirements; providing opportunities for public access to OPTN governance activities; and other administrative and logistical support and subject matter expertise.
3) Supporting the OPTN policy process and policy development committees and expert groups to address critical OPTN policy issues by: developing, revising, and maintaining OPTN bylaws, policies, standards, and guidelines for the operation of the OPTN; recruiting volunteers to serve on the OPTN policy development committees; documenting the OPTN policy development process; tracking policy development process metrics; reviewing the OPTN regional process; and hosting consensus conferences to solicit input from the transplant community and public on matters related to OPTN bylaws, policies, or operations.
4) Providing an OPTN electronic matching of donor organs to transplant candidates 24 hours per day, every day; ensuring real-time access to the electronic matching function for allocating deceased donor organs; developing innovative applications to enhance the matching functions; operating the OPTN Kidney Paired Donation Pilot Project (KPDPP); electroni cally managing all OPTN patient review board processes; and maintaining allocation decision rules.
5) Operating the Organ Center to facilitate organ placement by providing technical assistance to OPTN members 24 hours/day, 7 days/ week.
6) Monitoring OPTN member compliance and performance, quality improvement, and sanctioning, by: maintaining documentation describing the OPTN monitoring, performance improvement, and enforcement requirements; measuring the effectiveness of the processes used to identify compliance, encourage improvement, and determine sanctions; providing HRSA with an annual OPTN monitoring activity report on all OPTN members; reviewing and periodically reassessing OPTN membership applications, including submitting OPTN membership application forms for OMB clearance; developing new models for monitoring and improving OPTN membership performance through collaborative performance improvement structures; reporting to HRSA information about member performance that poses significant risk to patient health or public safety; and conducting special reviews of OPTN members as requested by the Secretary.
7) Collecting official OPTN data to support the operations of the OPTN and maintaining a data repository of all official OPTN data, which according to contract must be collected after submitting clearance packages for Office of Management and Budget (OMB) approval, collecting all official OPTN data through direct electronic transfer; integrating standard clinical data ontologies into OPTN data collection and operation of the OPTN, identifying and supplementing official OPTN data with information from external data sources, and collecting official OPTN data through survey methods.
8) Providing access to official OPTN data by: making standard analysis data sets and other data sets available to the scientific community and the public for research and analysis purposes; responding to data requests from HRSA and other components

within the Federal Government; responding to data requests from OPTN members and providing online access to OPTN- branded online data reports to members to improve system performance; and responding to data requests from the general public.

9) Coordinating OPTN policy development and analytic needs with the Scientific Registry for Transplant Recipients (SRTR) contractor through a formal written agreement for data transfer, and by coordinating activities and meetings with the SRTR contractor to discuss OPTN data issues, planning and participating in joint meetings with the SRTR contractor, and collaborating with the SRTR contractor on the development of the OPTN/SRTR Annual Data Report.
10) Maintaining and improving the OPTN website to be a comprehensive source of OPTN-related information for the public and the transplant community, which also must be securely configured.
11) Communicating about all activities of the OPTN with OPTN members, transplant professionals, transplant patients, living organ donors, donor families, media, and the general public by: developing a communications plan and a branding plan; developing OPTN educational materials for patients, the public, and transplant professionals; and informing HRSA and the SRTR of media inquiries.
12) Providing an OPTN patient services line to provide 24-hour toll-free information with English and Spanish capabilities.
13) Providing written updates and summaries on OPTN activity to HRSA as required for reports to Congress or other official reports.
14) Managing and maintaining OPTN records to retain functionality and integrity throughout the full records lifecycle, subject to the Privacy Act of 1974, including maintaining records identified in the OPTN System of Records Notice.
15) Executing special studies on topics identified by HRSA.
16) Meeting security and privacy requirements and safeguarding information and information systems by meeting Federal standards for protection, confidentiality, and nondisclosure of sensitive information; encryption of computing devices and information; complying with Federal Rules of Behavior, notifying HRSA of, and responding to, security incidents and privacy breaches; continuous monitoring of information security; permitting government access for security assessments; and adhering to security requirements for cloud services.

Federal appropriations constitute approximately 8–10 percent of the resources used to meet the obligations of the OPTN contract.

Question. On what activities are UNOS fees spent?

Answer. UNOS is a nonprofit nonstock membership corporation founded by the transplant community in 1984 to serve as the national transplantation network. With the tremendous growth in transplantation and to meet the broad responsibilities of the OPTN contract, UNOS has since grown to 450 diverse professional staff. The UNOS fee is one of the revenue sources for UNOS and those revenues are maintained in UNOS operating accounts where the fees are commingled with revenues from other sources including charitable donations, unrelated business income, and most significantly, costs reimbursed to the contractor under the OPTN contract. The UNOS fee makes it possible to provide enhanced services not required by Federal contract that respond to the community's needs and continuously improve the national transplant system. Examples of these UNOS enhancements include, but are not limited to:

- Data tools and analysis to help member institutions analyze and improve performance and patient outcomes.
- Innovative technology and research to improve the efficiency of organ offers, placement and transportation.
- Educational offerings and collaborative events to help transplant professionals grow their knowledge and skills.

General and administrative expenses are also covered by the UNOS fee, which include maintaining the infrastructure essential to serve as the OPTN contractor and which costs are not directly reimbursable under the OPTN contract.

The structure of a separate UNOS fee to provide enhanced services to the transplant community not covered by the OPTN fee represents an ongoing effective public-private solution to a public health challenge. Managed in the private sphere but overseen in the public, the U.S. organ donation and transplant system has demonstrated growth year over year that has led to nearly a million lives saved through transplant, more than any other country in the world.

Question. Are UNOS fees used to pay for activities disallowed under the Federal Acquisitions Regulations (e.g., lobbying expenses)?

Answer. UNOS's private funds are used for UNOS efforts, including our government relations work. Lobbying expenses are not an allowable cost for reimbursement under the Federal Acquisition Regulations and are never billed to the OPTN contract in compliance with HHSAR 352.203–70: Anti-Lobbying, which is incor- porated into the OPTN contract.

Question. Are any OPTN fees used to support OPTN/UNOS technology?

Answer. The National Organ Transplant Act (NOTA), 42 U.S.C. 273 et. seq. requires that the OPTN operate a national system to allocate organs using computer systems. Thus, the costs of operating the OPTN include the costs of operating a national system using computer technology to allocate organs, including updates to reflect changes in organ allocation policies, data collection, security, privacy, reliability, improvements and architecture. The OPTN contract requires the OPTN contractor to provide computer systems and software to meet the statutory obligations of the OPTN, as well as meet extensive Federal requirements for security, operability, privacy, and reliability. UNOS utilizes registration fees paid to the OPTN by transplant hospitals and appropriated funds paid to the contractor by HRSA to meet its technology obligations under the OPTN contract.

Question. Are any UNOS fees used to support OPTN/UNOS technology?

Answer. The OPTN contract requires the contractor to provide a computer system to meet all of the obligations of the OPTN organ matching and data collections functions for all organ types, while also meeting the extensive security and privacy requirements of the OPTN contract. The contractor's computer system must be in operation exceeding 99.9-percent availability, while being continuously updated by changes to organ allocation policies/algorithms approved by the OPTN board of directors. The government has never provided software or hardware to the OPTN contractor to meet these contract requirements.

UNOS pays its operating expenses and makes investments in technology from its operating account. The UNOS operating account receives funds from different sources but primarily from reimbursement of allowable costs under the OPTN contract, revenues from UNOS members paying the UNOS fee, charitable contributions, and unrelated business income. UNOS expenses are paid from its operating account, which include salaries and benefits for all staff;

general and administrative costs; and property, plant and equipment. Since UNOS was formed in 1984 by the transplant community, UNOS Information Technology staff developed, maintain and enhance UNOS software that it uses to power the OPTN and meet the obligations of the OPTN contract.

See Senator Cardin's first question.

Question. Please distinguish what aspects of the OPTN/UNOS IT system (e.g., hardware, platforms such as UNet, DonorNet, and TransNet, and code used to facilitate matching) were paid for using UNOS fees; which were paid for using OPTN fees; and which were paid for using appropriated funds awarded through the contract.

Answer. See question above.

Question. Please provide the amount spent on OPTN/UNOS IT from each of these three sources of funding for each year under the current contract for the operation of the OPTN.

Answer. Please see the below report of expenditures on the IT-related tasks under the current OPTN contract, which commenced with a partial year on April 1, 2019:

		Task 4—OPTN Electronic Matching	*Task 5—Collect Official OPTN Data*	*Task 9—OPTN Website*	*Task 20—Security and Privacy Requirements*	*Total*
Year 1	FY 2019 (Apr–Sep)	$12,114,912	$1,727,410	$106,806	$953,039	*$14,902,167*
Year 2	FY 2020	$26,567,255	$4,896,707	$264,113	$2,693,269	*$34,421,345*
Year 3	FY 2021	$26,216,727	$4,977,437	$323,871	$2,378,211	*$33,896,246*
Year 4	FY 2022 (Aug. YTD)	$26,210,887	$4,828,467	$231,152	$2,972,366	*$34,242,872*
	Total	*$91,109,780*	*$16,430,022*	*$925,942*	*$8,996,885*	*$117,462,629*

Question. In light of your misleading answer about taxpayer funding of the OPTN system and technology (since both HRSA funding and Medicare funding are from the taxpayer, as are funds from the other government sources such as the VA), how do you justify that the taxpayer should have to pay to buy back OPTN/UNOS technology in the event of HRSA electing different OPTN contractors?

Answer. With the passage of NOTA in 1984, Congress determined that the organ transplant network should reside in the private sector with appropriate oversight by the Federal Government. The OPTN contract requires the contractor to provide a computer system to meet the obligations of the OPTN organ matching and data collections functions for all organ types, while also meeting the extensive security and privacy requirements of the OPTN contract. The contractor's computer system must be in operation exceeding 99.9-percent availability, while being continuously updated by changes to organ allocation policies/algorithms approved by the OPTN board of directors. The government has never provided software or hardware to the OPTN contractor to meet these contract requirements. Through a cost-sharing contract, the government has exercised its discretion to utilize a contractor-owned, contractor-operated (COCO) system to meet the requirements of NOTA and the OPTN contract.

Question. Given that taxpayers have paid for this technology, how do you justify that UNOS refused to allow the USDS to inspect its code, making UNOS the first and only of nearly 100 agencies/contractors to rebuke such a request from USDS?

Answer. We appreciate the opportunity to address these concerns and believe it is important to establish the factual foundation for our response. As discussed above in more detail, since

1984, UNOS has developed and maintained its software that it uses to provide the services required by the OPTN contract and power the OPTN's statutory functions. The government has not provided software or hardware to the OPTN contractor and instead opted for a model where the OPTN contractor utilizes contractor-owned systems to meet the OPTN requirements specified by the government. UNOS has used a variety of funding sources to develop its software and it is inaccurate to state that taxpayers have paid for the UNOS-owned software and systems. For more information, please see our response immediately above.

We appreciate the opportunity to clarify that UNOS never received a request from the USDS to review our code. UNOS would have welcomed then—and still welcomes now—a meeting with USDS to have a focused review of our code, coding practices, code repositories, and other relevant information that could facilitate a more accurate understanding of our systems.

UNOS reiterated its willingness to undergo any additional review deemed necessary in an August 2, 2022, letter to the HRSA Administrator, so that we can discuss the significant factual errors about the OPTN IT infrastructure contained within the USDS report.[83] We would be pleased to have the opportunity to further clarify the facts for Congress, HHS and the USDS alike.

The HRSA team has consistently reviewed the performance and security of the OPTN IT system in great detail throughout our performance of the OPTN contracts, and their annual audit of our systems is currently underway. HRSA reviews all OPTN contractual requirements for compliance annually, as well as on a periodic basis throughout each year, and UNOS consistently meets or exceeds its contractual obligations.

Question. In response to The Washington Post article on UNOS's "refusal to turn over the full code," you stated that this was to "safeguard patient data"; as there should not be any patient data in the code itself, it is concerning that UNOS does not understand basic terminology. Can you clarify?

Answer. There is no patient data in our code. That being said, allowing broad access to any part of the system, regardless of whether it contains patient data, would introduce significant risk to system security. That's why UNOS works closely with HRSA to ensure access is given only to those with appropriate clearance. UNOS does, however, offer the opportunity for an on-site and fully secured review of the code.

We are pleased to share the full statement provided by UNOS to The Washington Post below as clarification.

USDS has never made a formal request to come onsite to review the code. As we've mentioned before, we would welcome USDS to visit UNOS, where we will provide an overview of our software, review matching function code, our coding practices, and how the code is managed and tested.

HRSA conducts annual audits of our system. We provide excerpts of code at their request if they identify areas of improvement during an audit. We also provide HRSA both before and after sections of code to show that the audit-identified improvements have been made.

Additionally, the OPTN contract requires that we regularly provide HRSA with extensive documentation, which includes decision logic used to implement the organ allocation policies.

---

[83] McCauley, Jerry, M.D., MPH. Letter to HRSA Administrator Carole Johnson. August 2, 2022. *https://unos.org/wp-content/uploads/20220802_UNOS-McCauley-Letter-to-HRSA-Administrator.pdf.*

This documentation is updated any time organ allocation policies change and is used by our software engineers when making any updates.

While the source code remains UNOS's intellectual property, we have still offered HRSA the opportunity to do an on-site review of our code repositories, but as of this writing, they have not taken us up on this offer.

We have struck an important balance: providing HRSA and other auditors the access they need to ensure the system's security while limiting wider access in order to safeguard patient data and protect UNOS' intellectual property.

Question. In light of concerns expressed by the Senate Finance Committee about the state of OPTN/UNOS technology, including but not limited to concerns identified by the USDS's report "Lives Are at Stake," please provide your total compensation for 2021 and 2022; the total expenditures for lobbying, marketing, and public relations for 2021 and 2022; and the expenditures for hardware and software maintenance in 2021 and 2022.

Answer. As reported on IRS form 990, total chief executive officer compensation for fiscal year 2021 was $734,490. The 2022 990 has not been prepared, but the chief executive officer compensation as of the September 30th pay stub was $627,634.

	FY 2021	FY 2022—Aug. YTD
Lobbying, Marketing, PR (UNOS expenses)	$296,129	$476,796
Hardware and software maintenance (OPTN and UNOS)	$25,584,244	$25,498,223

Questions Submitted by Hon. Todd Young

Question. Once an Organ Procurement Organization (OPO) is designated as on probation or not in good standing, how does UNOS evaluate when and how an OPO should be removed from probation or restored to good standing?

What corrective actions must occur for the OPO to get back in "good" standing?

Answer. The overall process is described in Appendix L to the OPTN bylaws. In general, the MPSC actively monitors the member's activity and documents progress toward process improvement. After the member has addressed the area(s) of concern and communicated to the MPSC's satisfaction the actions they have taken to meet performance standards, it will recommend to the OPTN board of directors that the designation be removed.

In the case of Member Not in Good Standing (MNIGS), the institution must remain in that status for a minimum of 9 months. It is also an option that the board may move the institution from MNIGS to probation for an additional period of time. Similarly, a member institution placed on probation must remain in that status for a minimum of 9 months before there is any consideration that it may regain full standing.

The corrective actions required for a member to demonstrate improvement and regain full member standing are specific to the issue(s) under review. The MPSC provides the member with notice of the areas where the member must document improvement, often with a specific set of milestones or metrics by which improvement will be assessed.

Question. In November 2020, CMS issued a final rule changing the methodology used to evaluate OPO performance. Based on 2018 data, CMS estimated that 22 of the 57 OPOs would fail the new outcome measures and be decertified. As the entity overseeing policy compliance, what steps is UNOS taking to improve OPO performance given the new performance measures?

Answer. The OPTN continues to believe that the best way to hold OPOs accountable for their performance is to develop an accurate, clear metric with a rationale that has been adequately justified. It is important to note CMS's metric is a comparative one, and each review period will always identify OPOs not in the top 25 percent as "failing" regardless of how many OPOs are in operation. Further, a comparative metric alone does not provide sufficient information on how well an OPO performs.

UNOS is committed to improving performance for OPOs and for the system as a whole. In addition to the OPTN MPSC's routine peer-review-based performance improvement work, already described in detail for the committee throughout the investigation as well as described on the OPTN website, the OPTN also provides other pathways for all member improvement. They include:

- *Collaborative improvement* (CI) projects designed to spread change in a targeted area of focus, involving transparent peer-to-peer sharing of successes and challenges in a collaborative environment. In an OPTN collaborative, members are part of a network with a common aim. With CI, effective donation and transplant practices can be gathered, shared and implemented by others for broad, collective impact.
- *Individual member-focused improvement* (IMFI) that involves working closely with an OPTN performance improvement support team and tailoring a project plan to meet specific quality improvement goals. IMFI also supports donation and transplant members by facilitating peer mentorship sessions with experienced leaders in relevant fields and delivering other services that can vary according to need.

More detail about these programs is available at https://optn.transplant. hrsa.gov/ professionals/improvement/.

The continued, accelerated growth in organ donation and transplant sustained over many years indicates that the U.S. system overall is strong. Notably, the volume of deceased organ donors has been steadily rising after a plateau of approximately 8,000 donors annually from 2006–2013. In 2021, nearly 14,000 deceased donors were recovered, the 11th straight year of growth.

While it is a commonly held misconception that the national opioid epidemic is the sole source of this growth, the data do not support this assertion. The number of donors from other natural causes, other injuries, and cardiovascular events has also continued to rise. The percentages of total deceased donors dying of drug intoxication, which includes but is not limited to opioid intoxication, was approximately 13 percent from 2016–2019, and then increased to 16 percent in 2020; this remained stable in 2021.

Regardless of the manner of death of an organ donor, OPOs and transplant hospitals have continued to increase performance for the last nine consecutive years in the number of deceased donor organs transplanted. Our community is grateful for the lifesaving gifts we've received from so many generous donors.

Question. What attention has UNOS given to the significant annual increase in organ discards? What plan does UNOS have to address and improve the organ discard rate?

Answer. While the decision whether to accept an organ for transplant belongs in the hands of transplant clinicians and their patients, UNOS and the OPTN have consistently provided system-wide tools, data and strategies to increase organ utilization across multiple modalities. A select few are below.

Policy Monitoring

All OPTN committees closely monitor the non-utilization ("discard") rate in organ allocation policy evaluation reports and have adjusted policies where possible to reduce their incidence. A recent example of this includes the 2018 implementation of allocation policies for dual and en bloc kidney offers, when data showed that these more complex organ offers were recovered but accepted at lower rates.

Data Tools

The kidney Offer Filters tool, discussed in detail in the NASEM report as an effective tool to decrease the time between offer and transplant, has shown a preliminary positive impact on the rate of kidneys recovered but not transplanted. Preliminary data following the national rollout of Offer Filters on January 27, 2022, show an approximate 5 percent decrease in the number of organs recovered for transplant but not transplanted. The OPTN Operations and Safety Committee sought public comment on ways to optimize the use of offer filters this fall.[84]

Transplant programs may utilize the Center Acceptance and Refusal Evaluation (CARE) report tool. The tool allows programs to see all of the outcomes for organ offers they accept as well as all of those they refuse. The CARE report is designed to help transplant centers adopt best practices and reduce the non-utilization rate by understanding their organ acceptance behavior and enhancing their ability to analyze acceptance patterns. The tool provides a visualization of organ rejection organ acceptance for specific types of donors as well as transplant-specific and aggregate outcomes so centers can learn what happened to the organs they turned down.

Performance Metrics

The MPSC Performance Metrics proposal, which was recently approved by the OPTN board of directors and which has begun to be implemented this summer, focuses on both pre-transplant as well as post-transplant patient data. With less emphasis placed just on post-transplant outcomes, acceptance behaviors are expected to change, which also may encourage more programs to transplant more complex organs that are otherwise refused.

---

[84] "Optimizing usage of kidney offer filters concept paper." OPTN Operations and Safety Committee. Fall 2022 public comment. *https://optn.transplant.hrsa.gov/policies-bylaws/public-comment/optimizing-usage-of-kidney-offer-filters/.* Accessed October 11, 2022.

Refusal Codes

In June 2021, the OPTN board approved a project to update OPTN "reasons for refusal" of organ offers made to patients. These revised codes were implemented in December 2021. Revising the list of refusal codes supports increased efficiency of the OPTN through better understanding of refusal behaviors, providing more robust data to develop improved allocation strategies to reduce cold ischemic time, reduce the number of non-utilized organs, and increase the number of transplants.[85]

Allocation Policy

In advance of the transition to the Continuous Distribution organ allocation framework beginning with lung in early 2023, the Utilization Considerations of Kidney and Pancreas Continuous Distribution Workgroup is studying the operational aspects of kidney and pancreas allocation that encourage optimization of kidney and pancreas utilization. The workgroup has a practical focus on utility and efficiency, and is composed of representatives from the OPO, Operations and Safety, Transplant Coordinator, Data Advisory, Kidney, and Pancreas committees, who provide experienced clinical and practical allocation perspectives. This workgroup is charged with developing recommendations for transitioning current utilization and efficiency optimization tools and ensuring that these tools function effectively in a Continuous Distribution framework.

Question. Please share the number of organs lost and/or delayed and the resulting loss of prospective transplants that occurred over the past year.

The data provided in response to this question is necessarily limited to only the small subset of organ transportation arrangements that were facilitated by the UNOS Organ Center, because the OPTN does not collect transportation data on a national, systematic basis.

It is important to note that transportation arrangements facilitated by the UNOS Organ Center are based on the transportation vendors and methods (driving, commercial aircraft, etc.) selected by the OPOs and transplant hospitals involved in the shipment. UNOS staff serve as a communication hub to connect those vendors with the senders and receivers of the shipments throughout the process. The vast majority of organ transportation arrangements are facilitated directly by the recovering organ procurement organization, and not by UNOS. As noted in a Kaiser Health News article, "Matters involving the transportation methods used by organ procurement organizations (OPOs) are arranged directly between OPOs and transplant centers."[86]

Between October 1, 2021. and September 30, 2022, the Organ Center assisted with providing deceased donor organ transportation arrangements for 1,727 of 35,319 deceased donor transplants (4.9 percent) performed in this same time period. Out of the 1,727 organ shipments, 70 had a 2-hour or more delay from the original estimated time of arrival, and 13 were transplanted at an alternate transplant hospital. Thirty-five organ shipments were not

---

[85] OPTN project to update refusal codes. https://optn.transplant.hrsa.gov/policies-bylaws/a- closer-look/project-to-update-refusal-codes/. Accessed October 11, 2022.

[86] JoNel Aleccia, "How Lifesaving Organs for Transplant Go Missing in Transit," *Kaiser Health News* (February 10, 2020), available at *https://khn.org/news/how-lifesaving-organs-for-transplant-go-missing-in-transit/* (accessed on February 26, 2020).

ultimately transplanted, but it is important to note that it is not possible to draw any absolute conclusions about the association between an incident that may have occurred in transit and the ultimate outcome of the transplant. There are many reasons why a transplant hospital may not ultimately transplant an organ it accepted for a recipient, including:

- Too much cold ischemic time (which may or may not be due to a transportation issue).
- The anatomy or appearance of the organ upon arrival (which may or may not be due to a transportation issue).
- A change in the health of the recipient that may make them unsuitable for the scheduled transplant.

The same reasons can also be true for organs without any "transportation issues." For all the same reasons (cold ischemic time, anatomy of the organ, health of the recipient) and many others not listed, the transplant surgery may still not occur.

Please see additional information about transportation in responses to Senator Wyden's seventh question and Senator Cardin's first question.

Question. Are there penalties or repercussions for OPOs or transportation companies if an organ is lost and subsequently discarded?

Answer. As provided by Federal law and regulation and the terms of the OPTN contract, the OPTN will review OPTN member institutions for compliance with OPTN obligations. "Transportation companies" including commercial airlines and couriers, are not members of the OPTN and therefore, the OPTN has no oversight or ability to impose penalties on those companies.

For OPOs, the OPTN has authority to investigate issues of potential OPTN policy noncompliance or issues involving patient safety. Of the OPTN adverse member actions resulting in either Probation or Member Not in Good Standing (MNIGS), none to date has specifically involved a sentinel event related to organ transportation. Such an issue, however, might be subject to OPTN review if the event or issue directly relates to OPTN Obligations or, in the opinion of peer reviewers, is a threat to patient safety.

Question. What process improvements has UNOS put in place to minimize lost organs?

Answer. UNOS developed its own organ tracking solution, in addition to the variety of organ tracking tools already available on the market. Because of this, UNOS has access to data for the OPO clients who use our tracking service, but not for all organs being transported. Since the product launched in June 2021, and as of September 2022, 5,628 shipments have been tracked, recently accounting for an average of 8 percent of all packaged organs. Clients on average track 30 percent of all their packaged organs. OPOs don't typically track organs such as hearts, lungs and livers because they are traditionally accompanied by the transplanting surgeon (accounting for 40 percent of all packaged organs). Other OPOs only track kidneys and/or livers that use commercial air and/or are exported from their service area. Currently, OPOs can choose the tracking system that best suits their needs.

Please see additional information about transportation in responses to Senator Wyden's seventh question and Senator Cardin's first question.

Question. In 2017, I asked UNOS for information about an OPO which it had recently placed as a "member not in good standing" as a result of patient safety endangerment issues. UNOS's response to me at the time, which was personally signed by Mr. Shepard, was that

UNOS could not share any of the documents I requested, but that UNOS "provides appropriate and highly effective oversight." Then, when Senators Grassley, Wyden, Cardin and I launched an investigation into these patient safety failures, UNOS changed its messaging to state that it actually does not consider itself responsible for OPO oversight at all.

How can Congress be assured there is "appropriate and highly effective oversight" when UNOS is unwilling to provide any documentation showing oversight is actually taking place—and when pushed, changes tactics to point fingers or deny UNOS's role in the oversight process?

Answer. Oversight of OPOs is shared between the Centers for Medicare and Medicaid Services (CMS) and the OPTN. The OPTN is charged with monitoring OPTN members, including OPOs, for compliance with OPTN Obligations as defined in the OPTN bylaws. These obligations include NOTA, the OPTN final rule, and OPTN policies and bylaws. Federal regulation,[87] the OPTN contract, and OPTN bylaws also require the OPTN to maintain a peer review process to promote quality assurance and performance improvement for all OPTN members, and this is the appropriate and intended role for the OPTN particularly with respect to OPOs where the OPTN's enforcement options are particularly limited. For example, the OPTN has no discretion whether to admit an OPO as a member of the OPTN nor does it have the authority to expel an OPO from OPTN membership.[88] The OPTN has requirements that OPOs must meet, and reviews OPOs for compliance with those obligations. When an OPO is found to be noncompliant with an OPTN obligation, the MPSC works collaboratively with the OPO to correct deficiencies, implement corrective actions, and improve the quality of services it provides.

The Centers for Medicare and Medicaid Services (CMS) has the most complete and extensive Federal regulatory oversight over OPOs. This includes granting licensure to operate and designation to serve as an OPO, and approving financial reimbursement. To the extent that the OPTN has oversight authority, as provided by Federal law and regulation and the OPTN contract, the OPTN addresses member compliance with OPTN obligations and, in the opinion of peer reviewers, issues which may affect patient safety and the quality of services it provides. This is by necessity a more limited scope, and with different enforcement mechanisms. OPTN "oversight" is not duplicative but rather, complements CMS's oversight authority.

Question. Will UNOS commit to sharing needed documents with appropriate oversight agencies to ensure thorough review and evaluation of adverse events in order to save lives and improve the organ donation and transplant system?

Answer. Yes. In an effort to support the committee's investigation, UNOS suggested several pathways for the committee to obtain the data it needs to conduct its work. These included offers to meet with investigative staff in person to review documentation, providing detailed but deidentified case information, and a suggestion that Congress request the Secretary for the information, because we are required to provide the Secretary with any information the Secretary requests. We would suggest these mechanisms for future requests as well.

UNOS is an organization that brings together all components of the nationwide organ transplantation community and has a compelling interest in preserving the sanctity of its highly effective peer review process. The medical peer review privilege between the OPTN and OPTN

---

[87] 42 CFR Sec. 121.10(b)(1)(i).

[88] "The OPTN *shall admit and retain as members* the following: (i) *All organ procurement organizations;*" 42 CFR Sec. 121.3(b)(1)(i) (emphasis added)

members is a reciprocal privilege; that is, both parties to the peer review process have an obligation to the other party to maintain the confidentiality of the communications and materials shared throughout the process. These mutual assurances of confidentiality ensure the candor and openness that is essential to an effective peer review process as envisioned in the Institute of Medicine Report, "To Err is Human: Building a Safer Health System."[89] Statements made and information provided by an OPTN member to the OPTN contractor and vice versa during any interview, hearing, investigation, or inquiry with the MPSC, as a peer review body, are made during the course of its confidential peer review process and with the understanding that these statements and information would also be protected from discovery under the medical peer review privilege. The OPTN bylaws provide assurances to OPTN members that information provided during compliance activities will remain confidential pursuant to medical peer review[90] and further exposes the OPTN contractor and its staff to personal liability for violating this peer review privilege.[91] In light of the OPTN's obligation to provide a peer review system and the widely recognized benefits of confidential medical peer review, UNOS provides aggregate data on system-wide compliance activities that demonstrate the OPTN provides appropriate and highly effective oversight when OPTN members are found to be non-compliant with OPTN obligations.

HRSA presently provides oversight of the OPTN on behalf of the HHS Secretary. The OPTN is required by regulation to provide the Secretary any information that may be requested by the Secretary (42 CFR 121.11(b)(iii)). The OPTN has always met this requirement and will continue to provide the Secretary any information that the Secretary prescribes.

Question. Organ Procurement Organizations (OPOs) are constrained from placing their own kidneys with national transplant centers and instead forced to wait for the Organ Procurement Transplantation Network system to place them. According to the Report of National Kidney Foundation Consensus Conference to Decrease Kidney Discards published in Clinical Transplantation, October 2018, the overall placement rate for high Kidney Donor Profile Index (KDPI) kidneys allocated through the Organ Center is 28 percent, which those with KDPI of 80+ have a placement rate of less than 15 percent. OPOs who work to place kidneys themselves,

have much higher placement rates. Why are OPOs penalized for placing the kidneys themselves?

Answer. The "Report of National Kidney Foundation Consensus Conference to Decrease Kidney Discards" published in *Clinical Transplantation,* October 2018, does not cite an overall placement rate for high KDPI kidneys or those with a KDPI of 80+ allocated through the Organ Center.

It's important to note that when this report was written, kidneys allocation was different than it is currently. Kidneys at that time were offered first within the OPO's Donation Service

---

[89] Washington (DC): National Academies Press (US); 2000. Available at: *https://pubmed.ncbi.nlm.nih.gov/25077248/* accessed October 11, 2022.

[90] OPTN Bylaws Article A.1 (A)(5)(B). "Any act, communication, report, recommendation or disclosure, with respect to any applicant or member made in good faith and at the request of the OPTN contractor and its representatives, anywhere and at any time, for the purposes described in (a) above are privileged to the fullest extent permitted by law as part of the OPTN medical peer review. The medical peer review privilege extends to any third parties who either supply or are supplied information and are authorized to receive, release or act upon the same."

[91] *Id.* at (c). "The immunity and release from liability provided in this section shall not apply to acts of willful misconduct by the OPTN contractor and its representatives."

Area (DSA), then regionally, and finally to the Nation. Once all potential candidates at transplant programs within the OPO's DSA and region had received and refused kidney offers, OPTN policy required the OPO to contact the Organ Center for assistance allocating the kidney. An OPO's placement rate of high KDPI kidneys at the local DSA and regional classifications is not comparable to the Organ Center's placement rate at the national classifications. The higher quality organs will be accepted and transplanted prior to offers at the national level. Kidneys that have been declined by the local DSA and region often have more extended cold ischemic times, abnormal biopsy/laboratory findings, and/or anatomical issues, making Organ Center nation placement attempts significantly more challenging.

Kidney allocation changed in 2021, and kidneys are now offered to transplant hospitals located within 250 nautical miles (NM) of the donor hospital and then to centers located over 250NM away from the donor hospital. OPTN policy requires the OPO to contact the Organ Center for assistance allocating a kidney once all centers within the 250NM classifications have declined. The same issues apply to these placements; higher quality kidneys are more likely to be placed within the higher ranked 250NM classifications, leaving the allocation of the harder to place kidneys to the Organ Center. Therefore, just as in the prior policy, placement rates between the OPO and the Organ Center are not comparable.

OPOs and the Organ Center use the same kidney match for placement. Successful kidney placement has three major components: (1) quality of the donor and organ,

(2) distance/logistical constraints, and (3) transplant program and transplant candidate requirements. If the OPO is following the rank order of the match, then holding all else equal, placement rates should be the same at the national classifications regardless of the entity that is making the offers. UNOS staff do not prohibit nor penalize OPOs that make national kidney offers. However, if made aware of a case, staff will educate them on the OPTN policy and the potential deviation.

The OPTN has pursued many projects from the 2018 NKF Consensus Conference recommendations. Below are just a few.

Recommendation: "Create expedited placement pathway to directly offer organs at risk of discard to small subset of centers that opt in to accepting these organs." "Center must sustain high rates of acceptance to receive offers."

In 2019, the Organ Center implemented a data-driven yearlong Kidney Accelerated Placement (KAP) project, which was very similar to the recommendation from the NKF Consensus Conference. During the KAP project, hard-to-place kidneys were offered to transplant programs that had a history of accepting them. The acceptance to transplant rate was slightly higher under KAP (72.7 percent versus 71.2 percent), although not significant. More information about the project can be found at:

- https://onlinelibrary. wiley.com/doi/epdf/10.1111/ajt.16859.

Recommendation: "Understanding the role of kidney biopsies in the evaluation of organ quality and impact on allocation/acceptance."

In June 2022 two policies related to biopsies were passed by the OPTN board of directors. The policies establish minimum kidney donor criteria requiring a biopsy and standardize the reporting and data collection of kidney biopsies. In addition to improving allocation efficiencies, these two policies will allow for further research around the impact kidney biopsies have on acceptance and transplantation rates. More information about those policies can be found at:

- o https://optn.transplant.hrsa.gov/policies-bylaws/public-comment/standardize-kidney-biopsy-reporting-and-data-collection/.
- o https://optn.transplant.hrsa.gov/policies-bylaws/public-comment/establish-minimum-kidney-donor-criteria-to-require-biopsy/

Recommendation: "Strengthen local OPO-transplant center cooperative QAPI efforts to reduce discard."

The OPTN created a collaborative improvement framework where members could share best practices and ideas for improvement. The primary aim of the Collaborative Innovation and Improvement Network (COIIN) was increasing transplantation with a particular focus on moderate to high Kidney Donor Profile Index (KDPI) kidneys. Favorable results were seen in both cohorts, and findings show that an increase in transplant rate and greater utilization of moderate to high KDPI organs were realized in many participating centers.[92]

Recommendation: "Develop and test measures of transplant center organ acceptance to help inform organ allocation."

In 2021, the reason for refusal of an organ list was updated.[93] Revising the list of refusal codes supports increased efficiency of the OPTN through better understanding of refusal behaviors. Offering members more options for reporting why an offered organ is refused provides more robust data to develop improved allocation strategies to reduce cold ischemic time and number of non-utilized organs well as increase the number of transplants.

Question. Why is UNOS so far behind in creating Application Programming Interface (API) software that electronically transmit data between hospitals/OPOs/transplant centers to UNOS without having to manually enter data into other databases first? What APIs currently exist? What is the process for their use? How many are entities in the system are using APIs?

UNOS launched the UNet application in 1999 with tools for users to transmit data electronically to avoid manual entry. As part of ongoing modernization, UNOS started a formal API program in 2016. Since that time, UNOS development and implementation of APIs has advanced and is increasing.

As of September 2022, 243 hospitals and OPOs use APIs to transmit or receive data. Our external APIs empower OPTN members to electronically:

- Manage donor data
  - o Demographics
  - o Vitals
  - o Medical and social history
  - o Clinical lab values
  - o Infectious disease testing results

---

[92] Wey, A., Foutz, J., Gustafson, S.K., Carrico, R.J., Sisaithong, K., Tosoc-Haskell, H., McBride, M., Klassen, D., Salkowski, N., Kasiske, B.L., Israni, A.K., Snyder, J.J. "The Collaborative Innovation and Improvement Network (COIIN): Effect on donor yield, wait-list mortality, transplant rates, and offer acceptance." *Am J Transplant.* 2020 Apr;20(4):1076–1086. *https:// pubmed.ncbi.nlm.nih.gov/31612617/.*

[93] Project to update refusal codes. OPTN Data Advisory Committee. Nd. https:// optn.transplant.hrsa.gov/policies-bylaws/a-closer-look/project-to-update-refusal-codes/.

  - Diagnostic test results
  - Urinalysis
  - Blood gases
  - Culture results
  - Medications and fluids
  - Human Leukocyte Antigens (HLA)
  - Kidney preservation data
  - File attachments (for images and source documentation)
- Manage candidate data
  - Demographics
  - Unacceptable antigens
  - Liver labs
  - Lung labs and functional status
  - Offer acceptances
- Report organ-specific data on patients and donors at key transplant milestones
  - Transplant Candidate Registration (TCR)
  - Transplant Recipient Registration (TRR)
    - Transplant Immunosuppression Data (IMR)
  - Transplant Recipient Follow-Up (TRF)
    - Transplant Immunosuppression Data during Follow-Up (IMF)
  - Deceased Donor Registration (DDR)
  - Living Donor Registration (LDR)
  - Living Donor Follow-Up (LDF)
- Calculate key transplantation scores
  - Calculated Panel Reactive Antibody Score (CPRA)
  - Model for End-Stage Liver Disease Score (MELD)
  - Pediatric End-Stage Liver Disease Score (PELD)
  - Lung Allocation Score (LAS)
- Report deceased donor referrals
- Retrieve donor hospital data
- Retrieve public reporting data

UNOS coordinates with OPTN members and EHR vendors prior, during, and after our own API development. This includes conducting community research to identify API development targets that OPTN members and their EHR vendors want to integrate with, maintaining regular communication and hosting town hall events with the community to describe upcoming offerings and changes to existing APIs, and collaborating with vendors and members throughout their implementations.

In addition to providing direct user assistance, we maintain a developer portal with detailed API documentation through our Google Cloud API Management platform, Apigee. We inform stakeholders of upcoming changes months in advance, provide them with specification details prior to implementation, and offer direct support throughout their own work.

Furthermore, we maintain our Beta Portal, an external facing, non-production OPTN System (UNet) environment that enables vendors and members to build and test their own systems against upcoming changes. Changes to existing APIs are deployed to Beta Portal 6–8 weeks prior to moving to production. UNOS regularly monitors Beta Portal activity to identify challenges developers are encountering. We also adapt our API roadmap to minimize the frequency an API experiences significant changes. These measures appropriately throttle our own development to provide stability for our customers (OPTN members end users) while still improving our technology.

The U.S. health-care system's unique complexity and fragmentation presents both a greater need for integration and a higher barrier to it, and that is reflected in current API adoption. UNOS recognizes that building APIs does not guarantee that transplant hospitals, organ procurement organizations and histocompatibility laboratories will use them. Decisions to adopt APIs go through software vendors as well as OPTN members' leadership, IT teams, and clinicians. These parties act in alignment with their own interests and constraints, and may choose to rely on historical solutions. Transplantation remains a small sector of health care, and in this respect, lagging API adoption and continued reliance on historical solutions are to be expected.

Nevertheless, UNOS is not a passive observer in this space. While OPTN members have not been mandated to use APIs, UNOS has taken measures to lead the community forward through the deprecation of previously developed solutions and standards. This includes the recent sunset of a tool to import candidates' unacceptable antigen data, which increased use of the corresponding API from 16 centers in January 2022 to 91 centers in September 2022. Similarly, UNOS is enforcing updates to API authentication protocols in 2022, ensuring that OPTN members consistently adhere to the most current cybersecurity standards for integration. In these cases, UNOS balances community readiness and value to the OPTN to set appropriate deadlines, similar to Congress and HHS's journey to retire ICD–9 from 2008 to 2015.

To further drive adoption, the UNOS API program has begun ramping up proactive engagement efforts with OPTN members. Staff are conducting direct outreach to OPTN members and EHR Vendors for API implementation based on their needs and their EHR vendors' capabilities, to assist with implementation and testing, and to drive continuous improvement for future API development, rollout, and updates. UNOS is also partnering with Accenture Federal, a consulting firm and tech leader, to expand and extend our API strategy to increase API adoption with plans to assist OPTN members with any implementation or testing needs, and driving process improvements to further streamline future adoption.

Question. What have you committed to investing in OPTN systems to bring them into the 21st century? What is your action plan, timeline and allocation of resources to do so?

Answer. Some of the key technology trends in the 21st century are Microservices, APIs, Cloud, Mobile, Big Data/Machine Learning and leveraging Agile methodology to build software.

In addition to implementing OPTN policy projects, since 2014, UNOS has leveraged these industry themes and never lost sight that the most important factor of successfully using technology is to focus on the customer.

With that in mind, to date we have invested in iterative modular development and automated testing while building an API platform, using Google Cloud's Apigee, that we can use to share data securely using RFC standards. We focused on modularizing our software through microservices. These web-based microservices are a foundation for all development as we build new solutions, seamlessly share data with external systems, and transform our production systems used by OPTN members to save lives. The illustration and summaries below depict some of the modernization efforts accomplished since 2016. In addition, the projects listed below the timeline are other OPTN Board of Directors or Member requested projects implemented during that time.

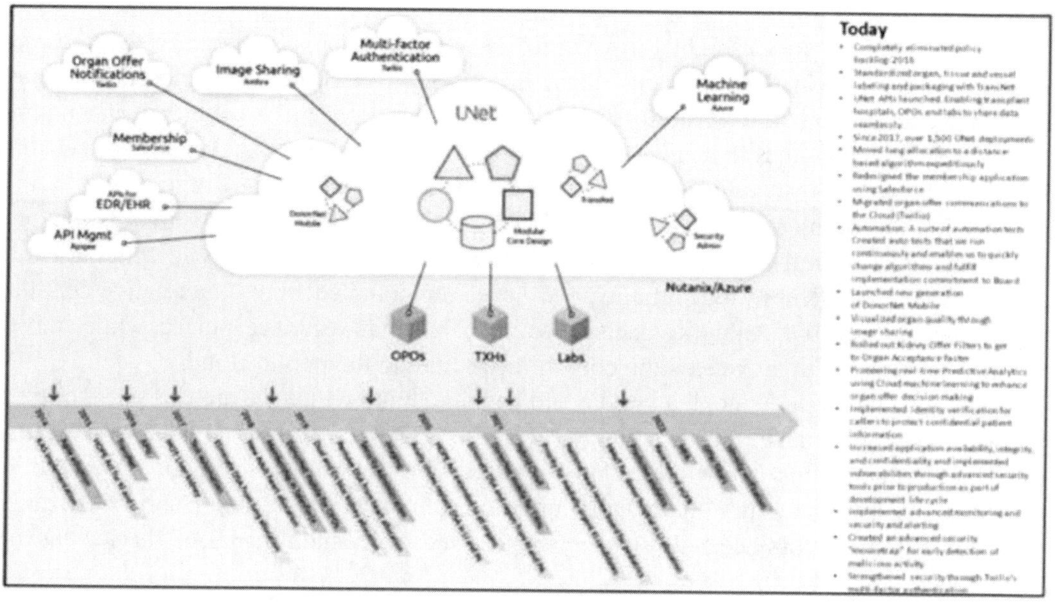

Technology Highlights Since 2016

In 2016, in addition to launching our APIs and Microservices efforts, UNOS developed and released reporting and analytics capabilities to help improve the quality, scope, and timeliness of organ offers for transplant centers and OPOs. Leveraging Big Data concepts, Hortonworks Connected Data Platforms, 100-percent open-source ApacheTM Hadoop and Tableau, transplant centers were given automated, detailed, and visually rich reports on all organ offers they received and the outcome if it was transplanted.

In 2017, UNOS developed a matching function test automation suite to conduct ongoing software testing to reduce project implementation time. This suite continues to be updated with every OPTN policy change or customer requested functionality enhancement. This was built on the open-source framework Selenium and gives us the robust capabilities to leverage coding to test all critical features.

In 2018, UNOS implemented and integrated with Salesforce.com leveraging their industry leading Software as a Service (SaaS) Customer Relationship Membership (CRM) platform to manage the OPTN Membership.

Also in 2018, a new reimagined and modernized version of the OPO mobile experience was released. This product was developed with critical input and prioritization by the OPO community and incorporated numerous existing and newly developed microservices.

We continued this journey in 2019, when we created a cross-departmental team that is focused on creating public cloud patterns that can scale our ideas and core infrastructure for the capabilities found in the public cloud. In parallel, we de veloped a new Security Administration application. The new application increased capabilities for OPTN site security administrators, leveraged microservices and features an immersive, modern user experience.

In 2020, UNOS implemented an integrated Clinical Image Sharing solution via integration with an industry leader, Ambra Health. This intuitive, feature rich DICOM viewer enables OPOs to upload organ donor clinical studies and allows transplant professionals to make more informed decisions.

Also in 2020, UNOS launched a new mobile, web-responsive experience for transplant hospitals to interact with DonorNet utilizing microservices. We collaborated closely with many transplant coordinators, administrators, and surgeons throughout the country using human-centered design techniques to create and test designs. This new design and experience enabled them to evaluate and respond to offers regardless of where they are at any time of day.

In 2021, we completed a transformation to a multi-regional hybrid cloud environment built using Nutanix cloud infrastructure and Microsoft Azure public cloud. Aligned with our cloud-first approach for all new functionality, we have implemented new cloud-native real-time capabilities in Predictive Analytics decision support for organ offer acceptance, while actively executing a roadmap to move existing core infrastructure to the public cloud.

To protect the organ matching system and patient data to which we are entrusted, over the last several years we made significant investments in security capabilities aligned with defense-in-depth and zero trust principles. Among these are robust authentication capabilities, application code vulnerability scanning, security log aggregation, correlation and visualization, industry leading endpoint detection and response, and distributed denial of service (DDoS) protection.

Resources Allocated

Since 2016, UNOS has invested more than 200,000 hours of resources into ongoing technology modernization efforts; we understand the importance of enhancing and securing the technology the OPTN members use to save lives.

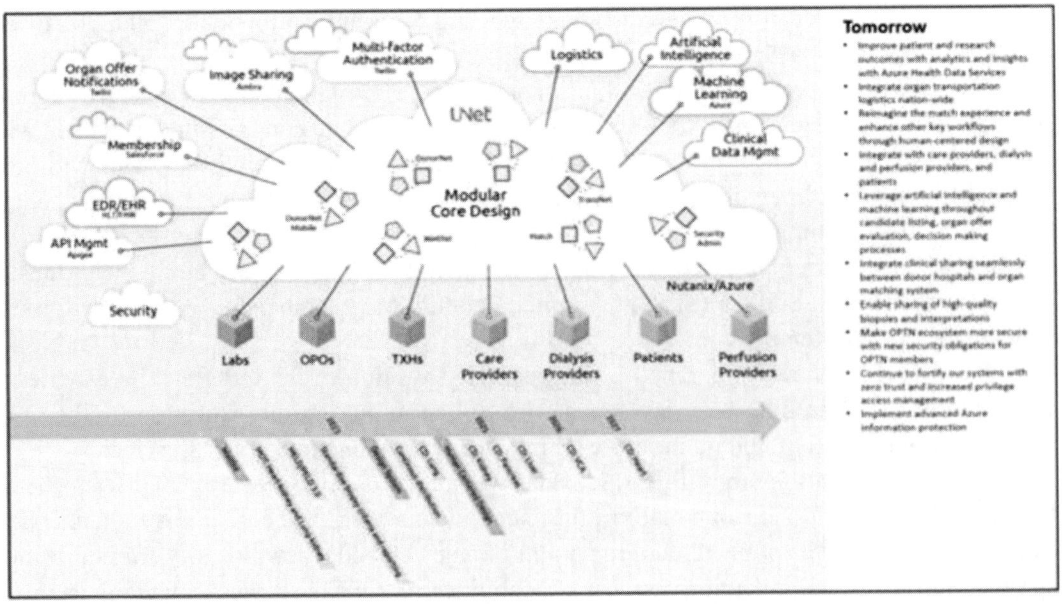

UNOS routinely documents and updates the OPTN Network Operations Oversight Committee (NOOC) and HRSA on improvement plans. Please see roadmap below, shared with the NOOC and HRSA, for planned improvements to the system.

The illustration below depicts continued improvements and innovation areas we envision and aim to implement over the next several years.

UNOS leverages microservices (internal-facing APIs) as part of its continued technology transformation into a modern microservices architecture. A number of internal system components already make heavy use of internal APIs, free of external dependencies, allowing UNOS to rapidly expand its footprint in this area. Through these efforts, we continue to mature our technology systems and practices.

Partnering with Leaders in Technology Innovation

A significant component of our strategy is leveraging or integrating leading technologies in areas beneficial to the transplant ecosystem. That is the reason UNOS has advanced the OPTN system with solutions utilizing open-source frameworks that include: Angular; Swift; Kotlin; and NodeJS.

This is extended with integrations offered by key Cloud SaaS providers: Twilio; Salesforce; Ambra; and Azure.

UNOS understands and has prioritized the use of opensource frameworks and created partnerships with dozens of recognized technology leaders to advance the capabilities of the OPTN system.

During the transformation of our technology, we have partnered with the Microsoft Tech for Social Impact team to align our vision with a reality we can bring to the transplant community. This partnership has also helped us make connections with other countries, share our learnings and assist them in using the public cloud for solving their problems.

Question. Why does it take 2-plus years to process a policy change at the OPTN, even when it is non-controversial and there is agreement on the needed change?

Answer. The OPTN must balance its requirements under the law, which includes involving multiple stakeholders during the policy development process and during public comment. Public comment, a critical aspect of the policy development process is required by NOTA (42 U.S.C. § 274(b)(2)(B)) and the OPTN final rule (42 CFR§ 121.4(b)(1)).

The time to process large allocation proposals has fallen over the last decade. For example, the revised kidney allocation system took over 9 years and liver distribution over 6 years. In contrast, the development of lung continuous distribution, which included an overhaul of the entire framework of the allocation system and member tools, took less than 3 years to develop.

Continuous advances in the science and practice of organ transplantation require ongoing refinement of policy that involves experts in the field as well as the public and the larger donation and transplant community. To ensure the best possible solutions for patients awaiting transplantation and for the donors whose precious gifts make that possible, the policy development process is:[94]

[94] OPTN Policy Development Process. https://optn.transplant.hrsa.gov/policies-bylaws/policy-development/#policy Process.

- Inclusive—encouraging participation by interested persons, organizations and the general public.
- Responsive—assessing and modifying policies to remain current with the field.
- Equitable—helping to ensure that all patients have an equal chance of receiving a suitable organ.
- Evidence based—making decisions based on extensive and valid scientific data and analysis.

The hundreds of volunteers who serve on OPTN committees that develop policy comprise highly experienced medical professionals, patients, and donor families. UNOS values the feedback of the whole community and strives to achieve consensus, which contributes to the time it takes to develop a policy.

Question. During the hearing, you referenced a rubric for matters referred to the Membership and Professional Standards Committee (MPSC)? Please provide the rubric.

Answer. The rubric, part of the MPSC's operational rules, is provided as part of this submission.

Question. What are you doing to ensure OPOs and donor hospital and transplant centers are aligned in their work? And what accountability measures do you have in place for transplant centers to align their efforts with those of OPOs?

Answer. UNOS brings together all stakeholders in the community to drive continuous improvement and increase transplant.

Our field is uniquely interdependent. Making the system more equitable and efficient requires regulatory agencies, OPOs, transplant centers and the approximately 6,000 donor hospitals in the U.S. to efficiently and effectively align their work toward our common goal of saving and enhancing lives. Many people, often in different parts of the country, collaborate at all hours of the day or night. This occurs nowhere else in medicine, and it requires our constant vigilance and care to assure that it is done well and that all facets of the system are accountable for its success.

Recent efforts by UNOS to better align work across the organ donation and transplant system and ensure the highest level of accountability include:

- A new performance monitoring system for transplant hospitals.
- Collaborative Improvement (CI) and Individual Member Focused Improvement (IMFI) projects that bring together transplant programs, OPOs and HRSA on quality improvement initiatives.[95]
- The incorporation of predictive analytics into the organ offer experience for adult deceased donor kidneys that is intended to impact acceptance behavior and increase organ utilization.

Every day, our community's collective efforts to provide exceptional clinical care, assure equitable organ allocation policies, and innovate to continuously improve move the system forward and save even more lives.

---

95 OPTN Collaborative Improvement. https://optn.transplant.hrsa.gov/professionals/improvement/collaborative-improvement/.

Prepared Statement of Hon. Ron Wyden, a U.S. Senator from Oregon

The last place anybody wants to hear about gross mismanagement and incompetence is in the business of saving lives. That's precisely and unfortunately what the Finance Committee meets to discuss today.

This morning's hearing is an update on an investigation Senator Grassley and I, along with Senator Cardin and Senator Young, have been conducting for more than 2½ years. It examines the network of dozens of organizations that manage organ transplants, and particularly the group that oversees and coordinates them, the United Network for Organ Sharing, or UNOS. We have reviewed 100,000 UNOS documents totaling more than a half-million pages.

Before I get to specific findings, I want to frame what we've learned as simply as possible. Far too many Americans are dying needlessly because UNOS and many of the transplant organizations it oversees are failing and seem uninterested in improving.

These issues involve an alphabet soup of acronyms and organizations, so I'll start out with a bit of background. A 1984 law created the first computerized system to match sick patients with the organs they needed. It was named the Organ Procurement and Transplantation Network. Somebody needed to manage that system for the entire country, so the government sought to contract an organization to run it. UNOS was the only bidder for that first contract in 1986. The contract has come up for bid seven other times. UNOS has won all seven.

Today the network UNOS oversees is made up of nearly 400 members, including 252 transplant centers and 57 regional organizations known as organ procurement organizations, or OPOs. Each OPO has a defined geographic service area. A family sitting in a hospital room thinking about donating a loved-one's organ doesn't have a choice of OPOs.

Those are the important terms to remember. When a kidney donated in Corvallis needs to get to a patient in Portland, that's where an OPO comes in. UNOS oversees the OPOs. As our investigation shows, UNOS does it very poorly.

Serious errors in the procurement and transplant system are shockingly common. Between 2010 and 2020, more than 1,100 complaints were filed by patients and families, staff, transplant centers, and others. The nature of those complaints runs the gamut. For example, in a number of cases OPOs had failed to complete critical, mandatory tests for things like blood types, disease, and infection.

Our investigation found one patient died after being transplanted with lungs that a South Carolina OPO marked with the wrong blood type. Similar blood-type errors happened elsewhere, and patients developed serious illness. Some had to have organs removed after transplant.

Another patient was told he would likely die within 3 years after an OPO in Ohio supplied him with a heart from a donor who had died of a malignant brain tumor. UNOS did not pursue any disciplinary action.

In a case from Florida, another patient contracted cancer from transplanted organs, and the OPO sat on the evidence for months.

In total, our investigation found that between 2008 and 2015, 249 transplant recipients developed a disease from transplanted organs. More than a quarter of them died.

Delivering organs has been another source of life-threatening errors. We found 53 such complaints between 2010 and 2020, as well as evidence that those were just the tip of the iceberg. In some cases, couriers missed a flight. In others, the organs were abandoned at airports. Some organs were never picked up. Many of these failures resulted in organs being discarded.

It's reasonable to assume that many more errors are going unreported. Why? Because filing official complaints with UNOS appears to accomplish zero productive oversight or reform. Organ transplant professionals repeatedly told the Finance Committee that the UNOS complaint process was a "black hole." Complaints went in, UNOS went quiet.

In interviews with the committee, UNOS leaders have dragged their feet, dodged tough questions, and shifted responsibility onto others. Investigations and disciplinary measures rarely amount to more than a slap on the wrist. Only one time— just once—has UNOS recommended that an OPO lose certification.

The bottom line is that the failures we've uncovered cost lives. Thousands of organs donated each year wind up discarded, including one in four kidneys. Yet according to Federal data, roughly 6,000 Americans die every year while waiting for an organ transplant.

This kind of mismanagement has a disproportionate impact on minority Americans. African Americans, for example, have a greater need for kidney transplants than those from other demographic groups.

The Centers for Medicare and Medicaid Services recently issued new standards for OPO performance, and more than a third of OPOs are failing to meet them. Fixing what's broken could substantially increase the supply of lifesaving organs available for transplant.

Finally, another area of the committee's investigation has examined the IT used by UNOS to run the transplant network. This system is outdated, mismanaged, and insecure. Using such decrepit tech to run the transplant network puts lives in danger and puts sensitive data at risk, and there is no apparent solution in sight. In a report issued last year titled "Lives Are at Stake," the U.S. Digital Service flatly concluded that UNOS did not have the technical capability to modernize the system.

I'll close on this. If you looked at the staff at UNOS and many of the Nation's OPOs, I'd wager the vast majority are hardworking people doing their best to save lives. The glaring issues uncovered in our investigation stem from leadership failures.

Our investigation is ongoing. It's clear this system needs reform badly. We're going to continue digging into issues at UNOS and the OPOs, as well as the policies that need changing at the Federal level. This is not a partisan subject. Everybody wants this system to work with as few errors as possible. Senators Grassley, Cardin, Young, and I are going to keep at it.

SFC OPTN Hearing
Exhibit O.148

Date: Thursday, March 1 2018 02:59 PM
Subject: Re: directed donation
From: Alexandra Glazier [redacted]
To: Brian M. Shepard [redacted]

Right.

But that said, if you needed surgery, I would not suggest you go under the knife with Alex Glazier, MD.

Alexandra K. Glazier, Esq.
President & CEO
New England Donor Services
[redacted]

On Mar 1, 2018, at 1:42 PM, Brian M. Shepard <[redacted]> wrote:

> [redacted] was on the phone.
>
> She said, "[redacted] tried to debate ALEX!"
>
> Her impression was that it did not go well for [redacted]
>
> **From:** Alexandra Glazier [[redacted]]
> **Sent:** Thursday, March 1, 2018 2:14 PM
> **To:** Brian M. Shepard [redacted]>
> **Subject:** Re: directed donation
>
> Really? I didn't copy [redacted] on my email. Did she say [redacted] was being a pest? Or that the mpsc was sideways?
>
> Alexandra K. Glazier, Esq.
> President & CEO
> New England Donor Services
> [redacted]
>
> On Mar 1, 2018, at 12:58 PM, Brian M. Shepard [redacted]> wrote:
>
> > [redacted] brought it up to me already, so I heard it from her.
> >
> > **From:** Alexandra Glazier [[redacted]]
> > **Sent:** Thursday, March 1, 2018 1:04 PM
> > **To:** Brian M. Shepard <[redacted]
> > **Subject:** Re: directed donation
> >
> > Keep in mind law is like sausage- it tastes great but you don't want to know how it's made.

SFC OPTN Hearing
Exhibit O.148

I think in the end the MPSC does a good job coming to a reasoned and appropriate result. Trust that there are enough experts from different backgrounds that will and do speak up that even if the path isn't linear ultimately we get there.

So I guess my message is: Be patient grasshopper.

And if you bring up this example (unless your staff tell you about it) it will seem like I'm complaining to you. Which I am. But my complaint is about [redacted] not the MPSC.

Alexandra K. Glazier, Esq.
President & CEO
New England Donor Services
[redacted]

On Mar 1, 2018, at 11:57 AM, Brian M. Shepard <[redacted]> wrote:

> I know you agree, but this whole thing drives me nuts. I don't know how to fill important positions with people who know what they're doing.
>
> Allowing the community to fill these jobs increases the community's belief in the validity of the outcomes. Even while it make MPSC more variable, or allocation policy less coherent. It's like putting your kids' artwork up at home. You value it because of how it was created rather than whether it's well done. Only in this case, we persuade ourselves that it's well done anyway.
>
> We've started to make some improvements in the process, and I know the goal can't be 500 of you, but I'm really struggling with how to do this better than we do now.
>
> **From:** Alexandra Glazier [redacted]
> **Sent:** Thursday, March 1, 2018 10:06 AM
> **To:** Brian M. Shepard <[redacted]
> **Subject:** Re: directed donation
>
> I did. And I was a bit sharp about it bc he started arguing with me. I shut it down.
> But he created enough confusion that other members asked for a summary of the law to understand if maybe the opo was legitimately confused bc its unsettled/unclear law.
> I offered to do that next mtg.
>
> **From:** Brian Shepard [redacted]
> **Date:** Thursday, March 1, 2018 at 9:57 AM
> **To:** Alexandra Glazier <[redacted]
> **Subject:** RE: directed donation
>
> Often wrong, never in doubt.
>
> What was the outcome? Did you straighten him out in public? Did [redacted]?
>
> **From:** Alexandra Glazier [redacted]
> **Sent:** Thursday, March 1, 2018 9:56 AM

SFC OPTN Hearing
Exhibit O.148

To: Brian M. Shepard <[redacted]
Subject: FW: directed donation

FYI–[redacted] told the MPSC this was unsettled law and maybe ok that the OPO skipped a whole bunch of people for 3 different organ allocations to comply with a donor family's request that all of their daughter's donated organs only go to the state the parent's live in (which wasn't even the state the donor lived in or where the donation occurred – not that is matters - but how crazy is that?)

From: Alexandra Glazier [redacted]
Date: Thursday, March 1, 2018 at 8:35 AM
To: [redacted]
Cc: [redacted] <
[redacted]
Subject: directed donation

[redacted]: This is settled under both federal law (Final Rule) and state law (the UAGA). The conclusion that federal law pre-empts state law is not necessary on this issue although there has never been a successful legal challenge to NOTA's pre-emption over organ allocation and while pre-emption analysis is always complex I believe its fairly clear.

Here is the UAGA provision (highlighted relevant language):

SECTION 11. PERSONS THAT MAY RECEIVE ANATOMICAL GIFT; PURPOSE OF ANATOMICAL GIFT.

(a) An anatomical gift may be made to the following persons named in the document of gift:

(1) a hospital; accredited medical school, dental school, college, or university; organ procurement organization; or other appropriate person, for research or education;

(2) subject to subsection (b), an individual designated by the person making the anatomical gift if the individual is the recipient of the part;

(3) an eye bank or tissue bank.

(b) If an anatomical gift to an individual under subsection (a)(2) cannot be transplanted into the individual, the part passes in accordance with subsection (g) in the absence of an express, contrary indication by the person making the anatomical gift.

(g) For purposes of subsections (b), (e), and (f) the following rules apply:
(1) If the part is an eye, the gift passes to the appropriate eye bank.
(2) If the part is tissue, the gift passes to the appropriate tissue bank.
(3) If the part is an organ, the gift passes to the appropriate organ procurement organization

SFC OPTN Hearing
Exhibit O.148

To: Brian M. Shepard <[redacted]
Subject: FW: directed donation

FYI–[redacted] told the MPSC this was unsettled law and maybe ok that the OPO skipped a whole bunch of people for 3 different organ allocations to comply with a donor family's request that all of their daughter's donated organs only go to the state the parent's live in (which wasn't even the state the donor lived in or where the donation occurred – not that is matters - but how crazy is that?)

From: Alexandra Glazier [redacted]
Date: Thursday, March 1, 2018 at 8:35 AM
To: [redacted]
Cc: [redacted] <
[redacted]
Subject: directed donation

[redacted]: This is settled under both federal law (Final Rule) and state law (the UAGA). The conclusion that federal law pre-empts state law is not necessary on this issue although there has never been a successful legal challenge to NOTA's pre-emption over organ allocation and while pre-emption analysis is always complex I believe its fairly clear.

Here is the UAGA provision (highlighted relevant language):

SECTION 11. PERSONS THAT MAY RECEIVE ANATOMICAL GIFT; PURPOSE OF ANATOMICAL GIFT.

(a) An anatomical gift may be made to the following persons named in the document of gift:

(1) a hospital; accredited medical school, dental school, college, or university; organ procurement organization; or other appropriate person, for research or education;

(2) subject to subsection (b), an individual designated by the person making the anatomical gift if the individual is the recipient of the part;

(3) an eye bank or tissue bank.

(b) If an anatomical gift to an individual under subsection (a)(2) cannot be transplanted into the individual, the part passes in accordance with subsection (g) in the absence of an express, contrary indication by the person making the anatomical gift.

(g) For purposes of subsections (b), (e), and (f) the following rules apply:
(1) If the part is an eye, the gift passes to the appropriate eye bank.
(2) If the part is tissue, the gift passes to the appropriate tissue bank.
(3) If the part is an organ, the gift passes to the appropriate organ procurement organization

SFC OPTN Hearing
Exhibit O.148

as custodian of the organ.

Here is the Federal Law which requires all organs to be allocated under the OPTN policies with an exception for directed donation if a recipient is named (consistent with UAGA):

§121.8 Allocation of organs.

(h) *Directed donation.* Nothing in this section shall prohibit the allocation of an organ **to a recipient named** by those authorized to make the donation.

Alexandra K. Glazier, Esq.
President & CEO
New England Donor Services – an affiliation of LifeChoice and New England Organ Bank
[redacted]

<image001.png>

SFC OPTN Hearing
Exhibit O.149

Date: Thursday, January 19 2017 09:37 PM
Subject: Re: Lung bio [redacted]
From: Alexandra Glazier <[redacted]>
To: Brian M. Shepard <[redacted]>;

LC can't say NEOB screwed up bc they are joint and severally liable to perform together.

In ten yrs you'll be 55. Too young to retire.
Politics perhaps?
Or the board will get smart and put golden handcuffs on you.

Alexandra K. Glazier, Esq.
President & CEO
New England Donor Services
[redacted]

On Jan 19, 2017, at 5:37 PM, Brian M. Shepard <[redacted]> wrote:

They're clearly less separate than [redacted], but what if LC told us that NEOB had screwed up entering lab results? At least, there'd still be a member to have a discussion with, which doesn't exist at [redacted]

I could support a limited category of members allowed to perform functions according to existing policies. 10 years from now, when HRSA is pushing MPSC to investigate some misuse of the machines, I'll be retired.

From: Alexandra Glazier [redacted]
Sent: Thursday, January 19, 2017 5:33 PM
To: Brian M. Shepard <[redacted]
Subject: Re: Lung bio [redacted]

Ha - excellent point.

But I would say the OPOs (members) and NEDS are one and the same - OPO functions are not outsourced. No contracts or service agreements.

Both OPOs are accountable to UNOS and as CEO of both I have control over operations/policies.

But you're right - it's not a totally bright line. Lawyer full employment act.

Alexandra K. Glazier, Esq.
President & CEO
New England Donor Services
[redacted]

On Jan 19, 2017, at 5:26 PM, Brian M. Shepard <[redacted]wrote:

I think there are other less-intrusive seeming contractors (offer screening centers) that perform duties required by policy, so it's not quite as clean as that, but I agree with the spirit. Does NEDS (not a member) perform any duties for NEOB or Lifechoice?

From: Alexandra Glazier [redacted]
Sent: Thursday, January 19, 2017 5:19 PM

SFC OPTN Hearing
Exhibit O.149

To: Brian M. Shepard [redacted]
Subject: Re: Lung bio[redacted]

Only UNOS members should be permitted to perform TX Ctr or OPO core responsibilities - the ones that are required by UNOS policy.

Yes, could and should be limited to that. UNOS cannot be overseeing device companies.

If such a device member violated UNOS policy, the consequences would include probation or member not in good standing. If that happened, the member device company could no longer perform the duties and therefore cannot participate in the system.

The privilege comes with duties.

Carrot and stick.

Alexandra K. Glazier, Esq.
President & CEO
New England Donor Services
[redacted]

On Jan 19, 2017, at 5:04 PM, Brian M. Shepard [redacted] > wrote:

> Good point. Ideally, we'd be able to create a membership category and policies that just focused on those core functions, which we understand and would be able to monitor. I'm just worried that the overgrown homeowners association that we run here will drag us into things we don't really understand. If you're right (and I grudgingly concede that you could be), the danger of going too far in one direction might be real, but might be causing me to overcorrect too far in the other.
>
> **From:** Alexandra Glazier [redacted]
> **Sent:** Thursday, January 19, 2017 4:26 PM
> **To:** Brian M. Shepard[redacted]
> **Subject:** Re: Lung bio[redacted]
>
> Not the same.
>
> Couriers are not responsible for core OPO functions required by specific UNOS policy.
>
> Unlike labeling which is.
>
> If a courier loses an organ, there is no UNOS policy violation.
>
> If a device company mislabeled an organ (let's say wrong ABO) - policy violation.
>
> You shouldn't want members to ever outsource core responsibilities. That creates the safety gap and compliance oversight issue.
>
> Alexandra K. Glazier, Esq.
> President & CEO
> New England Donor Services
> [redacted]
>
> On Jan 19, 2017, at 1:01 PM, Brian M. Shepard [redacted]wrote:

SFC OPTN Hearing
Exhibit O.149

I would think that holding OPOs responsible would be similar to the way you're responsible for couriers now. If a courier loses or damages an organ but has an otherwise solid record and the OPO shows they've worked with the courier to reduce the chance of recurrence, the MPSC isn't going to come crashing down. If you keep hiring the same courier over and over despite multiple issues, that's a preventable problem.

This particular contractor (perfusionists) clearly has a much greater ability to screw up, and we'll need a better way than we have now to review and correct them. They're not the only service contractor OPOs and tx centers use, though, and we seem to be able to manage the delegated responsibilities in other cases.

From: Alexandra Glazier [redacted]
Sent: Thursday, January 19, 2017 11:14 AM
To: Brian M. Shepard [redacted]
Subject: Re: Lung bio [redacted]

Yes, I agree with you and for those of us with our big boy pants on, we can handle that liability shift and stomach the possibility of being hauled to the MPSC for someone else's error because the benefit is worth the risk.

But there are many OPOs that may decide simply not to put themselves in that position. This will thwart wide adoption of what could leverage positive growth for the whole field.

And what will the MPSC do when the OPO has not violated any packaging/labeling policies but nonetheless there is a patient death bc the device company screwed up? Holding the OPO accountable for an agent's error would guarantee OPOs will not want to put themselves in that position (would you want to be publicly disciplined or have your contract to be cancelled based on another organization's error that you have no control over?).

So guidance from UNOS could be that the "responsibility" for labelling will be determined by the contractual relationship however, again, with no compliance jurisdiction over the device company, the contract is meaningless from the OPTN perspective.

This is a foreseeable gap in the system's safety net.

Alexandra K. Glazier, Esq.
President & CEO
New England Donor Services – an affiliation of LifeChoice and New England Organ Bank
[redacted]

<image001.png>

From: Brian Shepard <[redacted]
Date: Thursday, January 19, 2017 at 11:00 AM
To: Alexandra Glazier <[redacted]
Subject: RE: Lung bio [redacted]

I can't believe I'm even writing this, but I think we should trust the lawyers on this one.

In the long run, we need to determine whether to make these third parties members, but there's more to it that just saying so – what standards will they follow, how will we survey, how will MPSC evaluate if the only expertise is in a very small handful of perfusion centers. Our responsibility/inability to oversee histo labs is a constant pain in the ass.

SFC OPTN Hearing
Exhibit O.149

In the short run, though, I don't know why they aren't just an agent of one of the members. That might be an OPO that pre-emptively decides to improve the lungs before running a match, or it might be a center that's been allocated organs that wants to tune them up before they tx. There's going to be a contract or some written instructions that would make clear who the perfusionist is acting for. I don't see the upside in UNOS making a blanket statement that they're always an agent of the center or always an agent of an OPO.

UNOS could offer guidance that clarifies that custody is dependent on who's making the decision to perfuse. I think that's clarifying, others might think "it depends" is less than crystal clear.

In the meantime, trying to work on a technological solution to the re-labeling issue that doesn't have to wait for all of this to resolve.

Thanks.

From: Alexandra Glazier [redacted]
Sent: Thursday, January 19, 2017 10:25 AM
To: Brian M. Shepard <[redacted]
Subject: Re: Lung bio[redacted]

Hi Brian -

NEOB attempted to send lungs only once but it didn't happen for clinical reasons (and that was over a year and a half ago). We have very active lung programs here so we have not pursued.

The packaging concern is a chain of custody issue. After the lungs are repaired, [redacted] has to repackage according to UNOS policy and send back to accepting program. [redacted] states that they follow all UNOS policies but the concern is that if the lungs aren't packaged correctly, or labeled wrong, who is held responsible? Because they are not an OPTN member, would the OPO or receiving Tx center be responsible for that error (from the OPTN's perspective – us lawyers can shift any legal liability through contract).

[redacted] tells me the MPSC was considering this issue but hasn't come to resolution or discussed recently.

As you know, there are also concerns about the role device companies may play is allocation.

It's complicated but worth trying to resolve as these innovations will drive growth in organ availability.

Hope this helps,
Alex

Alexandra K. Glazier, Esq.
President & CEO
New England Donor Services – an affiliation of LifeChoice and New England Organ Bank
[redacted]

<image001.png>

SFC OPTN Hearing
Exhibit O.149

From: Brian Shepard <[redacted]
Date: Thursday, January 19, 2017 at 8:45 AM
To: Alexandra Glazier <[redacted]
Subject: Lung bio[redacted]

Do you ever ship lungs to [redacted]? Trying to better understand a TransNet packaging issue.

Thanks.

Brian Shepard
Chief Executive Officer

<image002.png>

Working together. Saving lives.

[redacted]

As of January 3, 2017, LifeChoice Donor Services and New England Organ Bank employees - now affiliated under New England Donor Services - will have a new email domain for their email addresses.
The new domain is: neds.org

As of January 3, 2017, LifeChoice Donor Services and New England Organ Bank employees - now affiliated under New England Donor Services - will have a new email domain for their email addresses.
The new domain is: neds.org

As of January 3, 2017, LifeChoice Donor Services and New England Organ Bank employees - now affiliated under New England Donor Services - will have a new email domain for their email addresses.
The new domain is: neds.org

As of January 3, 2017, LifeChoice Donor Services and New England Organ Bank employees - now affiliated under New England Donor Services - will have a new email domain for their email addresses.
The new domain is: neds.org

SFC OPTN Hearing
Exhibit O.149

As of January 3, 2017, LifeChoice Donor Services and New England Organ Bank employees - now affiliated under New England Donor Services - will have a new email domain for their email addresses.
The new domain is: neds.org

As of January 3, 2017, LifeChoice Donor Services and New England Organ Bank employees - now affiliated under New England Donor Services - will have a new email domain for their email addresses.
The new domain is: neds.org

Communications

Letter Submitted by Jaison M. Abraham

Hello, Honorable Senator(s),

For the record, I believe it is extremely unfair to blame United Network for Organ Sharing (UNOS) and OPOs for bad performance and poor outcomes. The allocation system may not be perfect but has evolved over the years. It will always be a continuous process to decrease disparities and better serve patients. Transplant Centers should also be held accountable. Programs that failed to evolve their practices are struggling more. The Senate committee selected AdventHealth, a non-academic center with one of the lowest organ offer acceptance rates and lowest 1M, and lowest 1Y outcomes in its Kidney and Liver Transplant programs, to provide witness testimony in its investigation. Though I do not believe the Senate intended to select a low-performing center to represent the transplant community—it did. I urge the Senate committee to look at a broader cross-section of the transplant community for better representation at future hearings.

The U.S. Transplant system is the most developed and successful in the world. Transparency is one of its strengths. As transplant administrators, we appreciate the efforts of the senate to improve the transplant system and are hopeful that the inquiry will elevate processes and improve care for the patients cared for by all of the centers.

Respectfully,
Jaison Abraham, MBA, LSSBB
Director of Transplant Programs UF Health Shands
Office: 352–594–5288
Web: https://ufhealth.org/transplant-center/

American Society of Nephrology

1401 H Street, NW, Suite 900
Washington, DC 20005

On behalf of the 37 million Americans living with kidney diseases, thank you for your efforts to improve the United States transplant system. ASN seeks to transform transplant care and applauds the Senate Finance Committee for investigating shortcomings of the Organ Procurement Transplantation Network (OPTN).

"ASN believes a strong and equitable transplant system is essential to meet the needs of the more than 800,000 Americans living with kidney failure. While a kidney transplant is the optimal therapy for most people living with kidney failure, transplantation remains out of reach for too many people. ASN is deeply concerned with reports of technology failures from the OPTN contractor that are contributing to the immense organ discard rate and shortage of kidneys for transplantation. ASN reaffirms our call for the OPTN contract to be modernized. The more than 21,000 kidney health professionals who comprise ASN are committed to creating a world without kidney diseases, including by transforming transplant care. ASN commends the Senate Finance Committee for continuing to drive improvements in transplantation and stands in partnership to ensure all Americans who could benefit have access to this critical therapy," said ASN President Elect Michelle A. Josephson, M.D., FASN in a press statement.

Of the more than 100,000 people currently on the transplant waiting list, there are nearly 90,000 people currently waiting to receive a kidney, the largest subset of anyorgan. Devastatingly, a national organ shortage means that 13 people die every day while on the kidney transplant wait list.

ASN believes that transformations are needed across the transplant system in order to meet the growing need for kidney transplantation, including at the level of the OPTN. This statement focuses on 4 policy recommendations that address challenges related to the OPTN, including:

- Modernize the OPTN contract by separating the IT infrastructure into a distinct contract.
- Address barriers to transplant access that promote or exacerbate inequities, including the use of race in the organ quality metric that guides allocation Kidney Donor Profile Index (KPDI).
- Streamline oversight of the U.S. transplant system by establishing an office of organ transplantation.
- Elevate transplant patients as partners in care, including by improving transparency regarding organ offers.

Modernize the OPTN Contract by Separating the IT Infrastructure into a Distinct Contract

The OPTN is a quasi-governmental government agency responsible for establishing organ transplant and allocation policy, conducting oversight and enforcement of transplant programs and Organ Procurement Organizations (OPOs), and maintaining an IT infrastructure to support transplantation. The OPTN contract has been held by a single not-for-profit organization, the United Network for Organ Sharing (UNOS) since the contract was created in 1986.

UNOS maintains an IT infrastructure, which UNOS claims to be proprietary despite being developed under a federal contract with tax dollars and user fees, to support wait-listing, organ allocation, sharing of donor information and data capture for regulatory oversight. As revealed by The Washington Post, stakeholders in government have expressed repeated concerns over UNOS continued use of antiquated systems for data capture and collection with no validation tools or interoperability features. The stakeholders, including the White House U.S. Digital Service, noted deep issues with transparency when reviewed by the service as well as major security vulnerabilities. Efforts to modernize these systems have been slow and ineffective, with changes in policy such as new organ allocation schemes taking as long as a year or more to implement.

Further, data are collected from different parts of the transplant system at the expense and labor of transplant centers and OPO staff, and then returned back to transplant centers and OPOs in the form of well curated dashboards (for a fee for national datasets), while some free reporting tools exist, they are often clunky and lack the depth of information provided in paid reporting tools. Despite being established through taxpayer- and user-fee-supported funding, The Washington Post reports that UNOS claims ownership of the system and would charge the American taxpayer $55 million to purchase the current IT system should it ever lose the contract.

This arrangement is unique as other important responsibilities in transplantation, such as the statistical and analytical support provided by the Scientific Registry of Transplant Recipients (SRTR), are structured as an independent contract. It is no surprise that stakeholders ranging from the White House U.S. Digital Service to a bipartisan group of HHS technology officers to the National Academies of Science and Medicine have all called for the IT infrastructure responsibilities of OPTN to be separated into an independent and competitive contract. Separating the IT infrastructure portion of the OPTN contract would align with other federal contracting protocols, increase competition, and drive innovation.

Address Barriers to Transplant Access That Promote or Exacerbate Inequity, Including the Use of Race in the Organ Quality Metric That Guides Allocation, Kidney Donor Profile Index (KPDI)

Kidney transplantation is the optimal therapy for most people living with kidney failure, yet kidney transplantation is not equally accessible for all Americans. For example, Black patients are less likely to be identified as transplant candidates, referred for evaluation to receive a pre-emptive transplant, and to complete the transplant evaluation. Black patients are also less likely to have the preferred living donor and less likely to be placed on the waiting list, while also being more likely to receive lower quality kidneys regardless of the age of the patient and length onthe kidney wait list, and have poorer transplant graft survival for a multitude of reasons that may include difficulties in access to care—a cyclical and compounding struggle that is nearly impossible to defeat without real identification and solution to racism.

Many of the policies needed to establish equity in transplant require cooperation between multiple stakeholders in the private sector and across different government agencies. However, one improvement is squarely in the purview of the OPTN contractor: removing the use of race in metrics related to organ allocation.

Race does not have any physiological relationship with the function of a patient's kidney, yet clinical decision support tools such as the estimated Glomerular Filtration Rate equation (eGFR) have included race adjustor variables, systemically overestimating the kidney function of Black patients and leading to reduced access to transplantation. On June 27, 2022, OPTN finalized a policy to remove race as a variable from eGFR, following the recommendation of the American Society of Nephrology and National Kidney Foundation and citing concerns that the variable was leading to a 16% overestimation of kidney function among Black patients.

Despite this welcome decision, OPTN is still allowing a race adjustment in the Kidney Donor Profile Index (KDPI), with no public plans to cease their use. The KDPI estimates the relative risk of post-transplant kidney graft failure of organs obtained from a deceased donor. The KDPI includes a race variable, automatically assigning lower quality to kidneys obtained from Black donors independent of biological factors, arbitrarily reducing the supply of donated kidneys and effectively turning away the gift of life from Black donors. Analyses from SRTR have demonstrated that removing a race variable does not alter the equation's predictability of graft failure or patient survival. Race variables should be removed from tools assessing biological factors, including the organ quality metric that guides kidney allocation, the Kidney Donor Profile Index.

Streamline Oversight of the U.S. Transplant System by Establishing an Office of Organ Transplantation

Oversight of the U.S. transplant system is currently divided between the Centers for Medicare and Medicaid Services (CMS), who oversee transplant programs, and the Health Resources and Services Administration (HRSA), who oversee OPTN and OPO contractors. This split responsibility leads to gaps in oversight, confusion in navigating the transplant system, and a regulatory framework that does not elevate patients to be true partners in care.

One glaring example of this confusion is the use of financial means testing to evaluate a transplant recipient's eligibility to receive a transplant. In 2020, Congress passed the Comprehensive Immunosuppressive Drug Coverage Act, effectively ending the need for kidney transplant recipients to pay for immunosuppressive drugs out of pocket and a commonly used justification for financial screening.

Both transplant programs, regulated by CMS under the Conditions for Coverage, and the OPTN contractor, regulated by HRSA under the OPTN final rule mandate that patient selection (CMS) and organ allocation (HRSA) must ensure fair and non-discriminatory distribution of organs, yet financial criteria are still used to screen low-SES people from access to transplantation, even if the patient is otherwise healthy and a good transplant candidate.

Establishing a unified office of organ transplantation at HHS would enable transplant policy to be built around people in need of a transplant as opposed to being built around regulatory silos. Broadly, transplant policy should be aligned with the primary goal of increasing access to kidney transplantation to the maximum number of patients with kidney failure while improving longer term post-transplant outcomes (particularly among our younger recipients) and quality of life (particularly among older recipients where long-term survival may not be the paramount goal).

Currently, regulations across kidney care, including for dialysis facilities, transplant centers, and OPTN are not aligned and do not recognize the role of all in facilitating a smooth transition of care for patients. As a result, there are silos of care that occur in the nephrology clinic, dialysis unit, and the transplant center that increase challenges faced by patients in achieving optimal patient care. Establishing a single office of organ and transplant policy would better encourage patient-centered regulation instead of the current framework which focuses almost exclusively on short-term patient outcomes. This shift would improve communications across silos of care (dialysis units, referring nephrologists, and transplant centers), encourage transplant centers to provide increased and timely access to evaluation and related testing, and encourage greater communication about wait-listed candidates among transplant centers and current care teams. Unifying oversight of the transplant system under a single office would ensure that patients' interests do not become lost in gaps of oversight.

Elevate Transplant Patients as Partners in Care, Including by Improving Transparency Regarding Organ Offers

ASN believes that patients should be informed partners in their care, and most patients want more rather than less information about their care. Unfortunately, the current transplant system does not emphasize this principle: most patients are currently unaware of organ offers that are declined on their behalf by their care team. This is particularly concerning given research has shown that 85% of all kidneys are declined at least once, and that the 10,000 people who die per year on the transplant wait list receive a median of 16 organ offers while waiting for an organ.

While real-time notifications of organ offers are likely not feasible, practical, or desirable, asynchronous communication of these offers are a potential option for improving patient engagement and elevating patients as partners in their care. IT systems could be developed to facilitate local EHR communications and increase transparency and communication between people waiting for a transplant and the transplant care team. and For example, informing patients at regular intervals (every three or six months) could help by improving communication between patients, transplant center and dialysis providers about patient preferences and priorities, and by helping patients appreciate the tradeoff between increased selectivity for organs and wait times for those organs.

Finally, it would be of considerable benefit for transplant centers to have effective tools to assess the implications of turning down an offer, just as much as patients need tools to assess the implications of accepting a higher-risk kidney compared to remaining on the transplant wait list. Above all, patients should be provided the opportunity to be true partners in their care, and transparency should be fostered in the transplant system to elevate patients to be informed decision makers wherever possible.

Conclusion

Again, thank you for addressing this high area of need in the transplant system. ASN stands ready to help address these challenges and transform transplant care into an accessible therapy for all Americans. Should you have any questions about this statement, please do not hesitate to contact Zach Kribs, ASN Manager of Congressional Affairs at zkribs@asn-online.org or 202–618–6991.

Sincerely,
Michelle A. Josephson, M.D., FASN President-Elect
Roslyn B. Mannon, M.D., FASN Chair, Policy and Advocacy Committee

Association of Organ Procurement Organizations

8300 Greensboro Drive, #L1–620 McLean, VA 22102
(703) 556–4242
https://aopo.org/

On August 3, 2022, the Senate Finance Committee held a hearing and released a report[96] entitled: "A System in Need of Repair: Addressing Organizational Failures in the U.S. Organ Procurement and Transplantation Network." The Association of Organ Procurement Organizations (AOPO) shares the Committee's goal of creating and maintaining a more equitable and efficient system.

The year 2021 marked the eleventh record year in a row for deceased organ donors and the ninth consecutive year of increases in the number of organ transplants nationwide.[97] We are actively working to ensure this upward trend continues. As part of that effort, we are committed to improvement and seek feedback from impacted individuals, communities, and other stakeholders.

AOPO agrees that by investing in new, promising technologies, aligning policies and metrics towards shared, system-wide goals, and establishing mutual accountability for participants in the organ donation and transplantation process, we can improve the efficiency and equality of our system and ultimately save more lives. To move forward, the Committee should endorse the findings from the National Academies of Sciences, Engineering, and Medicine (NASEM)[98] report which assesses where the system currently stands, delineates the role each stakeholder plays, and charts a path to a more equitable donation and transplantation system. We agree that continued improvements are necessary to advance care for patients.

Organ Acceptance Rates and Non-Utilization

The under-use of viable organs, leading to an increase in organ waste, is an urgent issue that all donation and transplant stakeholders must solve as it is a major contributing factor to the nationwide wait list exceeding 100,000 patients. According to research cited in the NASEM report, a person who dies on the wait list has, on average, been offered 16 organs. Unfortunately, transplant center acceptance rates are low, and one fundamental way to advance equity is by increasing acceptance rates for organs from older and more medically complex donors.

OPOs are currently engaging in groundbreaking technologies, pushing the bound-aries of what is possible. For example, lung perfusion technology can potentially rehabilitate and transplant up to two-thirds of lungs that would otherwise be unusable.[99] However, transplant programs are directly responsible for the patients in their care, and they decide whether to utilize organs that OPOs make available. In addition, transplant programs are evaluated based on survival rates that discourage them from taking on "riskier" patients or transplants.

At the hearing, specific cases of kidneys were discussed where the witness described declining an organ based on an assessment of its condition upon arrival. However, it should be

---

[96] *https://www.finance.senate.gov/imo/media/doc/UNOS%20Hearing%20Memo.pdf.*

[97] OPTN Press: "All-time records again set in 2021 for organ transplants, organ donation from deceased donors," *https://optn.transplant.hrsa.gov/news/all-time-records-again-set-in-2021-for-organ-transplants-organ-donation-from-deceased-donors/.*

[98] NASEM Publication: "Realizing the Promise of Equity in the Organ Transplantation System," *https://www.nationalacademies.org/our-work/a-fairer-and-more-equitable-cost-effective-and-transparent-system-of-donor-organ-procurement-allocation-and-distribution.*

[99] UNOS Press: "Companies at the Forefront of Organ Perfusion Technology," *https://unos.org/news/ insights/game-changers-at-the-forefront-of-organ-perfusion-technology/.*

noted that not all of these organs were discarded. In fact, one of the kidneys the witness rejected was re-allocated and successfully transplanted into a patient at another transplant program.

This example highlights the significant role that the variability in clinical practice by transplant center plays in organ acceptance practices. In fact, UNOS will now evaluate transplant centers by their acceptance rates and make that information available to the public. The acceptance rates are also affected not just by the donor's clinical factors but also by when the donor organ was recovered. The NASEM report cites research supporting the "weekend effect" as a reason for non-utilization, stating:

> There has been compelling research on the "weekend effect" for kidneys and livers. In SRTR data from 2000 to 2013, and compared with weekday kidneys, organs procured on weekends are significantly more likely not to be used . . . even after adjusting for organ quality. Program structure and staffing, particularly during weekends and in smaller programs, affects kidney use and ultimately affects a patient's chances of receiving a transplant. This is unacceptable for a lifesaving surgical procedure such as transplantation.[100]

High and increasing non-utilization of available organs is a significant problem involving all components of the donation and transplantation system. Between 2018 and 2020, the number of donor kidneys not transplanted increased by 34%,[101] partly due to low acceptance rates and high variability in acceptance practices across transplant programs. AOPO supports implementing a robust system to document the cause of every organ which is not utilized and the implementation of strategies to increase organ acceptance and minimize organ waste. For example, advancements in and the usage of screening tools could reduce the number of patients offered an organ with a known deferral, expediting the matching process and lowering the number of discards.

System Efficiency and Performance

The United States has the most effective system in the world for maximizing donation and transplantation. In the last 5 years, OPOs have increased the number of deceased organ donors by 35% and increased the number of recovered organs by 27%.[102] Although we are proud of the increase in the number of available organs for transplantation, there is more work to be done. AOPO concurs that improvements are necessary to advance care and equity for patients.

AOPO does note that the Senate Finance Committee report references the non-peer-reviewed Bridgespan report, which claims that more than 28,000 additional organs could be transplanted each year. AOPO submits that this is not validated and is conditioned upon certain circumstances which will not occur, including a 100% donation rate and 100% utilization of donated organs. Some organs are simply not safe for transplant.

---

[100] NASEM Report: "Realizing the Promise of Equity in the Organ Transplantation System" (pages 6–24), *https://www.nationalacademies.org/our-work/a-fairer-and-more-equitable-cost-ef-fective-and-transparent-system-of-donor-organ-procurement-allocation-and-distribution.*

[101] AOPO Report: "50,000 Annual Organ Transplants in 2026 Goal," based on OPTN data as of February 17, 2021, *https://aopo.org/wp-content/uploads/2022/03/AOPO50K-Campaign-Overview-03-29-2022.pdf.*

[102] AOPO Infographic: "U.S. Organ Donation and Transplantation Highlights," based on OPTN data as of January 30, 2022, *https://aopo.org/wp-content/uploads/2022-US-Donation-Highlights-Infographic-1.pdf.*

The Senate Finance Committee report also attributes increased donation and transplantation rates in recent years to increased suicides and opioid-related deaths. The study cited to support this claim is based on a dataset that includes all donors who had at any time in their life used an illegal drug or were reported as a one-time drug user by a family member. While the opioid epidemic impacted donation, it is far from the only factor. Much more significant are advancements such as donation after circulatory determination of death (DCDD), which has increased an unprece- dented 123% over the last five years, and organ preservation technologies extending the time between organ recovery and transplantation.

AOPO supports meaningful performance measurement that holds all system stakeholders accountable for reaching our shared mission of saving as many lives as possible. We are working with our member OPOs to meet the new performance metrics established by the Center for Medicare and Medicaid Services (CMS). In fact, several OPOs identified as having issues within the Senate Finance report have become top performing OPOs with a "Tier 1" status according to CMS's latest release of data.[103]

The report states that 22 out of 57 OPOs would fail the new outcome measures and be decertified. It is critical to understand that the new methodology used in evaluating OPO performance is a comparative measure defining the bar to "pass" as the top 25th percentile. Therefore, by design, the metrics can result in OPOs assigned to "Tier 2" and "Tier 3" categories being subject to possible decertification or competition, regardless of continued improved performance over the certification cycle.

Organ Evaluation

The Senate Finance Committee report shares that 249 recipients experienced disease transmission following an organ transplant or an error in blood typing, and 70 recipients died due to failures in the donation and transplantation system. Any death resulting from an error is tragic, and the system must ensure that when errors occur, they are reviewed and understood, and steps are taken to prevent them in the future.

Despite systems in place to prevent mistakes and best practices in place to identify the risk of transmission, the risk of disease transmission following an organ transplant is extremely low but will never be zero. The numbers reported by the Committee represent .03% of the 231,180 organs transplanted over the indicated seven- year period.[104] The numbers show that nearly 99.9% of transplants resulted in successful outcomes and did not result in illness or death due to infected organs. The minimal risk must be understood in the context of the extremely high risk of death from organ failure for patients not being transplanted.

Overall, organ transplantation is safe and the best treatment for organ failure. Patient safety is always of utmost importance to the OPO professionals working every day to save lives. All medical procedures have associated risks and complications, and OPOs work to prevent such adverse outcomes. OPOs conduct multiple tests for every organ donor to identify the potential for disease transmission and other safety issues. Many of these tests are guided by transplant

---

[103] CMS Quality, Certification, and Oversight Reports (QCOR): "OPO Public Performance Report," https://view.officeapps.live.com/op/view.aspx?src=https%3A%2F%2Fqcor.cms.gov%2Fdocuments%2F2021%2520OPO%2520Aggregate%2520Performance%2520Report.xlsx&wdOrigin=BROWSELINK.

[104] Based on OPTN data as of August 8, 2022, *https://optn.transplant.hrsa.gov/data/.*

centers when considering an organ for their patient to assess organ viability and donor match suitability.

The Organ Procurement and Transplantation Network (OPTN)/United Network of Organ Sharing (UNOS) requires a medical record review and donor risk assessment interview with the potential donor's next of kin to obtain a five-year history of illness and other social determinants of health. OPTN/UNOS also requires physicians to perform a visual examination and, if warranted, a biopsy of potential donor organs to identify risks. As an extra step to rule out undiagnosed cancers and other diseases, OPOs are actively working to routinely administer CT scans on patients that pose a known possible risk.

As part of organ evaluation, OPOs and hospital partners are also required to identify the potential donors' blood type to prevent organ rejection in the recipient. Some potential donors have experienced severe trauma requiring blood transfusions which can, in rare instances, impact the blood typing results. Therefore, OPOs and hospitals tasked with donor management and assessment must take extra precautions if the blood type test is unclear or has shown varying results. Following blood typing errors in recent years, new policies were implemented to prevent such incidences.

Organ Transportation

With mere hours to transplant life-saving organs after recovery, proper transportation is essential to the organ donation and transplantation process. OPOs are tasked with determining the safest and quickest way to transport donor organs. While even one organ lost or damaged in transport is too many, the transit incidents covered in this report are extremely rare,[105]10 and something OPOs have actively implemented mechanisms to avoid.

Post-9/11-rules prohibit OPO staff from taking organs through airport security and directly to an awaiting aircraft, which created a barrier to efficient commercial transport. In response, many individual OPOs use private aircraft, when possible, to avoid delays from restrictive commercial air travel schedules. OPOs also partner with charter, courier, and delivery companies to expedite the ground transportation of organs. Undoubtedly, additional tools from the OPTN to support transportation and track organs in transit will facilitate overall system efficiency and effectiveness. Federal Aviation Agency (FAA) regulations standardizing how airlines handle organ shipments would also improve efficiency and reduce travel-related delays.

It is noteworthy that in the interim, and as referenced during the hearing, OPOs are collaborating with companies offering organ tracking technology, which has helped improve transportation logistics and efficiencies between the donor hospital and transplant center. OPOs are also using TransNet, a barcode system, to automate the organ packaging and labeling process, ensuring that organs are transported to the correct recipient. When OPOs experience transportation issues, details are promptly documented and reported to OPTN/UNOS.

---

[105] During the hearing, it was stated that OPOs are 15 times more likely to lose, damage, or delay an organ in transport than a commercial airline does with passenger luggage. This appears to be based on a misunderstanding of a February 2020 *Kaiser Health News* article that examined shipments handled by UNOS. As the article correctly points out, UNOS only manages transportation for a small fraction of annual transplants. Regardless of the validity of the analysis concerning UNOS, our OPO members have not experienced adverse transportation incidents of the magnitude claimed.

In Conclusion

As the Committee is aware, the recent NASEM report includes several detailed recommendations focused on establishing a more effective and equitable system.[106] The recommendations align with AOPO's goal to achieve 50,000 annual organ transplants in 2026 by expanding collaboration with stakeholders, reducing health inequities, increasing organ utilization, and driving innovation and research. We welcome the opportunity to meet with Committee members and staff to discuss the report's recommendations and collaborate to identify changes to policies, practices, and programs that will help ensure the nation's organ procurement and transplantation system meets the needs of all patients.

We stand ready to work with our fellow stakeholders, Congress, and the Biden Administration to pursue the day when every donation opportunity results in lives saved.

Center for Fiscal Equity

14448 Parkvale Road, Suite 6
Rockville, MD 20853 fiscalequitycenter@yahoo.com

Statement of Michael Bindner

Chairman Wyden and Ranking Member Crapo, thank you for the opportunity to address this issue.

At first blush, the consideration of this issue by the Committee is puzzling until one draws the connection between Medicare and organ transplants, including establishing universal healthcare and funding it. Please see the following attachments, as well as the second part of this submission, for discussion of these topics.

Other than its impact on Medicare and affordable care, we are leery of any congressional involvement in this issue. Ideally, it is based on science and best regulated by medical professionals. Even without intervention, putting pressure on the system is ill-advised. With political pressure often comes pressure from donors. The beauty of the current process is that the ability to pay is not part of it. Of course, if there are abuses on this front in the current system, they should be looked into and dealt with by the Congress and this Committee.

Even with the best of motives, adjusting the process (even if flawed) does not resolve the issues facing organ transplantation. There are simply not enough organ donors and the system, which relies on voluntary donation for its legitimacy, would not be helped with economic incentives—especially as these would be more attractive to the poor. This borders on abuse. Not only do we exploit them in life, incentives would continue this exploitation in death.

Ultimately, the solution is better science. This is where government involvement can help and where issues of fiscal equity come in. Any treatment must be provided to all, regardless of

[106] NASEM Report: "Realizing the Promise of Equity in the Organ Transplantation System," *https://www.nationalacademies.org/our-work/a-fairer-and-more-equitable-cost-effective-and-transparent-system-of-donor-organ-procurement-allocation-and-distribution.*

the ability to pay. While the private sector may be helpful in developing treatments, government funded research would help the process and assure equity.

A promising solution is the use of retargeted stem cells, either grown on cartilage or injected into the sick organ. Both would render donation and its possibility of rejection to the realm of temporary solutions, as would artificial organs.

Research in this process can always be sped up with more government money for NIH. To make sure everyone can benefit from advancements, such as using 3D printing to create cartilage on which to grow stem cells both outside and inside the body, research and actual organ generation can be publicly funded. Public organ manufacture, because of its expense in every case, is likely better than relying on for profit medicine.

As we have stated before, most recently in March of this year, but also in 2019 and 2020, orphan drug research and manufacture should be owned and managed by the federal government. The same path can be taken for the development of cloned organs. If the government owned the process, profiteering would be minimized. To facilitate cooperation and speed the process, creation of a quasi-governmental enterprise would be useful. It would combine NIH, NSF, FDA. To repeat our previous comments on drug pricing:

> A main problem with high cost drugs, especially orphan drugs, is the high development costs and the cost of small batch manufacturing. This could drive the need to raise drug prices for mature drugs in order to subsidize the orphans, although some hikes are undertaken because no one can stop them. The solution for this is for NIH and the FDA to own the rights to orphan drugs and to contract out research and development costs as it does basic research, as well as testing and production.

Hospitals and doctors would still make reasonable profit, but the government would eat the risk and sometimes reap the rewards. NIH/FDA might even break even in the long term, especially if large volume drugs which were developed with government grants must pay back a share of basic research costs and the attached profits, as well as regulatory cost.

Another way to assure equity in the growth and distribution of cloned organs, health care reform is essential. Again, to repeat our comments from March:

> Universal coverage, starting with a public option under the Affordable Care Act, with eventual evolution to some type of single-payer system is inevitable. Unless we start building negotiation into the system now, we will give the drug companies a reason to oppose reform later.
>
> A public option will only pass if pre-existing condition reforms are abolished with public option enrollment being automatic upon rejection. The public option must be subsidized, replacing Medicaid for the disabled and those not requiring long-term nursing care. Long-term care should be removed from states and replaced with a new federal Medicare Part E.
>
> The profit motive, with the need to constantly increase profits to attract Wall Street investment or keep stock prices growing, will lead to an ever-increasing number of people who will be considered uninsurable, thus relying on the public option.
>
> Most health-care systems will provide services to both comprehensive insurance beneficiaries, the retired, the disabled and those with the public option. In other words, Medicare for All is our future, with the only exception being firms abandoning the system and providing their own doctors while making arrangements with local hospitals and specialists—essentially creating local HMOs.

The major issue here is funding, although more efficiency will reduce prices. Costs are already minimized by the for-profit and by governmental medical care (which often uses for profit networks). To repeat, with a shout THE ISSUE IS PRICE, NOT COST!

Thank you again for the opportunity to add our comments to the debate. Please contact us if we can be of any assistance or contribute direct testimony.

Attachment—Hearing on Pathways to Universal Health Coverage, June 12, 2019

There are three methods to get to single-payer: a public option, Medicare for All and single-payer with an option for cooperative employers.

The first to set up a public option and end protections for pre-existing conditions and mandates. The public option would then cover all families who are rejected for either pre-existing conditions or the inability to pay. In essence, this is an expansion of Medicaid to everyone with a pre-existing condition. As such, it would be funded through increased taxation, which will be addressed below. A variation is the expansion of the Uniformed Public Health Service to treat such individuals and their families.

The public option is inherently unstable over the long term. The profit motive will ultimately make the exclusion pool grow until private insurance would no longer be justified, leading again to Single Payer if the race to cut customers leads to no one left in private insurance who is actually sick. This eventually becomes Medicare for All, but with easier passage and sudden adoption as private health plans are either banned or become bankrupt.

The second option is Medicare for All, which I described in an attachment to June 18th and 19th's comments and previously in hearings held May 8, 2019 (Finance) and May 8, 2018 (Ways and Means). Medicare for All is essentially Medicaid for All without the smell of welfare and with providers reimbursed at Medicare levels, with the difference funded by tax revenue.

Medicare for All is a really good slogan, at least to mobilize the base. One would think it would attract the support of even the Tea Partiers who held up signs saying, "don't let the government touch my Medicare!" Alas, it has not. This has been a conversation on the left and it has not gotten beyond shouting slogans either. We need to decide what we want and whether it really is Medicare for All. If we want to go to any doctor we wish, pay nothing and have no premiums, then that is not Medicare.

There are essentially two Medicares, a high option and a low one. One option has Part A at no cost (funded by the Hospital Insurance Payroll Tax and part of Obamacare's high unearned income tax as well as the general fund), Medicare Part B, with a 20% copay and a $135 per month premium and Medicare Part D, which has both premiums and copays and is run through private providers. Parts A and B also are contracted out to insurance companies for case management. Much of this is now managed care, as is Medicare Advantage (Part C).

Medicaid lingers in the background and the foreground. It covers the disabled in their first two years (and probably while they are seeking disability and unable to work). It covers non-workers and the working poor (who are too poor for Obamacare) and it covers seniors and the disabled who are confined to a long-term care facility and who have run out their assets. It also has the long-term portion which should be federalized, but for the poor, it takes the form of an HMO, but with no premiums and zero copays.

Obamacare has premiums with income-based supports (one of those facts the Republicans hate) and copays. It may have a high option, like the Federal Employee Health Benefits Program (which also covers Congress) on which it is modeled, a standard option that puts you into an HMO. The HMO drug copays for Obamacare are higher than for Medicare Part C, but the office visit prices are exactly the same.

What does it mean, then, to want Medicare for All? If it means we want everyone who can afford it to get Medicare Advantage Coverage, we already have that. It is Obamacare. The reality is that Senator Sanders wants to reduce Medicare copays and premiums to Medicaid levels and then slowly reduce eligibility levels until everyone is covered. Of course, this will still likely give us HMO coverage for everyone except the very rich, unless he adds a high-option PPO or reimbursable plan.

Either Medicare for All or a real single payer would require a very large payroll tax (and would eliminate the HI tax) or an employer paid subtraction value-added tax (so it would not appear on receipts nor would it be zero rated at the border, since there would be no evading it), which we discuss below, because the Health Care Reform debate is ultimately a tax reform debate. Too much money is at stake for it to be otherwise, although we may do just as well to call Obamacare Medicare for All and leave it alone.

The third option is an exclusion for employers, especially employee-owned and cooperative firms, who provide medical care directly to their employees without third party insurance, with the employer making HMO-like arrangements with local hospitals and medical practices for inpatient and specialist care.

Employer-based taxes, such as a subtraction VAT or payroll tax, will provide an incentive to avoid these taxes by providing such care. Employers who fund catastrophic care or operate nursing care facilities would get an even higher benefit, with the proviso that any care so provided be superior to the care available through Medicaid or Medicare for All. Making employers responsible for most costs and for all cost savings allows them to use some market power to get lower rates.

This proposal is probably the most promising way to arrest health care costs from their current upward spiral—as employers who would be financially responsible for this care through taxes would have a real incentive to limit spending in a way that individual taxpayers simply do not have the means or incentive to exercise. The employee-ownership must ultimately expand to most of the economy as an alternative to capitalism, which is also unstable as income concentration becomes obvious to all.

Attachment—Tax Reform, Center for Fiscal Equity, December 7, 2021

Subtraction Value-Added Tax (S–VAT). These are employer paid Net Business Receipts Taxes. S–VAT is a vehicle for tax benefits, including

- Health insurance or direct care, including veterans' health care for non-battlefield injuries and long-term care.
- Employer paid educational costs in lieu of taxes are provided as either employee-directed contributions to the public or private unionized school of their choice or direct

tuition payments for employee children or for workers (including ESL and remedial skills). Wages will be paid to students to meet opportunity costs.

- Most importantly, a refundable child tax credit at median income levels (with inflation adjustments) distributed with pay.

Subsistence level benefits force the poor into servile labor. Wages and benefits must be high enough to provide justice and human dignity. This allows the ending of state administered subsidy programs and discourages abortions, and as such enactment must be scored as a must pass in voting rankings by pro-life organizations (and feminist organizations as well). To assure child subsidies are distributed, S– VAT will not be border adjustable.

The S–VAT is also used for personal accounts in Social Security, provided that these accounts are insured through an insurance fund for all such accounts, that accounts go toward employee-ownership rather than for a subsidy for the investment industry. Both employers and employees must consent to a shift to these accounts, which will occur if corporate democracy in existing ESOPs is given a thorough test. So far it has not. S–VAT funded retirement accounts will be equal-dollar credited for every worker. They also have the advantage of drawing on both payroll and profit, making it less regressive.

A multi-tier S–VAT could replace income surtaxes in the same range. Some will use corporations to avoid these taxes, but that corporation would then pay all invoice and subtraction VAT payments (which would distribute tax benefits. Distributions from such corporations will be considered salary, not dividends.

Tax Reform Summary

1) Employers distribute the child tax credit with wages as an offset to their quarterly tax filing (ending annual filings).
2) Employers collect and pay lower tier income taxes, starting at $100,000 at 7.2%, with an increase to 14.4% for all salary payments over $150,000 going up 7.2% for every $50,000 up to $250,000.
3) Shift payment of HI, DI, SM (ACA) payroll taxes to employers, remove caps on employer payroll taxes and credit them to workers on an equal dollar basis.
4) Employer paid taxes could as easily be called a subtraction VAT, abolishing corporate income taxes. These should not be zero rated at the border.
5) Expand current state/federal intergovernmental subtraction VAT to a full GST with limited exclusions (food would be taxed) and add a federal portion, which would also be collected by the states. Make these taxes zero rated at the border. Rate should be 19.5% and replace employer OASI contributions. Credit workers on an equal dollar basis.

Guidehouse, Inc.

1676 International Drive, Suite 800
McLean, VA 22102
guidehouse.com

Guidehouse appreciates the opportunity to submit a statement for the record to the Senate Finance Committee (the "Committee") on this critical public health issue. Guidehouse is a leading global provider of healthcare consulting services to the public sector, including the U.S. federal government, 40 U.S. state governments, and commercial markets providing broad capabilities in management, technology, and risk consulting. As a result of the services we provide across the entire health ecosystem, we are in a unique position to provide perspective across the various policies, governance, stakeholders, and technology influencing the OPTN. Our statement for the record includes two sections. The first section details our view on challenges and recommendations facing the OPTN with a focus on "Rebuilding Trust Through Policy and Governance Reform, Stakeholder Engagement, and Communications to Improve Quality" and "IT Modernization: Digital Twin Study and Impact with Performance Metrics." In the second section we detail our background, experience and previous related engagements to establish our qualifications in the tasks necessary to modernize the OPTN. We applaud the bipartisan support and ongoing examination by this Committee in its efforts to reform the OPTN to provide equity, transparency, and quality of care to save lives in an efficient and timely manner.

OPTN Challenges and Recommendations

Health Resources and Services Administration's (HRSA) released two Requests for Information, issued April 8, 2020, and April 8, 2022, but later modified and re-released on May 5, 2022, identifying required services to modernize and maintain the OPTN. Recommendations from the NASEM 2022 Report "Realizing the Promise of Equity in the Organ Donation Process," provided additional detail and prescriptive feedback for the OPTN. Based on this awareness of OPTN programming, Guidehouse provides the following lessons learned from implementing programs similar in scale and complexity for OPTN reform and modernization:

OPTN Operational Transformation: Rebuilding Trust Through Policy and Governance Reform, Stakeholder Engagement, and Communications to Improve Quality

Modernizing the OPTN requires rebuilding stakeholder trust through outcome focused policy and governance reform. We recommend HRSA and the OPTN to access a similar network of multi-discipline thinking and established partnerships for the OPTN to support national reform. We, along with additional partners, manage coalitions of the nation's existing medical research institutions and professional networks, including representation from Historically Black Colleges and Universities and other Minority Serving Institutions, can guide OPTN's health equity policy agendas and priorities. Part of this effort may include restructuring the OPTN Board, reassessing organ distribution criteria, and integrating quality control and evidence-based best practices with oversight management policies. The OPTN and government programs can leverage this expertise across health and medicine, gain access to unique and existing data resources, and realize valuable opportunities to collaborate with communities, including those underserved by current organ donation and transplant systems. Patient and provider engagement strategies must consider early on how cultural nuances influence communications outcomes, participation, implementation, and evaluation methods. Our Guidehouse and partnership programs engage racially and ethnically diverse stakeholders and keep them involved throughout the process. This is critical for the future of the OPTN network and helps to quickly identify and eliminate cultural biases. It is also an approach that helps minimize or avoid conflict of interest and rebuild trust with underserved communities.

Challenges: 20% discarded or unused; limited availability especially with underserved and minority communities, rural areas and Midwest states; status on the waiting list is a mystery.

Solutions: Increase targeted education with cultural appropriateness and community champions; create transparency with data and access to waiting list status; onboard patient advocates with hospital care transplant teams; maintain a Patient Advocacy Coalition and network of donors, recipients, and families; create additional opportunities to register as a donor besides the DMV (driver's license) including options with paired donations/living donors for kidneys through primary care providers.

In our experience assisting executive leadership teams launch system-wide, patient focused modernization initiatives in large health systems we have collected several lessons learned that are relevant to the OPTN. Accountability and transparency regarding tough decisions is necessary for optimizing change, building skills and redesigning processes that sustain success while focusing on measurable results and outcomes to address issues in real time. For the OPTN, we can apply these lessons learned from commercial industry best practices to align a redesign process with performance incentive models that drive accountability with the organ procurement organizations (OPOs). We also recommend partnerships, as recommended by the NASEM report, with the National Quality Forum and the National Academy of Public Administration to integrate oversight and monitoring standards with certified and contracted OPOs.

Increasing culturally appropriate and audience-segmented communication and education about organ donation and transplants is critical. The transplant process is less familiar and can be stressful to even the most informed patients. Having a better understanding through all phases of the process, especially from the patient journey perspective or the living donor perspective may encourage more donor registrations and accessibility to organs. Communication strategies need to be patientcentric and relevant to cultures and communities, especially with underserved communities and subpopulations. Using a "human-centered design" approach will engage patients who have already been through the process of donating or receiving an organ to inform new patients and families what they need to know prior to their journey. This approach can also highlight where challenges or bottlenecks in the process typically occur and where additional support may be needed.

Stakeholder engagement is also imperative when reforming the nation's OPTN. It is particularly important to maximize this engagement by diversifying partnerships and enlisting nontraditional organizations that can inspire community organizations among underserved populations to help recruit new organ donors. We have experienced success enlisting organizations to support clinical trial recruitment while building future workforces. Our vision for OPTN is to fully immerse the stakeholder voice into the OPTN Board through the formation and management of a virtual "roundtable" with ongoing feedback for the transplantation community through patient feedback and monitoring to provide quality improvement, influence and increase organ procurement, and represent diversity and inclusion across all OPOs.

IT Modernization: Digital Twin Study and Impact with Performance Metrics

Modernization of complex data collection systems in the 21st century requires the ability to model, represent, and evaluate inputs and outcomes of interdependent systems while interacting with the system's variables, dependencies, and connections. Led by Guidehouse's Chief Innovation Officer, Dr. Rod Fontecilla, Guidehouse understands that a real-time understanding of a complex network of people, places, policies, processes, and data is the first and most critical step towards achieving true data transparency and insight into the performance and quality metrics of that network and its individual components.

A unique concept Guidehouse proposes for HRSA and the OPTN is the "digital twin" virtual representation of physical entities such as devices, people, processes, or systems that use computer simulation, machine learning, reasoning, and real-time data to help organizations make model-driven decisions related to detection, prevention, prediction, and optimization.

Digital twins are more easily adaptable than their physical counterparts, as organizations can modify digital assets and assess the results without incurring the time or monetary costs needed to adjust physical assets. Digital twin architectures use data from the assets being modeled and from related systems, to provide a method of storing and providing access to that data, and track and organize that data so that it stays in sync with real-world data about the asset and other digital twins. Industries use digital twins to track assets, such as products, throughout their lifecycles. For example, a hospital might use a digital twin based on its emergency room attributes to simulate and evaluate their readiness (e.g., resources, infrastructure, processes) under different scenarios (e.g., infectious disease pandemic response, emergency due to civil unrest, or natural disasters etc.), to explore changes and predict outcome (i.e., improved readiness) prior to making changes.

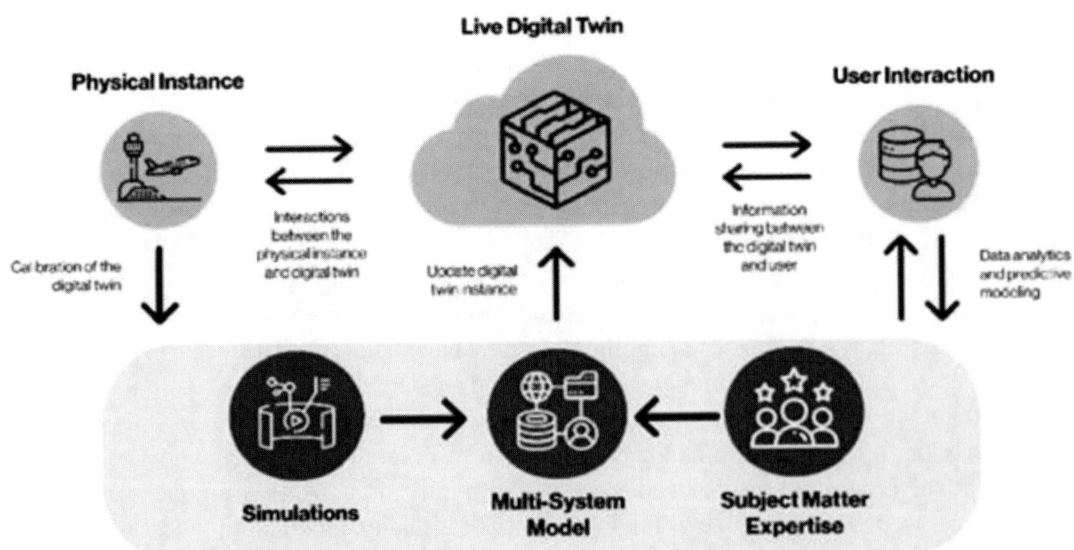

The digital twin concept was first introduced in 2002 for use in large manufacturing applications such as defense and aerospace engineering. Today's digital twins are accessible to any enterprise due to the scalable, cost-effective computing capabilities of the cloud. The level of maturity has driven commercial toolkits with cloud providers now offered at a price point that allows a broader set of use cases to use digital twins for enterprise applications. A digital twin's performance is driven by the effective use of cloud-based technologies for compute and storage, as well as the ability to ensure that the data is representative of live data in the field, so that data scientists and SMEs can more rapidly derive algorithms that ensure the simulations are operationally relevant.

Challenges: Conflict of Interest with the current OPTN Board and UNOS participation; lack of Quality Improvement monitoring.

Solutions: OPTN Board to be comprised of elected and credentialed members with backgrounds in medical research, bioinformatics, epidemiology, patient safety, transplant expertise; no engagement from the awarded contractor; equal representation from minority serving institutions and geographic diverse OPOs; use of evidence-based research and OPO performance metrics for decision-making; transparency of all OPTN Board communications and decisions.

Guidehouse proposes creating a digital twin of the OPTN to unite elements of the operational network environment (e.g., organ donor-specific, organ recipient-specific, processes related to procurement/logistics etc.) to inform HRSA performance metrics and impact of potential policy or process changes without changing the physical configuration of OPTN itself. Digital twins can incorporate relevant data, such as logistics, supply chain, physical and human resources, donor registration policy, recipient registration/wait-list practices, data collection and sharing, and social determinants of health. We propose a phased approach to simulate the behavior and future performance, as well as deliver real-time synchronization for data access, visualization, and dynamic decision making.

Background on Guidehouse

Guidehouse[107] is comprised of public and commercial health executives, strategists, actuaries, Ph.D.s, regulators, physicians, nurses, technologists, programmers, and consultants with direct experience modernizing IT systems and managing business operations for large scale health systems, including several of the U.S.'s largest transplant centers and the largest health system, Veteran's Affairs. We also provide expertise with finance and payer/insurance models, business process improvement, clinical transformation, and strategy for health equity and governance infrastructure that integrates transparency and performance metrics reporting. Examples of our related work to the OPTN include:

- Subject Matter Expertise: Edward Abraham, M.D., is a partner and executive physician leading and transforming academic medical centers, including healthcare delivery, finances, research, and educational programs. Most recently, he served as Executive Vice President for Health Affairs of the University of Miami and CEO of the University of Miami Health System, an academic medical center with more than $2.5 billion/year in revenues, 1,300 physicians, and 10,000 employees. He led the oversight of the Miami Transplant Institute, which has performed more organ transplants than any other center in the country. He served as Dean of two medical schools (University of Miami and Wake Forest School of Medicine), leading strategic planning initiatives including those around organ transplantation.

[107] https://guidehouse.com/capabilities/industries/healthcare.

- Public Sector Transplantation and Veterans: Guidehouse manages the VA's Office of Integrated Veteran Care, a national program that integrates healthcare services from the private sector for veterans for acute and chronic diseases where transplantation may be an option. Guidehouse supports VA in assisting with implementing the new Live Donor benefit and the Chimeric Antigen Receptor (CAR) T-cell therapy, coordinating with VA Medical Centers, VA Transplant Centers, community specialists, and the OPTN.
- Commercial Sector Transplantation and Business Process Improvement: St. Louis University Hospital engaged Guidehouse to evaluate and prepare responses to transplant contracts associated with payers. We developed a price transparency tool based on the provider files to create a comparative database of reimbursement by payer, plan, facility, geography, and service code. By integrating social determinants of health indicators, market share information, and hospital statistics, we detected trends in reimbursement for transplants.
- Medicare Claims with End-Stage Renal Disease (ESRD): We support contract work with the Centers for Medicare and Medicaid Innovation Center Business Services Group to identify, test, and evaluate new ways to improve care for Medicare beneficiaries with the Comprehensive ESRD Care model. This includes managing participant compliance and assessment of data collection and analysis of payment and service delivery.
- IT Infrastructure Modernization and Support: Guidehouse provides a full suite of enterprise IT services for a large, national defense contract including project management; application administration; application operations and maintenance support; cloud services planning and implementation; infrastructure management; ITSM implementation; and security operations, with 99.99+% availability. With 150+ full-time employees, including engineering, operations, and support personnel, the team securely designs, develops, and deploys all technical services for over 60 applications used by 150,000+ international users via 5,000+ hardware devices and serviced by 2000+ servers. Key modernization efforts have included server technology refresh, network upgrades, security compliant private cloud implementation, and converting the existing operating environment from traditional server-based infrastructure to a virtualized server environment with real-time backups and redundancy. These efforts, and other supported program initiatives, have led to multi-million-dollar savings on an annual basis.
- Modernizing IT for a Federal Health Research Agency: This agency required collations, analysis, and storage of large-scale datasets while using a wide range of digital tools for complex research processes. Guidehouse assessed the existing operating model and collaborated with the federal IT staff to develop a strategic roadmap to support the adoption of cloud technology, proactively mitigated risks, and defined critical processes to optimize IT operations and provide higher quality IT services for the agency. Our team also provided a change management strategy and training to support the maintenance of the new solutions.

Conclusion

We believe HRSA can reform and modernize the OPTN through a combined clinical and operational program transformation. This effort should focus on two major areas. First, rebuilding trust in the OPTN system by implementing a human centered approach to modernizing policy, governance, stakeholder engagement, and communications; and, second, accelerating technology implementations by using digital twins and performance metrics. Modernizing OPTN is essential for enhancing quality, optimizing distribution channels, and ensuring access for all patients involved with the OPTN. Thank you again for this opportunity to submit a statement for the record to the Committee on this critical public health issue.

For any further discussion or to answer any questions, please contact Steve Reynolds, Partner, Guidehouse Health, at (703) 258–2083 or sreynolds@guidehouse.com.

Letter Submitted by Suzanne Hughes

My kidney transplant date: June 15, 2022.

Summary: Received organ with inactive TB and active syphilis discovered post-transplant

I had been on the kidney transplant list since August 2020, and I received the call at 10:30 p.m. on June 14, 2022 that a kidney had become available, and I would need to take a flight the next morning for the transplant if I accepted this kidney. Per the call with the transplant nurse Cathy who is out of VA Portland (I am a U.S. Army vet, served 7 years in regular army and 2 years in reserves), the kidney was rated a 45 on the KDPI scale, which is a fairly good score. I was notified that the donor was positive for Hep C, but I knew the VA Portland had a good record of preventing transmission of Hep C post-transplant, and that I would be monitored. Since there were no other issues with the kidney and I am a difficult person to match with (I was told my body would reject 99 out of 100 kidneys), I accepted, and received the transplant on June 15, 2022 out of the Portland VA Hospital.

About 2 days post-transplant, I was visited by an infectious disease doctor, who told me that although most tests are completed prior to transplant, not all tests are back in time for the surgery. I was then told that in addition to Hep C, the transplanted kidney also was positive for TB, meaning the patient at one time had TB but it was not active TB at the time of the owner's passing. But in addition, the kidney also had active syphilis. My dismay and shock of learning about this was immense, even though every doctor assured me that it really wasn't a big deal, take the meds and move on. Obviously, I have not yet moved on.

Part of my career involves project management and research, and I approached my transplant the same way. I researched and read a lot of info prior to my transplant, and I had learned that nationwide the chance of me receiving an organ with an STD was 0.05%. So after receiving an organ with Hep C (known) and then also learning it had TB and syphilis, I was disillusioned with the organ transplant process. I still feel like I am waiting for another shoe to drop, even though the doctors assure me that all is well, and I should be grateful. One question a doctor did ask me is if I would have accepted the organ had I known about all of the issues with the organ, and I said I would not. I wish I had been provided a choice with all facts up front.

Currently I am being monitored and treated with meds to prevent Hep C, monitored for TB, and I have been tested and remain negative for syphilis. The treatment I received for syphilis is 3 LARGE intra-muscular injections in the rear end, and the shots are spread over 3 weeks. I cannot express how painful these shots are, and they result in a welt the size of a dollar coin that lasts 7 to 10 days. Now imagine you have a 12 inch incision on your belly from the transplant, and welts on both sides of your rear end, which means sleep was close to impossible due to the inability to find a comfortable position and pain.

I write to you in the hope that this does not happen to anyone else in the future. I was shocked to read some of the details on your investigation, and I think complications are either not being reported or are able to be cloaked under the privacy of organ donation. I certainly don't recall in my research seeing some of the stories that you uncovered. In addition to the above, I also had two other complications although not related to the donated kidney. One was leg numbness resulting in needing a walker to walk for one month, and I also developed bilateral DVTs most likely due to my limited mobility. Although this is not related to UNOS, I am hoping the hospital does list this as a complications so patients in the future have this info.

I thank you for allowing me to add my experience with the committee, and I hope for higher standards and oversight.

Best Regards,
Suzanne Hughes

Hypertrophic Cardiomyopathy Association

66 Ford Rd., Suite 213B Denville, NJ 07834
P: 973–983–7429
F: 973–983–7870
https://4hcm.org/

August 16, 2022
U.S. Senate
Committee on Finance
219 Dirksen Senate Office Building Washington, DC 20510–6200

Dear Chairman Wyden, Ranking Member Crapo, and Members of the Committee,

The Hypertrophic Cardiomyopathy Association (HCMA) respectfully submits this Statement for the Record in response to the Senate Finance Committee hearing on Wednesday, August 3, 2022, "A System in Need of Repair: Addressing Organizational Failures of the U.S.'s Organ Procurement and Transplantation Network." We commend the Committee for escalating the importance of the nation's organ donor and transplant system and its desire to improve upon the existing system to maximize the rate of organ donation in the country and maximize the rate of successful procurement and transplant of vital human organs.

HCMA was established in 1996 to serve the hypertrophic cardiomyopathy (HCM) spectrum disorder community. HCM is a genetic heart muscle disorder affecting one in 200 worldwide and presents with highly variable symptoms such as shortness of breath, chronic fatigue, life-threatening dysrhythmias, and the mental health challenges of living with a chronic illness. Approximately 5% require heart transplant. In a study published in 2010 in the United Network for Organ Sharing (UNOS) database, 1% of all heart transplants were given to HCM patients1. Today that number has grown to nearly 5% of all heart transplants, thanks partly to better disease management and timely listing for transplants. The age of transplant ranges from infants to those in their 70s. Kidney, lung, or liver transplants may also be necessary for these individuals.

On a personal note, I received a heart transplant at the age of 47 on February 2, 2017 due to complications associated with HCM and my sister, also afflicted with HCM, died of sudden cardiac death in 1995 and was a kidney and liver donor.

The current subject of this committee's investigation is of paramount importance to the HCM community and all stakeholders. In January 2016, I participated in a meeting held by UNOS on changes to the organ procurement process for donors and listing status for patients awaiting transplants. During this meeting, I inquired about UNOS' experience with what appeared to be inconsistencies among UNOS regions in the listing of an HCM patient in need of a heart transplant. HCMA pro vided guidance for listing HCM patients for heart transplant that were incorporated in 2018 to minimize inconsistencies in listing HCM patients for heart transplant.

HCMA wishes to alert the committee of a grave consequence of the lack of screening for HCM among potential heart donors. We know of at least two occasions when heart transplant recipients received hearts with hypertrophic cardiomyopathy. I am aware of another case in which a woman died from what was classified as tonsillitis complications. Later, her sister was found to have a diagnosis of hypertrophic cardiomyopathy. Upon communication with the OPO, it was confirmed that the individual had anatomy consistent with hypertrophic cardiomyopathy at her death. Yet, her heart valves were donated, and her family was never informed of the underlying disease process.

As a transplant recipient, a donor family, and an advocate on behalf of a community whose very lives rely on the safe, timely, and appropriate use of transplant medicine, I call on the committee to take appropriate action to ensure the highest standards are met when lives are on the line.

HCMA recommends the Organ Procurement and Transplantation Network (OPTN) be competitively awarded and the contractor be required to have in place an adverse reporting system that will capture these potential problems and others arising from the unknown consequences of donation. These reports must be transparent and timely.

HCMA recommends that governance of the OPTN, through government oversight and contractor performance, be conducted with utmost transparency and representation from all stakeholders in the organ donation and transplantation field. This includes donor families and recipients, both actual and those waiting. Government oversight of these actions is critical to the success of a robust, safe, fair, and sustainable system. Technology and systems used in the organ procurement process must be consistent, efficient, and not overly redundant.

Finally, HCMA encourages the committee to consider legislation that would adopt "opt-out" organ donor policies in the National Organ Transplant Act as in place in European nations.

Thank you for your time and attention and please contact me at lisa@4hcm.org should you have additional questions or I can be of assistance.

Sincerely,
Lisa Salberg
CEO and Founder

Ischemic Injured Organs and Limbs Foundation

2000 Kraft Drive, Suite 1208
Blacksburg, VA 24060

August 3, 2022
Hon. Ronald Wyden Chairman
Hon. Michael Crapo Ranking Member
U.S. Senate Committee on Finance

Ladies and Gentlemen,

I requested to appear before the Senate Finance Committee to present a different perspective of what needs to be done to eliminate the organ shortage and the security that is demanded to protect the personal identities of the organ donors, the donor families, and the transplant recipients. However, I became aware of this meeting on Monday, August 1, 2022. I will agree with this committee that UNOS has not been clear and open about the security of the current computerized system. UNOS, along with the OPOs, has also been very arrogant to the general public with an attitude that we know more than the general public about improving the organ donation rates in the United States. However, CMS is just as guilty when they have been contacted multiple times with ideas addressing how to increasing the number of viable organs for transplant. CMS's return comment to me was we control this monopoly and will not allow alternative OPOs to recover organs that go to the grave with trauma victims. HHS, along with the Division of Transplantation, are also just as guilty for refusing to listen to proposals that would exceed the new requirements for an OPO to be recertified. The Senate and the House of Representatives are also accountable because they control the budgets of these federal agencies. Jim Casey, the founder of UPS, stated, "you expect what you inspect." Have either the Senate or the House committees responsible for overseeing UNOS and the OPOs inspected what they have done since the Transplant Act of 1984 was approved? Since July 2020, I have been contacting the staff members of Senators Cardin, Van Hollen, Warner, Kaine, and Peters; as well as the House of Representatives' Raskin, Kildee, and Griffith. Their staff members have been kind and polite looking at our research numbers and were supposed to pass on the data to our elected officials but not one elected official has requested an appointment to see my data. Only Congressman Griffith has shown interest in our research data, and has met with my colleagues and myself at our Blacksburg, Virginia lab and his office twice in DC.

While attending the Ohio State University, majoring in perfusion, I was a work-study student in the dialysis and transplant programs performing preventative maintenance on the equipment. When I graduated in 1983, I worked full-time for the transplant program in the transplant research lab and the University based OPO. As I became more experienced in transplants, I learned to preserve kidneys on perfusion equipment, obtained organ consent, and assisted in organ recoveries. When there were no donor activities, I honed my skills in the transplant research lab; working on various projects from self-sealing dialysis grafts, xenotransplants, liver preservation systems, kidney preservation systems, and algorithms predicting kidney viability. 1993 moving to Washington DC to develop a Non-Heart-Beating trauma donor program, and in 1996 presented our data that led to a Federal law to preserve organs inside the cardiac dead trauma victim while the next-of-kin was located and gave permission for organ donation. 2000 established the Baltimore regional organ preservation lab for Johns Hopkins and the University of Maryland transplant programs and developed a new kidney preservation system. 2005 I went to the Army-Navy Transplant program to establish a limb preservation system for amputated arms and legs. To test the limb preservation hypothesis, I received Congressionally Directed grant W81XWH1120212, "Development of Room Temperature Human Organ & Tissue Preservation Technology." This grant set up the Army-Navy Transplant research lab in Bangkok, Thailand. 2016 I started collaborating with Dr. John Robertson to develop a more efficient cardio-emulating organ preservation systems for hearts, lungs, livers, kidneys, pancreas, small bowel, and amputated arms and legs. The system produces a cardiac QRS complex and the pressure Dicrotic notch waveforms. Raman Spectroscopy to monitor the preservation solution's chemistries, Infrared Imaging to provide a clear picture of the organ's vascular structure, and a filtration system that removes bacteria preventing infections, and reduces the need for antibiotics. In May 2022, the final prototype of the Robertson Cardio-Emulating heart, kidney, pancreas, small bowel, arm and leg systems are ready for the final system build-out. The room temperature preservation has been redeveloped to address the long ischemia time without oxygen, reduce the organ's metabolism, scavenger the cytokines and chemokines that are released due to the lack of oxygen, and vasodilate the vascular structure of the organs and preserve the organs for at least 24 hours.

In May 2021, the Ischemic Injured Organ and Limb (IIOL) Foundation was invited to participate in the first long-range FAA-authorized drone organ transportation project. We used a large kidney preservation system with 3D printed kidneys at the Ohio State Medical Center. Using a small Drone, we transported a box that contained blood and tissues specimens for cross-matching the organ donor and the transplant recipient from the OSU Medical Center to OSU airport. I drove the kidneys from the hospital to Don Scott airfield, where the kidney preservation system and the tissue typing material had arrived. They both were placed onto a remote-controlled helicopter to transport 30 miles northwest to a satellite hospital in Marysville, Ohio. Once at the Marysville airport, the kidneys and the tissue typing material were transferred to the Ohio State self-driving van for the 2 miles trip to the hospital. While drones were transporting the organs and tissue typing material, we were tracking them on our phone app, keeping track of the perfusion parameters and the location of the drones o an encrypted secure computerized program.

Background

Dr. Robertson and I were part of a collaborative team UNOS put together to submit a research project to the Chan Zuckerberg Initiative, which was not funded. However, we have been working with UNOS and the other collaborative universities to fund a more advanced transplant project. That will increase the number of transplants in the United States and address the past discriminatory practices of minorities and socioeconomically deprived individuals who are not eligible for the current transplant waiting list. Organs are in short supply, and the need for organ transplants will only increase over the next few years, primarily due to projected increases in the number of individuals with organ failure and chronic disease. Today more than 100,000 individuals are waiting for an organ transplant. Still, the number of patients on the National Organ Transplant Wait List does not encompass the entirety of organ failure prevalence across the United States. Approximately 800,000 Americans have an end-stage renal disease (ESRD), 6.2 million have heart failure, 5.5 million have end-stage liver disease (ESLD), and 16.4 million have Chronic Obstructive Pulmonary Disease (COPD). CDC estimates that over 3.1 million Americans are ineligible to be placed on the National Organ Transplant Waiting list. It is projected by 2030, over five million people in the US will require renal replacement therapy. We envision a future where there is no waiting list, and there is a lifesaving transplant for everyone in need. What science and technologies can be leveraged to address this anticipated surge in demand for kidneys and other transplantable organs? The organ transplant ecosystem must integrate living, brain dead, and cardiac dead human donors with the emergence of xenotransplantation and new technologies to manufacture organs and repair tissues in donated organs.

A more significant emphasis must be placed on the recovery, resuscitation, and validation of cardiac dead human organ donors. There are five different cardiac dead classifications: dead on arrival, those who succumb shortly after arrival at the hospital, those who are not brain dead but have no chance of survival and the family removes them from life support, brain dead patients who progress to cardiac death, and the patient that has either a cardiac arrest or respiratory arrest in a hospital with unsuccessful resuscitation attempt and pronounced cardiac dead. Since 2012 the Healthcare Cost and Utilization Project reported 661,000 annual hospital cardiac deaths. The American College of Surgeons trauma data has shown since 2010, and there have been an average of 200,000 cardiac deaths annually in the United States. The U.S. House of Representatives in the health and welfare subcommittee reported (February 2022), that since the beginning of the COVID pandemic, an average of 100,000 yearly opioid cardiac deaths along with an untold increased number of suicides.

The DMV Region consists of the states of Maryland, Virginia, and the District of Columbia. There are eleven adult and five pediatric Level I Trauma Centers, eleven adult Level II Trauma Centers, and nine adult Level III Trauma Centers in the DMV region. Because of the need to properly train staff at each Rapid Organ Recovery (ROR) unit, it was determined to establish ROR units at the six most active trauma centers in the DMV region. As more personnel are trained, ROR units will be expanded to the remaining trauma centers in the study region. Personnel may be assigned to two or more trauma centers in the rural areas of the DMV region.

ROR unit consists of Family Advocates (FA), Physician Assistants (PA), and Organ Recovery Technicians (ORT). FAs will be responsible for locating the next of kin, preserving forensic evidence, and obtaining organ donation consent. PAs will place the cannulas in the trauma victims and resuscitate the organs while waiting for authorization from the next of kin, assist with recovering the organs, and oversee the medical practices under the medical director's supervision. ORTs will operate the Rapid Organ Resuscitation system, correct and initiate resuscitation of abdominal and thoracic organs during consent, preserve the organs during recovery, and place the organs on individual organ resuscitation systems.

Training of the various ROR staff functions will consist of didactic and hands-on training. FAs will receive a minimum of six to eight weeks of training in forensic evidence identification, handling forensic evidence, identifying and locating the next of kin, obtaining organ donation consent, and identifying cardiac and brain dead organ donors. PAs will receive about four weeks of training in identifying and cannulating femoral arteries and veins in cadavers. PAs will also receive training in the chemical composition of the organ resuscitation solution and how to operate the various organ resuscitation systems, along with assisting in the recovery of the donated organs. ORTs will receive the most in-depth training for two to three years, receiving a Bachelor of Science degree before being eligible for certification. ORTs will learn transplant history, abdominal and thoracic organs anatomy and physiology, donor chemistry, monitoring the organs on the different organ resuscitation systems, transporting organs, Homeland Security and Transportation Security Administration rules and regulations for transporting organs on commercial airlines, and microbiology. We intend to initially train as many ORTs and get them hands-on experience in the animal lab as the Cardio-Emulating equipment is being prepared for FDA animal and human clinical trials.

Pilot Study Preliminary Data

The following tables show the potential number of cardiac dead deaths in the DMV Region. Table 1 shows the potential number of brain dead organ donors and the potential number of cardiac deceased organ donors. Table 1 shows the number of deaths reported by each hospital to the state's vital statistics department. Data from the Healthcare Cost and Utilization Project states that brain deaths were approximately 2% of the total cardiac deaths recorded annually in the United States.

Table 1. Mean death rates DMV region past 5 years

Hospital	City	State	Brain Dead	Cardiac Dead
Level I				
Shock Trauma UMMS	Baltimore	MD	30	1,200
Johns Hopkins Adult/Pediatric	Baltimore	MD	15	500
Washington Hospital Center/Children's	Washington	DC	15	575
George Washington	Washington	DC	15	525
Howard University Hospital	Washington	DC	10	375
Chipenham	Richmond	VA	12	400
INOVA Fairfax	Fairfax	VA	20	600
Children's Hospital Kings Daughter	Norfolk	VA	8	100
Sentara Norfolk	Norfolk	VA	15	525
Carillion Roanoke Adult/Pediatric	Roanoke	VA	10	375
VCU MC Adult/Pediatric	Richmond	VA	17	550
UVA MC	Charlottesville	VA	16	400
Level I Total			183	6,125
Level II				
Hopkins Bayview	Baltimore	MD	12	400
UMMS Capital Regional	Largo	MD	20	500
Sinai Hospital	Baltimore	MD	9	200

Table 1. (Continued)

Hospital	City	State	Brain Dead	Cardiac Dead
Hopkins Suburban Hospital	Bethesda	MD	10	275
Henrico Doctors	Richmond	VA	8	175
Lynchburg General	Lynchburg	VA	6	100
Mary Washington	Fredericksburg	VA	6	125
Reston Hospital Center	Reston	VA	4	225
Riverside Medical Center	Newport News	VA	5	175
Virginia Hospital Center	Arlington	VA	7	225
Winchester Medical Center	Winchester	VA	4	100
Level II Total			91	2,500
Level III				
Merritus Medical Center	Hagerstown	MD	4	125
UPMC Western Maryland	Cumberland	MD	4	100
Tidal Health Peninsula Hospital	Salisbury	MD	7	150
New River Valley Medical Center	Christiansburg	VA	6	125
Lewis Gale-Montgomery Hospital	Blacksburg	VA	4	100
Loudoun Hospital	Leesburg	VA	4	125
Southside Regional Medical Center	Petersburg	VA	3	75
Virginia Beach General	Virginia Beach	VA	3	75
Sentara Northern Virginia MC	Woodbridge	VA	3	80
Level III Total			38	955
Grand Total				9,580

Table 2 compares the Standard Acquisition Fee for the Brain Dead OPO versus the projected Cardiac Dead Standard Acquisition Cost. The Standard Acquisition Fee consists of evaluating the potential organ donor, recovering the organs, preserving the organs, transporting the organs to the transplanting hospital, personnel, office rent and utilities, various insurances, and other ancillary office costs. The Brain Dead OPO Standard Acquisition was taken from the "Milliman Research Report 2020 U.S. Organ and Tissue Transplants: Cost Estimates, Discussion, and Emerging Issues." The Cardiac Dead Standard Acquisition Fees are from the projected cost of the preservation systems, preservation solution, transportation, hospital recovery, personnel, office rent and utilities, various insurances, and other ancillary office costs.

Table 2. Comparison of the standard acquisition cost for BD OPO versus CD OPO

Organ	BD SAC	CD Pilot SAC	Difference (BD Savings)
Heart	$131,500.00	$59,500.00	$72,000.00
Single Lung	$110,100.00	$65,000.00	$45,100.00
Double Lung	$127,700.00	$68,000.00	$59,700.00
Liver	$104,200.00	$65,000.00	$39,200.00
Kidney	$113,900.00	$58,500.00	$55,400.00
Pancreas	$113,900.00	$61,000.00	$50,800.00
Total	$699,200.00	$377,000.00	$322,200.00

Collaborative Team Approach

A solution to the organ shortage is at hand, but only if we work together. This collaborative, diverse team of regional university partners will work for the creation of a Bio Hub focused on enhancing and expanding the existing organ transplant ecosystem. This endeavor will bring together powerhouses across the transplant community with a regional focus centered within the region. The collaborative team consists of the United Network for Organ Sharing (UNOS), Virginia Tech, University of Virginia, Virginia Commonwealth University, Old Dominion University, and Wake Forest University. This collaborative group presents unique scientific and scholarly strengths across every facet of organ and composite tissue transplants.

UNOS: is a private, non-profit organization that serves as the United States organ transplant system (Organ Procurement and Transplantation Network [OPTN]). UNOS collaborates internationally with transplant organizations in Canada, the United Kingdom, Europe, France, and Australia.

Virginia Tech (VT): brings decades of experience designing and fabricating organ preservation systems for abdominal, thoracic, and amputated limbs. VT's focus has been on resuscitation of ischemic injured organs and limbs utilizing predictive analytics, sensing technologies, and algorithms to predict organ viability. VT's expertise in multimodal machine learning, medical imaging, data quality, visualization, and data fusion, augmented reality and geospatial systems make them a strong partner in the group's efforts to enhance and expand the existing organ transplant ecosystem, especially in cardiac dead organ donors, with a seamless transition to new technologies maximizing equitable patient access and outcomes. The VT team combines the expertise of organ preservation and transplantation engineers with specialists in multimodal predictive data analytics, augmented and virtual reality-based visualization systems, and transplantation "hardware" prototyping.

University of Virginia (UVA): is one of the oldest transplant programs in the United States, focusing on transplantation research, ischemic-reperfusion injury, engineering, and applied science, translational medicine, social and decisional analytics, system science and advanced computing, mathematical and biocomplexity, visual and decision informatics, and engineering in medicine. UVA's transplant research lab offers cutting technology and innovative methods to explore novel opportunities to eliminate end-stage organ diseases, optimize donor organ health, and dramatically improve transplant patients' outcomes.

Virginia Commonwealth University (VCU): Is one of the country's most extensive liver and kidney transplant programs, with expertise in reducing minorities and socioeconomic disparity, and unique protocols to utilize Hepatitis C, HIV, and COVID donor organs in successful transplants. VCU's transplant laboratory uses molecular biology and cell culture models in standard and extended criteria donors and cardiac dead donors for therapeutic interventions.

The Virginia Modeling, Analysis, and Simulation Center (VMASC) is an enterprise center of Old Dominion University (ODU): the advanced analytics, geospatial analytics, machine learning, and artificial intelligence methods analyze data collections from the community and stakeholder-led efforts, environmental assessments, and curating of social, environmental and medical information to determine various outcomes from the collected and analyzed data.

Wake Forest Institute of Regenerative Medicine (WFIRM): is pioneering regenerative medicine technologies to improve human health. These technologies aim to enhance the human body's intrinsic regenerative ability to repair after damage, rendering marginal organs transplantable and enabling the manufacturing of body parts that will replace functionally impaired organs and tissues. WFIRM scientists are currently working to create organs and tissues, developing therapeutic cell treatments for over 30 areas of the body. WFIRM is the coordinating site for the Armed Forces Institute of Regenerative Medicine II, with 35 participating institutions throughout the United States. WFIRM recently received a significant award from the Defense Threat Reduction Agency for their "Body on a Chip" project to develop a miniaturized system for human organs that mimics the body's responses to harmful agents and develop potential therapies.

Air Space Link: Northern Virginia company building small drones and contracts with the FAA for routing drone flights in the United States. Has developed small drone technology to transport blood and specimens for transplant histocompatibility and serology testing. Air Space Link's expertise will allow for developing and implementing drone transport of organs and tissues and obtaining FAA certification.

MOOG Aerospace, a Division of MOOG Incorporated: is located on the Virginia Tech campus. Large drones up to helicopter-size remote-controlled aircraft to transport the deceased body to an organ recovery center or transport multiple organs from a donor hospital to a regional organ preservation lab.

Revivicor: is a biotechnology company that has developed a unique line of pigs that are compatible with humans to increase the supply of organs for human transplants Revivicor provided the pig heart for the first Xenograft, pig to human, transplant in January 2022. Revivicor brings expertise in developing xeno-transplantable organs for humans that cannot be matched with a deceased organ donor.

Space Link: is a secure communication network located in Northern Virginia utilizing Medium Earth Orbit (MEO) satellites. Collaborating with Space Link will allow for more rapid communication between regional organ preservation labs, UNOS, the organ center, organ recovery teams, and the transplanting teams. This system will ensure that personal data will be transmitted with clear and concise information about the recovered organs to the transplanting team. Space Link solves the security problem, and the data is encrypted, so there will be no Personal Information, Privacy Issues, or HIPPA violations when sharing data between multiple locations, thus allowing for more placement and delivery of organs around the United States.

From Bench to Bedside

In the first two years of funding, this collaborative research between the university programs will develop algorithms to evaluate the organs before transplantation. Share secure computerized organ perfusion data so multiple transplant centers can simultaneously evaluate organs. Expeditiously distribute the organs to the appropriate transplant recipient. Collect and analyze pre and post-transplant data and predict the survival length of the transplanted organs. In order to implement the findings, a central location, either the VT campus in Crystal City or Falls Church, is the most central location for the trauma centers and the transplanting hospitals involved in the DMV pilot study. The Cardiac Dead Pilot program in the DMV Region will use the 1996 Federal to recover and resuscitate organs from all Maastricht cardiac dead classification. If the hypothesis proves true at the end of the DMV cardiac dead pilot program, we will expand the cardiac dead trauma victims program nationwide. By having a nationwide Cardiac Dead OPO complementing the Brain Dead OPOs, we anticipate in five years a minimum of 50,000 Cardiac Dead organ donors and 12,000 to 15,000 yearly Brain Dead organ donors, providing a potential of 300,000 to 400,000 yearly organ transplants. As the programs become more acceptable, we believe there will be over 200,000 Cardiac Dead organ donors and close to 35,000 to 40,000 Brain Dead organ donors annually. Thus, allowing Revivicor to continue its research and obtain FDA clearance to transplant xenoallographs into individuals who cannot receive a human organ transplant because of rare antibodies that do not match an organ donor.

Table 3. Potential of cardiac dead organ donors in the DMV pilots study

Hospital	Yr. 1	Yr. 2	Yr. 3	Yr. 4	Yr. 5
Level I					
Shock Trauma	120	180	180	180	180
Johns Hopkins Adult/Pediatric	0	60	60	60	60
George Washington	0	60	60	60	60
Washington Hospital Center/Children's	60	60	60	60	60
Howard University	0	36	60	60	60
Chipenham	0	0	36	48	60
INOVA Fairfax	60	120	120	156	156
Children's Hospital Kings Daughter	0	36	36	60	60
Sentara Norfolk General	0	60	84	84	120
Carillion Roanoke	0	36	60	60	60
Virginia Commonwealth Adults/Pediatrics	60	60	84	84	84
University of Virginia Adult/Pediatric	60	60	84	84	84
Total	360	768	924	996	1,044
Level II					
Bay View	0	48	48	60	72
UMMS Capital Regional Medical Center	60	60	72	72	84
Sinai Hospital Baltimore	0	36	48	48	60
Suburban	0	60	60	72	84
Henrico Doctors Hospital	0	0	36	48	60
Lynchburg General	0	36	48	60	72
Mary Washington Hospital	0	0	36	48	60
Reston Hospital Center	0	0	36	48	60
Riverside Medical Center	0	0	36	48	60
Virginia Hospital Center	0	0	36	48	48
Winchester Medical Center	0	0	36	48	48
Total	60	240	492	600	720
Level III					
Merritus Medical Center	0	0	36	48	60
UPMC Western Maryland	0	0	36	48	48
Tidal Health Peninsula Hospital	0	0	0	36	36
New River Valley Medical Center	0	36	36	48	48
Lewis Gale-Montgomery Hospital	0	36	36	48	48
Loudon Hospital	0	0	36	48	48
Southside Regional Medical Center	0	0	36	36	48
Virginia Beach General Hospital	0	0	36	36	48
Sentara Northern Virginia Medical Center	0	0	36	48	48
Total	0	72	288	396	432
Grand Total	420	1,080	1,704	1,992	2,196

Development and Utilization of Drone Technology

The DMV region is one of the worst areas for traffic delays in the United States. A small drone is needed to transport blood and organs from the donor hospital to regional histology and serology labs. Transporting the specimens to the proper laboratories more expeditiously will allow the lab results to be obtained sooner, thus decreasing the time to start the organ placement. Once the donor and the recipients are identified for each organ, especially if recipients are determined before the organ recovery procedure is initiated, the organs need to be resuscitated and prepared for transportation to the regional preservation lab. Because of the potential of eight organs being recovered from one donor and transported to the regional preservation lab, larger drones will be required to transport the organs. As more Cardiac Dead Organ Donors become standard practice, the need to have a regional recovery center added to the regional organ preservation lab will expedite organ recoveries and placement. Having both the recovery center and the preservation lab located up to 250 radial miles from the trauma centers would require larger drones for the more extended transportation of donors and organs.

Secure Communications for all Transplant Parties

One of the biggest complaints from transplant surgeons concerning the recovery teams is the lack of clear communication. The Bio Hub proposal will address this significant problem that leads to many discarded organs because of long preservations time and unclear documentation of recovered organs outside the transplant team's home region between the organ recovery team and the organ transplanting teams. Utilizing the Bio Hub collaborators, computer science engineers, and scientists to develop a secure communication link to share real-time data. There needs to be a partner organization to transmit and share real-time data securely. The addition of Space Link (an MEO satellite provider) allows for UNOS, the regional organ preservation labs, and the transplanting hospitals to share real-time data about the recovered organs with each team member. Another major problem with the current organ center's sharing policy is the wasted time placing the cadaveric organs because transplant programs do not trust the existing data transmitted to the potential recipient hospitals. By simultaneously utilizing real-time encrypted donor information to all potential recipient hospitals so the transplant programs can decide whether to accept the organs. Then creating a cue for which recipients will receive the organs can be done more expeditiously than in the current system. This same system will have pre-signed consents for all potential recipients accepting Cardiac Dead organs for a transplant. The potential transplant recipients will have all their blood work, health exams, and vaccines maintained at a current status or be placed in an inactive status until the transplant centers have the potential recipient missing data brought current. Using secured, rapidly transmitted data at Terabyte speed will make the data system more user-friendly and efficient. Allowing for the transportation of organs around the United States to the closest match donors and recipients is an exciting benefit of this proposal.

As Dr. Robertson and myself work with UNOS to set up the collaboration between the multiple universities to address the concerns of this Senatorial Committee, we have seen the UNOS staff members' awareness of past mistakes and an interest in becoming more accountable for their past actions. I believe submitting this Statement for the Records will hold UNOS responsible to the Senate and the House of Representatives during this five-year proposal. I look forward to presenting a more in-depth presentation of our data for this proposal to the Senate Finance Committee and addressing your questions. I also ask for your support in funding this proposal through the American CARES Act 2.0 and hold us accountable for the annual milestones for this funded project.

Respectfully,
Frederick A. Gage Director

Letter Submitted by Michael G. Ison, M.D., MS et al.

U.S. Senate
Committee on Finance
219 Dirksen Senate Office Bldg. Washington, DC 20510–6200

Organ transplantation provides the opportunity for improved life for patients with end-stage organ disease. Recently, there has been attention to adverse outcomes of the organ procurement and transplantation processes in the United States. While these reports may be viewed as alarming, it is critical to place them within the context of the overall risk of end-organ disease and transplantation. As prior chairs of the Disease Transmission Advisory Committee (DTAC) of the Organ Procurement and Transplantation Network (OPTN), a volunteer position, we have a unique understanding of many of the relevant issues. We write as practicing physicians, engaged in the care of transplant recipients and involved in the transplant community.

Recent media attention and Senate hearings have highlighted transmission of disease from the organ donor in 249 people of whom 70 have died. While these numbers may seem high and the details of specific cases may seem shocking, they must be placed within the context of the absolute number of transplants performed annually. End-stage organ disease has significant risk of death and illness; more than 50% of people with advanced liver disease die within 3 months of diagnosis. From 2008 through mid-2015, the period that the Senate reported on, 174,338 individuals underwent transplantation, placing the rate of unexpected disease transmissions at 0.14%. During this same time, the deaths attributed to disease transmission only account for 0.09% of the 74,253 total deaths that occurred in patients transplanted during this period. Importantly, the types of diseases transmitted as well as the rates of disease transmission and death are nearly identical to those reported by other countries that track donor deaths such as France where transplantation oversight is managed by a government agency, Agence de la Biomedecine. The fact that results under the UNOS oversight of organ vigilance and donor screening are similar to those under the French system suggests that these outcomes are part of the known risks associated with transplantation.

The OPTN DTAC was established to develop an organ vigilance system in the United States. The group represents a unique collaboration between the various transplant communities, including transplant center and organ procurement professionals, and key government agencies, including HRSA and the Centers for Disease Control and Prevention (CDC). Since its inception, the DTAC has strived to be transparent, sharing key findings through regular presentations and publication of current data. The program's success has made it the model emulated as other countries sought to establish similar programs.

This organ vigilance work has helped keep transplant patients safe, maintaining a low rate of disease transmission whilst fostering an increase in transplant volume amidst the challenges of a pandemic. UNOS has encouraged DTAC to be nimble, updating testing parameters for organ donors based on continuous assessments of patient experience. We have seen similar updating in other committees of the OPTN, where the need to be proactive remains a high priority. The pandemic is an especially good example of how this constant process of reassessment allows for the maximal safe use of donors. Data on testing and disease transmission risk have been reviewed and guidelines updated throughout the pandemic. As a result, transplantation in the US not only returned to pre-pandemic rates but grew to record numbers despite the ongoing impact of SARS–CoV–2.

Organ transplantation is incredibly complex and limitations exist as to what can be known about any donor within the time available between a donor becoming eligible to donate and organs being placed into their grateful recipients. Optimal donor assessments must always balance risks with benefits to ensure maximal use of potential donated organs. The landmark Institute of Medicine article "To Err is human" recognized that rather than assigning blame, processes need to be developed to prevent errors or minimize harm. Similarly, through lessons learned as part of organ vigilance programs, we continue to strive to improve our systems and processes. Unexpected disease transmissions and other adverse events will always occur no matter what system is in place, but putting these into context is critical. Thankfully they occur rarely and when recognized, systems implemented by UNOS, refine the processes further in a non-blaming fashion to improve survival of all transplant recipients. While every system requires continuous quality improvement, the implication that the current system has failed to promote patient safety as relates to disease transmission—or that an alternative administrative structure or contractor would result in a safer system—is not supported by our experience.

Michael G. Ison, M.D., MS
Northwestern University Feinberg School of Medicine,
Chicago, Illinois 340 E North Water St., Unit 2210, Chicago, IL 60611

Emily Blumberg, M.D.
Perelman School of Medicine at University of Pennsylvania, Philadelphia, Pennsylvania
3400 Spruce St., 3 Silverstein Suite E, Philadelphia, PA 19104

Michael Green, M.D.
University of Pittsburgh School of Medicine, Pittsburgh,
Pennsylvania 3705 5th Avenue, Pittsburgh, PA 15213

Dan Kaul, M.D.
University of Michigan Medical School, Ann Arbor, Michigan 3116 Taubman Center,
Ann Arbor, MI 48109

Marian Michaels, M.D.
University of Pittsburgh School of Medicine,
Pittsburgh, Pennsylvania 3705 5th Avenue, Pittsburgh, PA 15213

Cameron Wolfe, M.D.
Duke University School of Medicine, Durham, North Carolina
Hanes House, Room 150, Trent Drive, Durham, NC 27710

Mississippi Organ Recovery Agency

4400 Lakeland Drive
Flowood, MS 39232
PH 601–933–1000
FAX 601–933–1006
https://msora.org/

August 17, 2022
U.S. Senate Committee on Finance
Dirksen Senate Office Bldg. Washington, DC 20510–6200

Re: Mississippi Organ Recovery Agency's Statement for the Record on Senate Finance Committee Hearing of August 3, 2022, entitled "A System in Need of Repair: Addressing Organizational Failures of the U.S.'s Organ Procurement and Transplantation Network"

Dear Members of the Senate Committee on Finance,

On behalf of the Mississippi Organ Recovery Agency (MSOP), I thank the Committee for its dedication to improving the organ procurement and transplantation system. During the above-referenced hearing (Hearing) on August 3, 2022, the Committee represented that the goal of the hearing was to create a more equitable and efficient organ donation and transplant system. We greatly appreciate the Committee's willingness to work to engage with the stakeholders to improve the system to ensure as humanly as possible that every organ is given the best chance to save a life.

In conjunction with the Hearing, the Committee released a memo entitled "Staff Memo on Organizational Failures of The United States Organ Procurement" (Memo) along with exhibits. Page 11 of the Memo references a "Courier Case" involving Mississippi Organ Recovery Agency (MSOP), and states that "[o]n February 25, 2017, two incidents were reported to UNOS where the courier service requested by the OPO did not arrive in time to get the organs to their flight." Appendix F to the Memo provides additional documentation related to the events. I write to provide information to clarify the situation identified.

With regard to the incidents on February 25, 2017, it is important to clarify that MSOP facilitated the donation of the right, but not the left kidney. The right kidney was offered by MSOP and accepted by AZMC. According to the courier, when the courier arrived at our local airport, the commercial airline company agent refused to accept the kidney for the flight to Phoenix via Dallas. Also, according to courier, even though the right kidney arrived within the parameters of acceptance for acceptance for the flight, the airline agent refused to put it on the flight. The courier immediately notified the UNOS Organ Center. UNOS, in collaboration with the courier company, then identified another commercial airline company to fly the kidney to AZMC, AZMC declined the kidney due to the later arrival time on the new flight, even though the new flight departed only fifteen (15) minutes later than the original flight. The right kidney was then quickly accepted by the transplant center that had also accepted the left kidney. Both the right and left kidneys were then placed on the same flight to the new transplant center on a different commercial airline company flight. Both kidneys arrived in a safe and timely manner to the transplant center that accepted both kidneys. However, according to the accepting transplant center, on arrival and after further evaluation, unfortunately the effects of the donor's history of hypertension and diabetes had damaged the kidneys to the point they were not transplantable.

In spite of the transportation challenges in this case, MSOP worked diligently with the courier and UNOS to ensure that the organ was quickly placed with another transplant center and transported expeditiously. In spite of these efforts, ultimately, the discard in this case was within the discretion of the transplant center.

MSOP recognizes the urgent need to address organ discards and supports the statement made by AOPO on August 4:

> AOPO encourages a robust system to trace the cause of every organ discard to better determine the reasons for organ declines by transplant centers and develop strategies to minimize organ waste and increase organ acceptance. With the discard rate trending upward this year, this is an urgent issue that all donation and transplant stakeholders must solve for all the patients on the waiting list.

More broadly, MSOP also agrees with and strongly supports Senator Wyden's statement that the system should work with as few errors as possible. However, in order to effectively reduce or eliminate those errors and meaningfully transform the system, the policies and practices of all donation and transplant partners should be considered. As Senator Wyden acknowledged in his opening statement, UNOS oversees nearly 400 members, including 252 transplant centers and 57 OPOs. The focus of the Hearing was on the "failures" of the government Organ Procurement Transplant Network (OPTN) contractor, UNOS, and Organ Procurement Organizations. Notably absent from this discussion is any reference to transplant centers or their policies. OPOs and transplant programs are equally integral to the system. If the system is to be comprehensively reformed, all partners' policies must be considered.

In addition to OPOs and transplant centers, the above-referenced incident highlights the numerous partners, whether members of UNOS or otherwise, whose practices affect the ultimate outcome of a successful organ recovery and transplantation. In addition to this event, others of the "Transportation Failures" referenced in the Memo appear to have been completely outside of the control of UNOS, the organ procurement organization, or the transplant program. MSOP suggests that policies should be developed to ensure that all partners, including transportation partners, maximize protection of these precious life-saving gifts.

The Mississippi Organ Recovery Agency has been and always will be striving to be the best possible organ procurement organization in the United States of America. We welcome any meaningful and comprehensive improvements to the system to ensure that ALL stakeholders are held accountable.

Sincerely, M. Kevin Stump President/CEO

National Down Syndrome Society

1155 15th Street, NW, Suite 540
Washington, DC 20005
800–221–4602
www.ndss.org

U.S. Senate Committee on Finance
219 Dirksen Senate Office Building Washington, DC 20510 6200

Dear Chairman Wyden and Ranking Member Crapo:

On behalf of the Down syndrome community, we wish to thank you for holding a hearing on addressing the organizational failures of the United States' organ procurement and transplantation network. We look forward to working together to address this critical issue, particularly as it affects individuals with intellectual and developmental disabilities. As you consider improvements to the system, we urge you to recognize that the lives of individuals with disabilities have equal value to the lives of people without disabilities, so they deserve equal access to organ transplants. We ask that you advance meaningful solutions to address systemic discrimination against individuals with disabilities found at all levels of the organ procurement and transplantation network.

Organ transplants are a key part of our nation's health care system. They save lives every day. Unfortunately, people with disabilities have consistently been denied organ transplants in the United States based on unfounded assumptions on their quality of life and ability to comply with post-operative care. This is in direct violation of the Americans with Disabilities Act, Section 504 of the Rehabilitation Act of 1973, and Section 1557 of the Affordable Care Act, which prohibit discrimination on the basis of disability.

Despite these existing overarching protections, real-world discrimination persists. The National Council on Disability (NCD) recently reviewed applicable federal and state laws, the disability-related policies of various organ transplant centers, and policies of the Organ Procurement and Transplantation Network and issued a report in September 2019.[108] The report found that people with disabilities are frequently denied access to organ transplants based on written and unwritten policies excluding people with disabilities as organ transplant candidates, even in the nine states that, at the time, had state laws in place prohibiting such practice. Furthermore, some medical professionals even refused to evaluate a patient's medical suitability for organ transplant because of their disability.

In our community, the threat of discrimination in organ transplantation presents a real-world danger. About 50% of all people born with Down syndrome have congenital heart disease, which often requires heart surgery and, if unsuccessful, can lead to the need for transplantation. Last year, NDSS learned of Zion Sarmiento, a baby born in June with Down syndrome in Florida. Zion had a congenital heart defect and underwent multiple surgeries, but ultimately, he needed a transplant to survive. Despite Florida having passed a state-law

[108] National Council on Disability. (2019). Organ transplant discrimination against people with disabilities. Retrieved from https://ncd.gov/sites/default/files/NCD_Organ_Transplant_508.pdf.

prohibition of disability discrimination in organ transplantation, effective July 1, 2020,[109] Zion was unable to access a transplant and tragically passed away in October. He was less than four months old.

While progress has been made since NCD issued their report, including the passage of laws in 34 states,[110] this patchwork does not adequately ensure individuals with disabilities are protected because the organ transplant ecosystem, as a whole, is firmly interstate. We therefore strongly urge the Committee to support consideration and passage of the Charlotte Woodward Organ Transplant Discrimination Prevention Act (S. 3301), which would prohibit discrimination against people with disabilities who need organ transplants, upholding, clarifying, and building upon rights established in the Americans with Disabilities Act of 1990, Sec. 504 of the Rehabilitation Act of 1973, and Sec. 1557 of the Affordable Care Act. This commonsense legislation is bipartisan in both chambers (with H.R. 1235) and has no fiscal impact.

NDSS is eager to partner with you as the Committee explores and develops meaningful policies to improve the nation's organ transplant ecosystem, including protecting the civil rights of individuals with disabilities. For more information, please contact Bartholomew N. Devon, senior director of public policy, at *bdevon@ndss.org*.

Sincerely, Kandi Pickard
President and CEO

The National Down Syndrome Society (NDSS) is the leading human rights organization for all individuals with Down syndrome. NDSS envisions a world in which all people with Down syndrome have the opportunity to enhance their quality of life, realize their life aspirations, and become valued members of welcoming communities.

National Kidney Foundation

30 East 33rd Street New York, NY 10016

Statement of Sharon Pearce, Senior Vice President, Government Relations

The National Kidney Foundation (NKF) respectfully submits our statement for the record on behalf of the 37 million individuals in the United States, 1 in 7 adults, estimated to have chronic kidney disease (CKD).[111] The prevalence of kidney failure is expected to increase dramatically, possibly exceeding one million people who may need access to the transplant

---

[109] Florida CS/HB 1179 (2020), *https://www.myfloridahouse.gov/Sections/Bills/ billsdetail.aspx?BillId=69420.*

[110] National Down Syndrome Society. (2022). *Organ transplant discrimination state laws.* Retrieved from *https://www.ndss.org/advocacy#p_health.*

[111] Centers for Disease Control and Prevention. *Chronic Kidney Disease in the United States, 2021.* Centers for Disease Control and Prevention; 2021.

wait list by 2030.[112] There are not enough deceased or living donor organs to meet current or future needs creating a public health emergency that needs immediate attention. Although 24,669 people received a kidney transplant in 2021, far too many are still waiting. Many never access the transplant wait list or learn that a transplant is an option. There are over 100,000 individuals on the transplant wait list, and more than 90,000 are waiting for a kidney.

NKF is fiercely committed to holding the transplant system accountable for the ethical stewardship of organs as a precious, life-saving resource. NKF's transplant policy agenda seeks to implement policy changes, payment reforms, legislative solutions, quality measurement, and oversight activities that:

- Maximize the number of kidneys procured and transplanted;
- Minimize the number of kidneys discarded;
- Enhance the transplant process to become more transparent and patient-centric; and
- Drive continuous performance improvement across the transplant system.

The United Network for Organ Sharing (UNOS) has been the sole contractor of the Organ Procurement and Transplantation Network (OPTN) contract—without competition—since 1986. In its nearly 40 years of providing oversight of the organ donation and transplant system, UNOS has witnessed the continuous growth of the wait list, which comprises almost 106,000 organ failure patients currently waiting for a kidney transplant.[113] UNOS is acutely aware that supply is not meeting demand. The OPTN goals should include transparency, equity, and efficacy of organ donation and transplantation practices.

A vital responsibility of UNOS is to provide oversight to the nation's organ procurement organizations (OPO). As revealed in recent congressional investigations, life-threatening inefficiencies and inequities in the transplant system are directly related to OPO underperformance. OPOs are the only transplant stakeholders with the privilege and responsibility of recovering organs from deceased donors for transplant. The lack of oversight is a catastrophic disservice to patients. Transplant centers and OPOs are left to their own devices and tools to sort out logistics of organ and patient transportation leading to inefficiency, wasted expense and directly leading to increased discards.

We have made many recommendations to the Centers for Medicare and Medicaid Services (CMS), Health Resources and Services Administration (HRSA), Organ Procurement and Transplantation Network (OPTN), and Scientific Registry for Transplant Recipients (SRTR) on strategies to improve the organ donation and transplant system, which are summarized below.

1) Improving Organ Procurement and Increasing Organ Donation

Immediate data transparency: OPOs collect organ donation data that is currently inaccessible to the public. As an entity whose sole purpose is to serve the public, it is a disservice to patients needing transplantation, organ donors, and donor families who make

---

[112] McCullough K.P., Morgenstern H., Saran R., Herman W.H., Robinson B.M. Projecting ESRD Incidence and Prevalence in the United States through 2030. *J Am Soc Nephrol.* 2019 Jan;30(1):127-135. DOI: 10.1681/ASN.2018050531. Epub 2018 Dec 17. PMID: 30559143; PMCID: PMC6317596.

[113] National data—OPTN *(hrsa.gov).*

the selfless decision to donate their loved one's organs. The following metrics (at a minimum), currently captured by all OPOs, should be made publicly available for quality assurance, performance improvement, and stratified by gender, race, ethnicity, age, zip code for health equity purposes:

- Number of organ referrals.
- Number of braindead donors.
- Number of donation after cardiac (DCD) donors.
- Missed organ referrals.
- Conversion rate.
- Approach rate.
- Consent rate.
- Percentage of first-person consent.

Regulatory consequences for OPOs failing to respond timely to donor hospitals to evaluate potential organ donors: When donor hospitals make a referral for a patient who is not automatically clinically ruled out as an organ donor, the OPTN contractor should require OPOs to make every effort to elicit a timely onsite response for an evaluation.

Regulatory consequences for missed organ referrals: Donor hospitals should face repercussions for missed referrals of potential organ donors. When a hospital fails to notify an OPO of a potential organ donor, critically ill patients continue to wait for a life-saving organ transplant. Further, families lose the opportunity to continue the legacy of their loved ones through the selfless gift of organ donation, and the wishes of the person who has designated their desire to donate their organs are unfairly forfeited.

Staffing to reflect the DSA (Donor Service Area) community: The OPTN contractor must call for OPOs to recruit, hire, and train staff representing the diverse racial, ethnic, and cultural communities they serve. Diversity, equity, and inclusion should be reflected across all departments within the OPO, including executive leadership, OPO professional staff, the clinical teams that interface with donor hospitals, and the teams that work with potential donor families.

Transportation: Organ transportation delays and inefficiencies have life-threatening consequences for waiting patients. It is unacceptable that donated organs are discarded due to transportation pitfalls after donors and donor families have made the selfless decision to donate organs. Examining challenges in the transportation system and identifying policies, best practices, and strategies to mitigate cold ischemia time that results in organ discards is imperative.[114]

Consent training: Reducing disparities and ensuring that each donor and their families are respectfully considered and supported during the donation process must be a standard upheld by all OPOs.[115] OPO staff must be adequately trained and equipped to approach families of all races, ethnicities, socioeconomic backgrounds, and religious beliefs for organ donation. OPOs

---

[114] Cooper M., Formica R., Friedewald J., et al. Report of National Kidney Foundation Con- sensus Conference to Decrease Kidney Discards. Clin Transplant. 2019;33(1):e13419. doi:10.1111/ctr.13419.

[115] Guadagnoli E., McNamara P., Evanisko M.J., Beasley C., Callender C.O., Poretsky A. (1999). The influence of race on approaching families for organ donation and their decision to donate. American Journal of Public Health, 89(2), 244–247. https://doi.org/10.2105/ajph. 89.2.244.

should be held accountable for instituting donor family communication best practices, especially around recognizing and eliminating implicit bias, ensuring racial equity, and delivering trauma-informed care.

Donor management and patient safety: The OPTN contractor must assess and improve the clinical knowledge of OPO staff to maximize organ recruitment and transplantation. This includes perfusing organs and donation outcomes after cardiac death (DCD) and braindead (BD) donors and organs. Patient safety during organ recovery and transplantation must never be compromised, and documentation of adverse events should undoubtedly be documented, reported, and reviewed to determine the cause and need for remedy.

2) Reducing Deceased Donor Kidney Discards

In partnership with CMS, HRSA, and other stakeholders, the OPTN contractor should implement regulatory changes, payment policy adjustments, and quality improvement initiatives to incentivize OPO and transplant center practices that could reduce discards as recommended by NKF's 2017 Discard Consensus Conference:[116] Such recommendations include:

- Begin the organ allocation process earlier in the donor evaluation phase.
- Improve communication between OPO and transplant surgeons—The Kidney Allocation System relies on an electronic communication platform, DonorNet, that limits verbal communication between the OPO and transplant center. The exclusive use of DonorNet without collaborative conversations between the OPO and transplant center contributes to decreased organ utilization.
- Accelerate virtual crossmatching and send early prospective crossmatch samples.
- Require frequent QAPI meetings with OPOs and transplant centers to review and analyze data and investigate root causes for low organ transplant rates.
    - Secure "local backups" to mitigate the possibility of a kidney discard.
    - Increased patient-centricity around organ offers may reduce kidney discards.
    - The OPTN contractor should consider creating an algorithm that recommends which patient group receives specific organ offers (ex., determine which patient group would benefit most from a particular organ offer to mitigate "list diving" and reduce organ discards).

Risk aversion in the transplant system is a significant contributor to kidney discard and devastating for patients depending on a life-saving kidney transplant. NKF has urged CMS to develop new reimbursement mechanisms that incentivize transplant centers to list high-risk patients, accept less-than-perfect organs for transplant, and adopt innovative therapies and technologies. New transplant center performance measures should be designed to reduce risk-aversion.

Patients have an essential role in improving risk aversion and reducing discards by making their wishes clear to their care teams. Patients are often less risk-averse than their surgeons and centers. As they spend more time on the wait list, they may accept an imperfect organ that still

[116] Cooper M., Formica R., Friedewald J., et al. Report of National Kidney Foundation Consensus Conference to Decrease Kidney Discards. *Clin Transplant.* 2019;33(1):e13419. doi:10. 1111/ctr.13419.

confers clinical value compared to dialysis. Transplant centers, nephrologists, and dialysis facilities must regularly consult patients to assess and refine their transplant goals. Increasing utilization is closely linked to reimbursement, transparency, and improved organ acceptance practices. However, it begins with a patient-centered approach to understanding the waitlisted patient's goals and preferences. Transplant programs should also promote shared decision-making with inactive wait-list patients.

Place urgent attention on the role of organ transportation in organ discards: Changes in the allocation system have resulted in more organs being transported across the nation than ever before. Dependence on commercial flights presents several challenges for transplantation that contribute to avoidable discards. Organ recovery usually occurs in the late hours when donor hospital operating rooms are less busy and when there are fewer commercial flights. Every hour a recovered organ waits to be transplanted, cold ischemia time (CIT) increases, decreasing the likelihood of transplantation. Federal regulations no longer allow organs to fly in the cockpit with the pilot, only as cargo, which exacerbates CIT. Kidneys with too much CIT are discarded and represent a potential life lost on the wait list. Deceased kidneys are a scarce resource; inefficiencies in air travel should never be a reason for organ discard.

3) Making the Transplant Process and Experience More Transparent and Patient-Centered

Patients on the wait list receive many organ offers; however, the transplant center often declines organ offers on behalf of their patients without their knowledge or consent. Increasing organ utilization is closely linked to reimbursement, transparency, and improved organ acceptance practices. However, it begins with a patient-centered approach to understanding the wait-listed patient's goals and preferences. Transplant programs should never lose sight of promoting shared decision- making with patients. Patient-centricity should be a priority for every regulatory agency that oversees the organ donation and transplant system, as patients should always have the option to be active participants in shared decision-making with their healthcare team.

There is a need for organ donation and transplant stakeholders to implement additional patient-centric process measures, including bi-annual reports to patients on organs offered and declined on their behalf and annual conversations between patients and their care team regarding patient preferences and tolerances for accepting or rejecting imperfect organs. In addition, if, through this process of shared decision-making, transplant programs and candidates discover either donor or recipient characteristics that would result in universal organ decline, we encourage transplant programs to utilize the organ filters now better optimized to minimize allocation of unacceptable offers resulting in increased cold ischemia time and slowing identification of the appropriate recipient and potential organ discard.

4) Improving System Performace

Harmonizing regulatory agency oversight: NKF supports policies that remove silos, improve operations, drive system-level performance, and increase equity. CMS, UNOS, HRSA, SRTR, and the Joint Commission share oversight of the organ donation and transplantation system. This fragmented oversight contributes to communication, process, and alignment gaps. NKF advocates for one HHS-level office that would provide overall management of the transplant ecosystem to mitigate deficiencies that result from a lack of cohesion and accountability. It is of the utmost importance that performance standards among the regulatory agencies that oversee organ donation and transplantation are aligned in both process and implementation. Misaligned measures only muddle behavior rather than direct it towards shared goals.

Modernizing the technology infrastructure: NKF supports two separate contracts for the Information Technology (IT) Infrastructure and one for other OPTN priorities. The current IT architecture is outdated and fraught with inefficiencies that impair organ donation and transplantation, such as OPO and transplant center communication, wait-list management, and organ allocation. Patients face life-threatening consequences because the UNOS technology is not sophisticated enough for efficient organ distribution. For example, nearly one in five kidneys is offered to a deceased person still on the wait list because the transplant center is unaware that the patient has died, and deceased candidates receive a median of 4 organ offers before being removed from the wait list.[117]

The OPTN contractor should not own any technology associated with the organ donation and transplantation process. Separating the two contracts allows OPTN to leverage significant improvements in information technology and mitigate the risk of disruption to the donation and transplant process.

Mandating transparency: Data transparency of organ donor hospitals, OPOs, and transplant centers must be prioritized to improve organ allocation processes. The lack of data transparency creates significant barriers to care and inequities for the entire population that could benefit from transplantation. Data collected from OPOs and transplant centers are outdated, inadequately audited, incomplete, and self-reported, making it impossible to develop modern quality measures, specifically for steps in the pre-transplant process. Patients need real-time data, or as close to real-time as possible, to make informed decisions about transplantation. The current delay in data does not accurately portray the current state of organ donation and transplantation.

NKF was deeply troubled by OPTN's announcement about adding 35,000 verified deaths to the standard analytical files. This adjustment illustrates the failure of the current system to capture data from a range of sources and cross-reference it to ensure maximum efficiency. Further, OPTN's announcement lacked urgency or even recognition of the gravity of data inconsistencies and their implications for transplantation-related research. This incident reinforces the critical need for transparency and the need to separate the IT contract from other OPTN requirements to ensure that patients and the system benefit from the cutting-edge technologies that can eliminate these inconsistencies and inefficiencies. HRSA must also determine how death data is collected and verified with the OPTN contractor and CMS to mitigate an error of this magnitude in the future.

Enhanced wait-list management: The transplant wait list is poorly maintained because of inconsistent communication between transplant centers, dialysis facilities, and patients or caregivers due to the current antiquated IT architecture. Patients on the wait list are frequently unaware of their wait-list status—active or inactive—and receive little or no information from the transplant centers. This absence of communication among patients, their dialysis facilities, and transplant centers represents a failure of the OPTN to improve communication between

---

[117] Husain S.A., Winterhalter F.S., Mohan S. Kidney transplant offers to deceased candidates. *Am J Transplant.* 2018 Nov;18(11):2836–2837.

various stakeholders in transplantation, resulting in inefficient allocation and the perpetuation of silos of care.

Health equity: Prejudice and implicit bias are common elements of OPO practice. Beliefs that people of color will not donate perpetuate patterns where hospitals are less likely to refer prospective donors to the OPO. In studies, Black/African American families have declined donation because of insufficient time to process and discuss important issues and a lack of sensitivity and empathy during the approach process.[118] Research has also found that OPOs are more likely to approach White families over Black/African American families.[119] NKF strongly opposes race-based adjustments to the OPO metrics and suggests that OPOs adopt best practices to overcome bias and prejudice on the ability of families to donate their loved one's organs. For example, hiring staff that represents the communities they serve and implementing frequent training on cultural sensitivity, diversity, and inclusion to improve conversations with non-White populations about donation.

A kidney transplant is the optimal treatment for end-stage renal disease. Still, Black/African American people are disadvantaged at every step of the transplant process and have poorer graft outcomes.[120] Organ failure patients desperately need an equitable transplant ecosystem. Justice, fairness, equity, and transparency are values our organ donation and transplant system need, and patients deserve. Federal agencies that oversee the organ donation and transplant system must uphold these values to influence public confidence in our organ donation and transplant system. Regardless of demographic characteristics or socioeconomic status, every person should have the right to access the national transplant wait list.

Amplifying the Patient Voice

As a patient advocacy organization, NKF is proud to uplift the voices of the patients we have the honor to represent. Improvement of the organ donation and transplantation system should not occur without patients learning what they need and want for the success of their transplant journey. When presented with the opportunity to comment on how to improve the current transplant system, we received the following responses from patients:

Improve communication — "Ensure that transplant centers have adequate resources and staff to support their patients with consistent and effective communication. Patients deserve to know when they are listed for transplant and the actions they can take to maintain optimal health on the wait list. Centers must alert patients of their wait-list status when they become listed and made inactive or delisted. Physicians, Advanced Practice Providers, Nurses, Transplant Coordinators, Social Workers, and other transplant center staff that interface with patients should adequately and compassionately share the reasons for an inactive status with patients and why they have been delisted."

---

[118] Siminoff L.A., Alolod G.P., Gardiner H.M., Hasz R.D., Mulvania P.A., Wilson-Genderson M. A Comparison of the Content and Quality of Organ Donation Discussions with African American Families Who Authorize and Refuse Donation. *J Racial Ethn Health Disparities.* 2021;8(2):485–493. doi:10.1007/s40615–020–00806–7.

[119] Guadagnoli E., McNamara P., Evanisko M.J., Beasley C., Callender C.O., Poretsky A. The influence of race on approaching families for organ donation and their decision to donate. *Am J Public Health.* 1999;89(2):244–247. doi:10.2105/AJPH.89.2.244.

[120] Norton JM, Moxey-Mims MM, Eggers PW, et al. Social Determinants of Racial Disparities in CKD. *J Am Soc Nephrol.* 2016;27(9):2576–2595. doi:10.1681/ASN.2016010027.

Include the patient as part of the care team — "Clear and timely communication between the transplant team and patients can promote shared decision-making should be afforded to each patient. Transplant centers have complained about patient compliance; if transplant centers want improved cooperation from patients, they should prioritize shared decision-making."

Promote cultural sensitivity — "Clinical and non-clinical transplant center staff must practice cultural sensitivity and inclusivity to decrease patients' risk of falling through the cracks due to language barriers and cultural misunderstandings. Transplant centers need appropriate communication strategies and mechanisms to relay messages with non-English speaking patients to prevent patient isolation and poor outcomes."

Address patients' mental and emotional well-being— "Organ failure is scary. Dialysis creates added stress and anxiety. Dialysis patients face various challenges—healthcare complications, lethargy (too tired to participate in common daily activities), lack of social support, and depression, to name a few. Patients experience a general fear when faced with organ failure and the prospect of their mortality. Organ donation and transplant surgery are overwhelming to think about. Transplant centers could assuage these feelings by communicating with their patients in as close to real-time as possible about what to expect during the process (not just once, but reminders throughout would be helpful)."

Conclusion

The National Kidney Foundation has been fighting kidney disease for over 55 years and works tirelessly to improve outcomes for kidney patients and patients at risk by emphasizing prevention, early detection, and CKD management to slow or stop the progression of kidney disease. We are also committed to increasing access to kidney transplantation and improving patient choice of high-quality, patient-centered options to treat kidney failure. Kidney care is fraught with disparities. We will continue to advocate for policies that prevent barriers, biases, and prejudices that prevent all patients from receiving the care they rightly deserve.

We welcome any questions about our recommendations and to improve the American organ donation and transplant system. Please contact Morgan Reid, Director of Transplant Policy and Strategy (morgan.reid@kidney.org), or Lauren Drew, Director of Congressional Relations (lauren.drew@kidney.org).

Thank you for your consideration.

Organ Donation Consortium

975 F Street, NW, Suite 400–A Washington, DC 20004 odc@organ.org

August 5, 2022
U.S. Senate Committee on Finance
219 Dirksen Senate Office Bldg. Washington, DC 20510–6200

Chairman Wyden, Ranking Member Crapo, and Members of the Committee:

The Organ Donation Consortium (the "ODC"), comprised of five of the nation's leading organ procurement organizations ("OPOs") and collectively representing almost 38 million Americans, applauds the work of the U.S. Senate Committee on Finance (the "Committee") addressing organizational failures of the U.S. Organ Procurement and Transplantation Network ("OPTN"), including severely lacking technology and its impact on our ability to save lives through organ donation and transplantation. We formed the ODC in part to address such failures and gaps left by many in the donation and transplantation ecosystem. Our strategic focus is fully aligned with the Committee's work as well as with many of the key recommendations, particularly those concerning health equity, organ utilization and the modernization and integration of state-of-the-art heath information systems, found in the report of the NASEM Committee on a Fairer and More Equitable, Cost-Effective, and Transparent System of Donor Organ Procurement, Allocation, and Distribution.

The ODC's strategic focus is on technological innovations and integrations, cross-sector stakeholder collaboration, and transparent accountability. With the open integration of systems among all stakeholders—donor hospitals, OPOs, and transplant centers, as well as the OPTN—we have set out to save more lives through donation and transplantation while:

- Eliminating health disparities in donation and transplantation;
- Increasing the number of organs made available for transplant;
- Eliminating the unnecessary discard of transplantable organs;
- Reducing inefficiencies and errors in the donation process;
- Improving quality through the donation process;
- Reducing the time it takes to shepherd a life-saving organ from donor to recipient;
- Reducing costs in the donation system; and
- Providing a framework for the consistent and reliable collection of data for performance measurement of all stakeholders that make organ donation and transplantation possible.

No one is above scrutiny in these matters, including OPOs, hospital systems, transplant centers, and those overseeing this work, including the OPTN, and the ODC stands ready to assist in the development of further reforms and technological innovations to achieve significant improvements in organ donation and transplantation for all Americans.

Sincerely,

Janice F. Whaley
President and CEO
Donor Network West
San Ramon, California

Diane Brockmeier
President and CEO
Mid-America Transplant
St. Louis, Missouri

Kelly Ranum
President and CEO
Louisiana Organ Procurement Agency
Covington, Louisiana

Bradley L. Adams President
Southwest Transplant Alliance Dallas,
Texas

Ginny McBride
Our Legacy
Orlando, Florida
Executive Director

Organ Procurement and Transplantation Network Patients Affairs Committee

August 2, 2022
Dear Members of the Senate Finance Committee,

As the leaders of the OPTN Patients Affairs Committee (PAC), we are reaching out to share our experiences on the committee that we believe indicate a systemic failure of UNOS to serve patients as the OPTN. This is all the more urgent in light of investigative reporting from The Washington Post.[121]

Antiquated technology and an apathetic culture cause patients to languish with incomplete and often incorrect information, and leave people to die every day on the list. OPTN PAC members have raised these points often with UNOS leadership, and have seen our calls for reform ignored. We have been aghast at the absolute failure of UNOS to operate the practice and business of transplant, and to acknowledge— much less effectively serve—patients who are waiting and dying on the organ wait list.

On July 28th, in preparation for the upcoming August 3rd Senate Finance Committee hearing into UNOS, PAC leaders received an email from UNOS CEO, Brain Shepard, referring to your investigation, in which he makes four assertions that UNOS has shared with the Committee.

We wish to correct the record for your urgent consideration.

Shepard: "Our IT system remains safe, secure and routinely meets and surpasses federal standards."

The Washington Post reported "The system for getting donated kidneys, livers and hearts to desperately ill patients relies on out-of-date technology that has crashed for hours at a time and has never been audited by federal officials for security weaknesses or other serious flaws."

We hope the Committee asks UNOS how many patients have died due to the inability to match organs during downtime, as well as other technological inefficiencies such as data error due to manual entry, as well as how many patient life-years have been lost due to delays in

[121] https://www.washingtonpost.com/health/2022/07/31/unos-transplants-kindeys-hearts-tech- nology/.

organ transportation. That said, given the lack of transparency in the UNOS tech system, it is difficult to imagine anyone at UNOS could answer this question with any confidence.

Shepard: "We have worked together as a community to improve the transport of organs with innovative, evidence-based products."

The UNOS transportation record on organs is woefully—and fatally—inadequate, as outlined by investigative reporting from Kaiser Health News[122] —as well as cases brought before the Senate Finance Committee. Put simply, UNOS operates as an antiquated, closed system that keeps out external innovators that could help patients with better tools and services.

Shepard: "Our committees and staff are proud to work collaboratively with all members to serve as partners in improvement."

PAC members have often sought—and not received—clarity on how patient input is used. When PAC takes clear positions (such as the need to fast-track proposed changes to using eGFR results to list people of color), UNOS has refused to act. Compare this to a recent UNOS fast track process that addressed a hardware defect in a mechanical heart that went through in less than a month. Black patients deserved this kind of speedy remedy when eGFR was proven to have racial bias. We also note Washington Post[123] reporting that UNOS's policy making processes have been so divisive that they have "spark[ed] open conflict" among OPTN members.

Shepard: "The system we are all so honored to be a part of just surpassed 41,000 transplants in 2021, while continuing to expand equitable access to transplant."

UNOS obscures its underperforming record behind recent increases in organ donation rates that have resulted from tragic spikes in opioid overdoses, gun deaths, and car accidents, including second-order effects of the COVID pandemic, not from UNOS's own performance. See the former U.S. Chief Data Scientist making this point in MedPage,[124] and research in the Journal of the American Medical Association[125] finding that, after controlling for public health trends and scientific advancements which have increased the size of the donor pool, organ donation rates have not even kept pace with population growth.[126]

The alarming revelations in The Washington Post (antiquated technology; covering for failures of organ procurement organizations; and lack of cooperation with the government, even devolving to UNOS having "threatened to walk away") lead us to believe that UNOS has proven itself incapable of functioning as the OPTN.

We ask that you ensure that the federal government makes the fast-approaching contracting OPTN cycle competitive for the first time since the original OPTN contract was awarded in 1986, opening critical functions up to best-in-class innovators across the country; and we implore you to ensure that UNOS does not hold patients hostage in the process.

We urge you to continue with your oversight and institute urgent reforms that will literally result in lives saved.

---

[122] https://khn.org/news/how-lifesaving-organs-for-transplant-go-missing-in-transit/.

[123] https://www.washingtonpost.com/national/health-science/liver-transplant-rules-spark-open-conflict-among-transplant-centers/2019/05/16/91b37f84-781c-11e9-bd25-c989555e7766_story. html.

[124] https://www.medpagetoday.com/opinion/second-opinions/98363.

[125] https://jamanetwork.com/journals/jamasurgery/article-abstract/2771051.

[126] https://bloomworks.digital/organdonationreform/assets/PDF/donation-increase.pdf.

Signed,
Garrett Erdle
Chair, OPTN PAC
Living Kidney Donor, Alexandria, VA
Molly J. McCarthy Vice Chair, OPTN PAC
3-time Kidney Transplant Recipient, Redmond, WA

Chris Yanakos
Former Member of OPTN PAC
Living Liver Donor, Caregiver and Donor Family Member, Pittsburgh, PA

Steve Weitzen
Region 2 Representative, OPTN PAC Heart Recipient, Randolph, NJ

Calvin Henry
Region 3 Representative, OPTN PAC Lung Recipient, Dacula, GA

Lorrinda Gray-Davis
Region 4 Representative, OPTN PAC Liver Recipient, Yukon, OK

Julie Spear
Region 8 Representative, OPTN PAC Donor Family Member, Boulder, CO

Eric Tanis
Region 10 Representative, OPTN PAC Liver Recipient, Gary, IN

Paragonix Technologies, Inc.

222 Third Street
Cambridge, MA 02142
https://paragonixtechnologies.com/

August 16, 2022
U.S. Senate Committee on Finance
219 Dirksen Senate Office Building Washington, DC 20510–6200

Dear Chairman Wyden, Ranking Member Crapo, and Members of the Committee,

Paragonix Technologies, Inc. ("Paragonix") respectfully submits this Statement for the Record in response to the Senate Finance Committee hearing on Wednesday, August 3, 2022, A System in Need of Repair: Addressing Organizational Failures of the U.S.'s Organ Procurement and Transplantation Network. We commend the Committee for escalating the importance of the nation's organ donor and transplant system, and its desire to improve upon the existing system to maximize the rate of organ donation in the country and maximize the rate of successful procurement and transplant of vital human organs.

Paragonix Technologies, Inc. is a medical device company headquartered in Cambridge, MA, that designs, produces, and markets organ transportation devices that preserve human organs intended for transplant during the journey between the donor procurement facility and the transplant recipient center. Paragonix is a leader in providing FDA-cleared devices for the transportation and preservation of all solid organs: heart, liver, lung, kidney, and pancreas. Since its commercial launch in 2020, Paragonix devices have preserved over 2,200 donor organs.

We also recognize the benefits of the Recommendations provided by the Senate Finance Committee following the Hearing on August 3, 2022. In particular, we would like to offer support and solutions towards improvements in the methods, tracking and data reporting of organ transportation systems, highlighted as one of the most pressing concerns voiced at the Hearing. We refer to the following specific recommendation:

VIII. Recommendations

Increase transparency and accountability for chain of custody and transportation of organs procured for transplant by providing for public reporting, as appropriate, on the status of organs in transport."

(https://www.finance.senate.gov/imo/media/doc/UNOS%20Hearing%20Confidential%20Memo%20(FOR%20RELEASE).pdf)

Improvements in the Method, Tracking, and Data Reporting of Organ Transportation Systems

For nearly 5 decades, the most common form of organ preservation (i.e., storage during transport between donor and recipient) has been ice-cold storage in simple non-medical grade, non-regulated containers (e.g., plastic coolers, cardboard boxes, food storage tubs, etc). This method is fraught with complications and potential hazards and lacks any regulatory oversight consistent with updated methods and needs.

This is an extremely outdated approach to the storage of organs during transport, yet remains embedded in current OPTN Policy (sections 16.3.E.i. and 16.3.E.iii):

> An outer container of corrugated plastic or corrugated cardboard, with at least 200 pounds burst strength, that is coated with a water-resistant substance." (OPTN Policy, Section 16.3.E.i) . . . "If a member of the organ recovery team is accompanying the organ to the potential transplant recipient's transplant hospital, the organs and tissue typing material may be transported in a cooler. A cooler may be reused only if it is properly cleaned and sanitized and all labels from previous donor organs are removed." (OPTN Policy, section 16.3.E.iii)

These policies describe a method of cold storage using coolers or disposable cardboard boxes filled with ice to cool the organ and thereby reduce the metabolic demand of the organ. This ice-based method has been ensconced in the transplant field to the point it thwarts innovation and progress. It also is not reflective of the technological advancements and clinical advantages of mechanical preservation systems.

Admittedly, this ice-based method provides an inexpensive approach to organ preservation; however, it poses serious risks to the patient and is difficult, nearly impossible, to standardize. In short, the ice-based method of transporting organs is outdated, potentially harmful, and does not reflect current methods of storage recognized and cleared by the FDA.

A multitude of potential harms have been noted, including: (a) freezing injury of organs as a result of organs becoming frozen due to an ice-based method of preservation, (b) uneven cooling of the organ tissue and violations of FDA-regulated temperature requirements of preservation solutions, (c) lack of standardization due to a variability in composite, type, and strength of packaging materials; (d) the inability to know the biocompatibility of the material that touches the organ; (e) potential tissue injury due to erratic movements or vibrations during manual handling; and (f) the lack of knowledge of the real-time changes in temperature during transport, one of the most important parameters in organ preservation that directly impacts organ function post-transplant.

With these limitations in mind, Paragonix makes the following recommendations regarding transporting organs for transplantation:

A) OPTN Policies should require, and organ procurement and transplant programs should adopt, the use of FDA-cleared and regulated preservation systems.

In contrast to non-regulated containers used during organ transport (e.g., plastic food containers), FDA-regulated devices require rigorous review and validation prior to gaining market clearance for use in a healthcare setting. This includes design verification, electronic safety review, thermal qualifications, ship testing (for clinical use conditions), sterile validations, sterile barrier qualifications, biocompatibility testing, etc. None of these requirements are made of retail, commercially purchased storage containers, posing unknown risks to patients. For example, retail coolers used for transporting organs are not required to demonstrate they are safe for physical contact with human organs, nor are they validated to maintain a consistent, documented temperature.

The 2020 Consensus Statement of the International Society of Heart and Lung Transplantation states, "[T]here are some new technologies for packaging . . . that prevent direct contact of the ice with the "myocardium [which] may cause freezing. . . and is undesirable because freezing and thawing cause irreversible cellular damage." In short, transplant professionals recognize the advantages possible in newer technologies, such as mechanical preservation systems that offer temperature control.

Using our own technology, Paragonix has shown the clinical and economic value of mechanical and controlled preservation of organs over uncontrolled cold storage on ice through studies conducted with data from the GUARDIAN registries (NCT04141605, NCT04930289 for lung, NCT05082077 for liver). In particular, the GUARDIAN Heart registry collects and evaluates various clinical effectiveness parameters in patients with transplanted donor organs that were preserved and transported within the Paragonix SherpaPak- Transport Systems and those that were transported using simple ice storage. Data collected by 17 transplant centers for approximately 800 patients was presented at the International Society for Heart and Lung Transplantation in April of 2022 (Leacche et al.). In a propensity-score analysis, the authors showed improvements in the function of donor hearts post-transplant using controlled mechanical preservation when compared to simple ice storage in several important areas, including statistically significant:

(i) fewer complications within 24 hours post-op of the transplant, as evidenced by a 72% reduction in severe primary graft dysfunction,
(ii) improved post operative care as evidenced by a 39% reduction in post-transplant mechanical circulatory support, 66% reduction of the use of intraaortic balloon pumps, and a 60% reduction in ECMO or temporary VAD requirement, and
(iii) improved long-term benefits, as evidenced by a 68% mortality reduction at 1 year.

These clinical findings were noted even at extended total ischemic times (i.e., long transport times).

GUARDIAN registry data has also been analyzed to evaluate post-operative cost differences from improvements in clinical outcomes and their associated reductions in clinical interventions, with a total average savings of tens of thousands of dollars per patient when a Paragonix system was used to transport a donor heart.

In summary, the requirement to use an FDA-regulated preservation system will ensure that the most current approaches using technology that is validated specifically for safe use in organ transplantation is consistently utilized across all organ procurement and transplant programs. Paragonix recommends that those organ procurement organizations (OPOs) and transplant programs that currently do not utilize an FDA-regulated mechanical preservation system develop a plan to adopt this method of organ transport by 2024.

B) OPTN Policies should require, and organ procurement and transplant programs should adopt, the use of FDA-cleared and regulated preservation systems that continuously collect data on the temperature of the preservation solutions used during transport of the organ and have such data incorporated into the donor record.

The lowering of an organ's metabolic demand during transport using hypothermic storage is another critically important concept in organ preservation. Again, however, current OPTN policies do not require temperature data to be collected or reported.

The lack of temperature data makes it difficult to ascertain organ viability. Rapid temperature decreases to below freezing temperatures have been observed in multicenter clinical studies as well as preclinical studies that show average organ temperatures during ice cooler transportation below 2 °C and below 0 °C (Horch et al., Transplant Proceed 2002; Hendry et al., J Thorac and Cardiovasc Surg 1989; Michel et al. Ann Transplant 2014; Michel et al. Ann Transplant 2015; Ingemansson et al., Ann Thorac Surg 1996; Mankad et al., J Thorac and Cardiovasc Surg 1992; Keon et al., Ann Thorac Surg 1988). Organs such as the liver, lung, and kidney frequently are exposed to prolonged (several hours) temperatures at freezing, below, or just above freezing. The consequences of frozen preservation solutions, and of exposing a donor organ to temperatures at or below freezing, poses undue harm and injury to the organ and potentially leads poor patient outcomes.

Even in Dr. Locke's insightful testimony in the August 3 hearing, she highlighted the issue of receiving frozen kidneys. In her written testimony, she writes of receiving a kidney "as hard as a rock, like an ice cube you could put in your drink," where she was forced to discard the selfless gift of a donor and inform the potential recipient they would have to remain on the wait list.

Although this data is currently not collected on a routine basis, the FDA recognizes the importance of temperature regulation in its review and approval of all preservation solutions used during transport. For example, the Belzer UW® Cold Storage Solution, used to "flush" the organ's vasculature and provide cold storage of kidney, liver, and pancreas organs, has an Indication for Use (IFU) that reads: *Belzer UW® Cold Storage Solution must be cooled to 2° to 6 °C (36° to 43 °F) prior to use . . . Administration of Belzer UW® Cold Storage Solution, at the recommended temperature, will effectively cool the organ and lower its metabolic requirements.* Similar IFUs for other solutions state: "do not freeze" and "do not use if frozen." Thus, it is well recognized that temperature control is a key necessity in organ transportation systems, and should be continuously monitored and recorded.

C) OPTN Policies should require OPTN members to develop written protocols for recording temperatures during transport, including corrective actions for deviations from recommended temperature ranges.

Paragonix recommends that OPOs and transplant centers develop written protocols and/or regulations to collect data regarding the temperature of preservation solutions. Additionally, Paragonix recommends the placement of corrective actions should the monitored temperature be observed lower or higher than required by the labeling of the FDA-cleared preservation solution. Transport temperature data would be easy to obtain, does not require any laboratory testing or interpretation of findings, and is consistent with the growing use of innovative mechanical technologies used in organ transport. There would be no inherent additional burden on the OPO or transplant program to collect this data. This data can be analyzed to review the likelihood of temperature control during the transportation of organs and its impact on post-transplant organ function.

D) OPTN policies should be developed to require the tracking of organs during transport.

Of considerable concern, the inability to track an organ with any confidence during its transport between donor and recipient was voiced repeatedly at the Senate Finance Committee Hearing on August 3, 2022. Sadly, many noted the comparison to a consumer's use of DoorDash, "who knows where my food is," and the lack of similar tracking abilities in something as critical as organ transportation.

Paragonix wishes to call attention to the newer technologies that can easily and aptly track organs during transport with confidence and accuracy. In developing its own tracking system, the Paragonix App allows users of the Paragonix organ preservation systems to (1) utilize Bluetooth technology for pairing with Paragonix organ preservation systems for real-time monitoring and data collection; (2) monitor GPS tracking so organs are not misplaced or lost; (3) log key clinical events in real-time to minimize communication between coordinator and transplant hospital; and (4) rely on HIPAA compliant communications platforms to keep all parties informed in real-time. This type of technology simplifies an enormous amount of work, time, and resources traditionally expended by personnel. It eliminates outdated, subpar methods of tracking organs, streamlines the process more efficiently across the country, ensures a consistent and readily available "picture" of the organ during transport, and minimizes the risk of an organ being lost.

Tracking systems that provide similar advantages should be routinely used by OPOs and transplant centers and, if not standardized, at a minimum include a baseline number of capabilities that eliminates the chance that organs will be lost or misplaced during transport.

E) OPTN Policies should require, and organ procurement and transplant programs should adopt, the collection of "ischemic time" data during organ transport.

The transplant community has historically placed considerable emphasis on the donor organ's "ischemic time"—the time between the cross-clamp of blood flow to the donor organ and the *in situ* reperfusion in the recipient. Organ allocation policies have been based, in part, on unique ischemic times for each organ type; however, the actual time the organ spends within an organ preservation device is not documented. OPTN policies should require data collection and reporting of "ischemic time" during organ preservation and transport. This data should be part of the donor record.

In closing, Paragonix appreciates the opportunity to provide this Statement for the Record to be officially entered into the Senate Finance Committee's record. It is deeply concerning that challenges exist in the transportation of human organs for transplant that can be readily eliminated by improvements in transportation protocols that are reviewed and regulated by the FDA and accessible to all within the field.

Please contact me at lisa@paragonixtechnologies.com with any additional questions regarding our concerns and recommendations.

Respectfully,
Lisa Anderson, Ph.D.
President and CEO

Science in Donation and Transplant

791 Alexander Rd.
Princeton, NJ 08540

August 16, 2022
U.S. Senate Science in Donation and Transplant
791 Alexander Rd.
Princeton, NJ 08540

Committee on Finance
219 Dirksen Senate Office Building Washington, DC 20510–6200

Chairman Wyden and Ranking Member Crapo,
Thank you for this opportunity to respond to the issues raised during the August 3, 2022 presentation concerning the United States' Organ Procurement and Transplantation Network

before the Senate Finance Committee. Our organization, Science in Donation and Transplant (SID&T), shares the commitment of the physicians, patient advocates and donation professionals who labor daily to make the miracle of transplant work. This commitment includes the study of ways to improve the nation's system of altruistic organ donation and transplant, a system which is, already and without question, the best opt-in system in the world. SID&T understands that the foundation of a system based on altruism is public trust. We are concerned that certain actions of the Senate Finance Committee, and the process of one-sided vituperative attack, risks damaging this trust, and that this attack is not designed to further the goals of system improvement, but rather engenders mistrust and threatens the peer-reviewed scientific evidence based quality-enhancing processes.

Congress recently charged the National Academies of Sciences, Engineering, and Medicine (NASEM) to examine and recommend improvements to research, policies, and activities related to deceased donor organ procurement, allocation, and distribution.[127] The congressional language requested that the report include recommendations to update the Organ Procurement and Transplantation Network's (OPTN's) policies and processes. NASEM took up this challenge and issued its report earlier this year, making targeted recommendations for further study, not only of the OPTN, but of the OPOs and transplant centers and physicians that make the miracle of transplant a reality. The Senate Finance Committee hearing, the report for which was drafted before the hearing was even held, added nothing to the worthwhile and serious project of NASEM to save more lives, more equitably. Instead, it damaged efforts to ascertain quality in an irresponsible effort to diminish the public's trust in a system, which while imperfect, is in need of support, not constant, privately orchestrated attack. If there was an interest served by this hearing, it was not the public's interest, or the interest of even a single patient on the waiting list.

The purpose of the "hearing" (which to be fair was more of a public flogging), was for Chairman Wyden and Senator Grassley to voice their concerns about the government contractor serving as the nations' Organ Procurement and Transplantation Network (OPTN). United Network for Organ Sharing ("UNOS") is the private non-profit entity that has been designated to serve as the Network for the last thirty-eight years. Federal oversight of UNOS' organ transplant policies is conducted by the Health Resources and Services Administration ("HRSA"), an agency within HHS (see 42 U.S.C. § 274c). The "hearing," apparently intended as an expose´ of gross failures, instead demonstrated the wisdom of Congress in 1984 when it put the complex issues of organ donation and transplantation policy in the hands of a non-profit representative member organization, made up of experts, and not into the political sphere.

Experts in healthcare, such as peer-selected UNOS leadership know how to review, evaluate, and assess factual claims. They also know how to utilize data on frequency, severity and trends. Most importantly, they know how to conduct reviews of facts in a manner best calculated to obtain those facts, design better outcomes, and protect the confidentiality of the patients involved. The Senate Finance Committee's process and report flouted all of these standards and practices, decimating its own statutory construct for a peer review system in order to spew a few out-of-context sound bites designed not to improve quality, but presumably to score media headline points. Having already gnawed one leg of the table, by flogging the

---

[127] Realizing the Promise of Equity in the Organ Transplantation System (The National Academies of Sciences, Engineering, and Medicine Consensus Study Report, 2022), *https://nap.nationalacade mies.org/catalog/26364/realizing-the-promise-of-equity-in-the-organ-trans-plantation-system*

network of non-profit OPOs, the second leg has now been chewed to a nub. According to the Committee, the next leg will be the Executive Branch. We will see if transplant centers and hospitals, as the fourth leg, will also be cut off, leaving no institution left for the public to rely on to ethically obtain organs from the altruistic deceased and their families, and equitably share them nationally. The only solution proposed to correct the "failures" of the world's most successful system seems to be closure and de facto replacement by new, preferably technology-based entities, and the entry of large for-profits into Americans' most intimate moments.

While there are real problems to be addressed, by serious and knowledgeable policy makers, the Senate Finance Committee seems to prefer overlooking the remarkably few errors over several years, the significant gains in organ donation and transplant, and ways for improving the existing donor transplant infrastructure. The report on which the hearing was based was released to the press, the non- UNOS participants and others prior to the hearing, but was withheld from UNOS, its membership, and the public until after the spectacle, eliminating any opportunity to correct errors, provide context or correct misleading contents. This process underscored the nature of the hearing as an effort to sling mud, rather than to gather or examine facts.

Rather than discuss the recommendations of the Congressionally mandated and financed NASEM report, including the need for a lengthy and fact-based examination of the OPTN's IT capability, the Senate Finance Committee instead shared stories concerning medical errors investigated by UNOS, without context, comparison or recommendation about how another, different process would have changed any of the incidents. While SID&T believes that any error is too many, we support the process of peer review and corrective action that is the bedrock of all healthcare quality efforts. UNOS' role is not to "close poor performers", but rather to investigate and remediate the causes of errors, in order to prevent them. While UNOS can recommend to HRSA that action be taken against an OPO or transplant center, its statutory role is not primarily punitive, but rather policy-making and prophylactic. Public stoning, like the Senate Finance Committee meeting, has never fixed a process error. By punitively revealing materials that were openly shared in a peer review process, and sharing more than the minimum necessary facts about these materials, Congress undermines the peer review process created by the National Organ Transplant Act created; a process that has saved more lives than any other nation's donation and transplant system.

The OPTN is a membership organization that was established to be "operated by the transplant community [. . .] with oversight by HHS." It is governed by a Board of Directors that is made up of representatives from transplant centers, physicians, organ candidates, donors, and recipients, along with organ procurement organizations ("OPOs"), voluntary health associations, and members of the general public. Members include OPOs, transplant hospitals, and other institutions or individuals with an interest in organ donation. Each of the witnesses paraded before the Finance Committee admitted to being UNOS members, and each of them was unquestionably granted an equal voice in policy decisions and processes. What the Committee failed to share with the public is that most of the individuals testifying are also engaged in litigation against UNOS, due to policy disagreements between their private hospitals, and UNOS' representative members.[128]

---

[128] *See e.g., Adventist Health Sys./Sunbelt, Inc. v. United States Dep't of Health and Hum. Servs.*, No. 320CV00101SMRSBJ, 2021 WL 973455, at *20 (S.D. Iowa Mar. 12, 2021), aff'd, 17 F.4th 793 (8th Cir. 2021) in which both Mr. Friedman's employer (Adventist) and Dr. Locke's hospital (University of Alabama) sought to enjoin national organ allocation policy, and where the Court ruled "This case demonstrates exactly

SID&T does not have a comment on the wisdom or equity of the policy position that UNOS' membership and HRSA approved, a policy determination that has thus far been sanctioned by the courts, but we note that presenting members engaged in active litigation against the nation's plan to equitably allocate organs as being representative of the transplant community as a whole was at least disingenuous, and could be seen as disqualifying in any real "hearing". These witnesses had conflicts of interest that, at least, needed to be disclosed.

The risks of political actors engaging themselves in issues of complex policy and healthcare systems without objective guidance were on full display during the hearing. For example:

1) Although UNOS, a private non-profit entity, is currently the contract holder for the nation's OPTN system, they will presumably be in a competitive bidding posture against other private entities in the near future. This hearing taints the process of public contracting by injecting political pressure into what should be a fair bidding process based on legal processes and measurable deliverables.
2) The Committee spouted facts and figures without context or analysis, as though numbers have an independent magical meaning. When discussing healthcare outcomes, stating that 70 deaths occurred is profoundly misleading without the context of the number of successful transplants over those seven years, which in this case is over 230,000. It is also meaningless without the context of medical error rates in general.[129] Any health care outcomes reviewer would acknowledge that the numbers compare extremely favorably to overall death rates due to medical error (0.03% for deaths due to donation and transplant system errors, compared to 9.5% for medical error rates overall). If the point of the hearing was fact-finding, or general concern, as opposed to lobbying for a new private contractor, this point would have been shared.
3) The Senators, both in the report and in Committee, devoted much time to stating that of the complaints submitted, too few were forwarded to HRSA for decertification. Again, this presumes that referral for decertification is the best or most appropriate response to a complaint, rather than review, investigation, peer review, root cause analysis and monitored effective corrective action. It also assumes that all complaints are within UNOS' scope of action, and meritorious. Again, without context, such facts are meaningless, worth less than anecdotes. Health care quality does not arise from the recounting of stories, it arises from close analysis of the cause of mishaps, and full-throated participation from the professionals involved, including doctors, nurses, OPO

why judicial review of agency action—particularly that based on scientific expertise, complex data modeling, and detailed statistical analysis—should be made in a slow, deliberate, and cautious manner. Plaintiffs raise genuine policy disagreements [but] they do not reach the high threshold required to block the enactment of a federal regulation. [. . .] The short time frame under which the Court is asked to rule on Plaintiffs' claims weigh strongly against [. . .] second-guessing the technical expertise of a scientific body." Where the courts were leery of second-guessing technical expertise, the Senate Finance Committee had no apparent problem with allowing one side of a policy dispute to rail against the other without the burden of evidentiary rules or the ability to cross-examine. *See also, Callahan v. United States Dep't of Health and Hum. Servs. Through Azar,* 434 F. Supp. 3d 1319, 1327 (N.D. Ga. 2020) in which a hospital affiliated with Ms. Brockmeir's OPO sought unsuccessfully to enjoin the nationwide implementation of UNOS and DHHS' policy for allocating donated livers.

129 According to a study by Martin Makary of Johns Hopkins, 9.5 percent of all deaths each year in the U.S. stem from a medical error. Thus, as unacceptable as a single death due to error in transplant system processes is, the rate of deaths due to transplant error is indicative of high quality, not failure. *See Medical error—the third leading cause of death in the U.S.*, BMJ 2016;353:i2139, *https://doi.org/10.1136/bmj.i2139* (Published May 3, 2016).

professionals and others. UNOS promises that those who participate in fact-sharing will be protected, because this is how quality is done in America.

Perhaps the worst thing accomplished by the Senate Finance Committee in its presentation was the assault on health care quality by its unnecessary violation of basic tenets of peer review and quality. The Senate requested, and eventually obtained, the peer review privileged material entrusted to UNOS under federal law. In managing the OPTN, UNOS has established a Membership and Professional Standards Committee (MPSC) that, among other things, conducts quality assurance and peer review of OPTN members, and reviews events that are identified as a risk to patient safety, public health, or the integrity of the OPTN. Participation in the quality assurance and peer review process is mandatory for continued membership in the OPTN. In reporting the results of its "investigation," the Senate Finance Committee bared these sensitive materials to the public eye in a manner and scope that served no public purpose; there was not a single point made or scored that could not have been made without revealing sensitive data.

The purpose of peer review protection is to ensure the very transparency that the Committee states that it is trying to achieve, and that Congress mandated as it passed such laws as the UNOS enabling statute and the Healthcare Quality Act. With a single publication, the Finance Committee broke the trust of the hundreds of witnesses and evaluators who have participated in UNOS' standards' committees over the years, and damaged the ability of this organization or any other quality review organization in the future to do its job. As any health care provider can tell you, revealing such information as patient age, gender, diagnosis and date of death, all identifying factors which could easily lead to public identification of donors or recipients violates both law and basic privacy. This breach served no public purpose except to cast aspersions on some but not all of the participants in the chain of events leading to possible medical errors. Again, without the full story, expert involvement and explanation, the citation of these ten incidents serves no purpose but to re-state cases which have already undergone complete review and disposition. Every medical professional would agree that medical errors happen, and that improvements in process are always possible. Reiterating this conclusion in this hearing and report does nothing to further quality, transparency or trust. It is merely sensationalizing the very real tragedies of the patients who were injured, while adding nothing to the journey toward quality.

Furthermore, the line of questioning related to access and equity was simply hypocritical because a number of the Senators doing the questioning had long since written letters to the Department of Health and Human Services asking to expedite Trump Administration regulations that will decertify OPOs and leave system vacuums in the organ donation and transplant ecosystem, particularly among high risk populations.

We all have a shared desire to improve organ donation outcomes through a more accountable, more equitable, and more productive organ transplantation system. The NASEM report has provided us with the tools to achieve these goals for all the patients and families who need the system to work to its full potential. We owe it to them to heed the consensus advice of our scientific community. We look forward to working with you to follow the science and build the stronger, fairer transplantation system that America deserves.

Sincerely,
Anthony Pizzutillo Chair

Letter Submitted by Amy Silverstein

Living with a transplanted heart for 34 years has allowed me to experience first-hand the history of the organ transplant system in all its aspects, almost since the inception of the UNOS contract.

Over these decades, I've dug deep into the workings of transplant from the inside out, giving back to the community by serving as an elected patient representative on the UNOS board (and executive committee) for six years, as well as an appointed patient rep on committees of professional transplant organizations—the American Society of Transplantation (AST), the American Society of Histocompatibility and Immunogenetics (ASHI), and the Scientific Registry of Transplant Recipients (SRTR). I have also written articles for transplant medical journals, as well as two transplant-centered books that have been published by major publishers. Given my substantial and uniquely lengthy experience in transplantation, I feel a responsibility to share my insights with the Committee in the wake of yesterday's ground-breaking hearing.

What it's Like on the Waiting List

My transplant peer and friend Cal Henry did a wonderful job answering your questions on this issue. I'd like to offer some additional food for thought. Here's what it's like on the heart wait list.

I was a 24-year-old, second-year law student at NYU School of Law when, from out of nowhere, I developed heart failure. The doctors said it was a virus and all would resolve in about 6 months. But 6 months later, I was rushed by ambulance to Columbia Presbyterian Hospital in New York City, having had an episode of ventricular fibrillation that nearly ended my life. I spent the next 2.5 months at Columbia, waiting for a donor heart. I was told that in order to get to the top of the heart waiting list (where it's most possible to get a donor heart), patients generally need to have a 2-week life expectancy. I was in that precarious zone. I was that sick. And yet, I waited 2.5 months for a donor heart, hospitalized and dying.

The defibrillator cart careened into my room with gruesome regularity. A swarm of physicians had the terrible task of trying to prevent my heart from giving out. One morning, I flatlined—lost breath and pulse for a good long time. I woke to the sound of crying nurses, one of whom kept calling my name through tears, "Amy! Amy!"

Being on the heart transplant waiting list is an experience no one should ever have—watching and feeling one's own death. I experienced my heart dying increasingly by the day. I lost my ability to get out of bed (even to go to the bathroom) because it would set off another deadly arrhythmia attack. I lost my breath: my lungs became like two balloons poked with holes. At 24, I came to know death as much as any living person can.

And most affectingly, to this day, I carried and carry the trauma that comes with waiting desperately at the top of the heart transplant waiting list.

To think that there was inefficiency, ill management, greed, mumbo jumbo transportation glitches, and other slipups in the organ donation/procurement system that might have elongated the intense illness and trauma I experienced on the waiting list—is horrifying. To think that I might have had my chest burned by defibrillator paddles for additional days or weeks due to systematic failures—I shudder. And I know many heart recipients who have been or are currently in as desperate a position as I was: they shudder, too.

Please keep wait-listed heart patients in mind when getting tough on UNOS and OPOs.

The Gratitude Problem

But of course, there is a happy ending to my wait-list story: I received a heart. And this part of the transplantation is, I believe, a major factor in why and how UNOS, OPO's (and other system aspects of transplantation) have been able to perpetuate their failures so well and for so long. I think of it as "the gratitude problem". It is a phenomenon in transplant that did not come up at the hearing, but was a constant underpinning, nonetheless.

Every transplant saves a life. Every transplant moves a patient from organ failure to organ function. Every transplant delivers a patient from death's door to life's promise. It's wonderful.

I can tell you—you lie down on the operating table, and you cannot catch your breath, and you wake up hours later with pink cheeks and toes (both had been gray from oxygen deprivation), an appetite (which had disappeared), and an incredible sense of being full of air and light. The death is gone. You are full of life. And enormous gratitude and awe for the donor whose pulse has now become your own. A pulse that saved you. Two weeks later, you're hiking. Six weeks later, I was jogging.

And you're told by everyone you know: It's a miracle! And you find yourself saying all the time: I'm so grateful!

Miracle and *grateful* become your transplant mantras. There's a problem with this.

Transplant is not a miracle. It is the result of science and medicine. And there is nothing miraculous about the life expectancy post heart transplant: after my transplant in 1988, I was told if I was luckiest lucky, I might eke out 10 years with my transplanted heart (the statistics are still pretty much the same, 34 years later). And I soon found out that the transplant medicines have serious side effects that impair everyday life—and they also cause secondary diseases like diabetes, high blood pressure and cancer. Worst of all, it became clear that these immuno-suppressive medicines, for all their side effects and drawbacks, do not work to protect transplanted organs long term.

I bet you didn't know this, senators.

Transplant is a wonderful medical intervention. But it is no miracle. Everyone I know who received a transplant around the time I had mine in 1988 is long gone. And I know donor families who are bereft because the donated organs of their loved ones lasted only a few years. Patients and donors alike are aware that transplant is no miracle. And yet society expects us to speak the miracle mantra at every turn.

This makes for a silent, non-complaining transplant community of patients. How dare we criticize UNOS or OPO's when we are living miracles? How dare we voice our frustrations about antiquated transplant medications and the gross underfunding of transplant research by the NIH and FDA when it's a miracle that we are alive?

If there is anything miraculous about transplantation, it's this: organ donation. That families or others can rise above their incredible grief to donate an organ or organs at the most terrible moment of their lives is, I believe, a miracle in humanism.

And this, too, acts as a silencer of patients' complaints: it would be ungrateful to say something is wrong with the way transplant works—administratively, clinically, medically.

Have you ever heard a transplant patient say transplant life is incredibly hard? Debilitating? Frustrating? Heartbreaking? Cancerous? Deadly? Or that complacency in transplant research/science has maintained the status quo with the same antiquated, dangerous transplant medicines just where they've been for the last 34 years, and the lack of FDA and NIH funding has stymied progress?

Before yesterday's hearing, had you ever heard a transplant recipient say the transplant system is a mess or that they deserve better than the current system?

I rest my case.

Transparency

The hearing raised issues about UNOS' Membership and Professional Standards Committee (MPSC) with regard to citing and censuring troubled or failing OPOs. I'd like to point out another issue with the MPSC.

MPSC is tasked with managing low performing or failing transplant centers as well. Last year, the head of the MPSC rallied my committee at the AST in hopes that we might post a comment in the public record in support of some changes to MPSC rules. My committee was not satisfied with the changes. Namely, it was apparent that patients still would have no way of knowing if their transplant center was in serious or even dangerous violation of transplant center safety rules. It seemed to me notable that when we go to restaurants, we see the safety grade posted in the window (which allows us to gauge whether to, say, have the seafood salad), but we know nothing about our transplant centers. In many areas, there are several transplant centers to choose from; patients, thus, need information to transparency to make an informed decision about where to entrust their survival.

The MPSC chairman responded to my comment by saying "Some things have to stay behind the curtain." When I pushed and asked why, he said something like, "Patients don't need to know how the sausage is made."

I told him that I am alive for 34 years post-transplant precisely because I have made it my business to know exactly how the sausage is made—and to make my sausage choices very carefully. To which he replied that the information found on the SRTR should suffice. But see, it doesn't.

There is no way for patients to know if the transplant center they're choosing for their care is failing or in serious violation of transplant regulations.

Transparency is crucial to transplant health and well-being. But, again, patients don't dare ask for it. They're miracles, after all. And they are expected to be nothing but grateful. They have the seafood salad they're served and hope for the best.

Thank You, Senate Finance Committee

I watched yesterday's hearing while texting with a transplant friend—a kidney recipient who has had 3 kidney transplants over the last 31 years (again transplant does not last long). We shoveled popcorn into our mouths and drank root beer, and we shared with each other our feelings: aghast, excited, sad, thankful.

We have been waiting a long time for what we call "truth in transplant." The "miracle and gratitude" mantras attached to transplantation have put a veil over the whole system. It takes courage and grit to stand up to it (as the speakers yesterday attested to). My transplant friend and I have had to shore up ours to speak up about the various issues I've mentioned in this long comment. We've been rebuffed and rebuked at times. We've also made some inroads.

As we see it, UNOS/OPOs is a crucial start of the process of seeking, revealing, and attending to "truth in transplant."

We hope to live long lives with good quality. We hope to help all patients do the same. To honor our donors, we must help these donor organs live on and on. Thank you for your part in addressing the systemic aspects of our quest.

Amy Silverstein

Starzl Network for Excellence in Pediatric Transplantation

4401 Penn Avenue Faculty Pavilion, 6th Floor
Pittsburgh, PA 15224
https://starzlnetwork.org/

August 16, 2022 Chairman Ron Wyden
Ranking Member Mike Crapo
U.S. Senate Committee on Finance 219 Dirksen Senate Office Building Washington, DC 20510–6200

RE: Statement of University of Pittsburgh Medical Center (UPMC) in response to August 3, 2022, Full Committee Hearing, "A System in Need of Repair: Addressing Organizational Failures of the U.S.'s Organ Procurement and Transplantation Network"

Dear Chairman Wyden and Ranking Member Crapo:

We are writing on behalf of the families and pediatric transplant providers of the Starzl Network for Excellence in Pediatric Transplantation *www.starzlnetwork.org.*

The Starzl Network is a consortium of leading pediatric liver transplant centers across the United States—including centers in California, Colorado, Florida, Georgia, Illinois, New York, Ohio, Pennsylvania, Texas, Virginia, and Washington State. The Network closely integrates the patient and family voice along with transplant professionals and other collaborators to increase transparency, develop and share best practice, and improve outcomes for children undergoing transplantation.[130] The Network recognizes that delivering the best care possible is an urgent task and adopting policies which align with and enable such practice will benefit the whole of the transplant community. Thus, we applaud the Committee for highlighting the voices of transplant patients and their families in their recent hearing. Incorporating the

---

[130] Perito E.R., Squires J.E., Bray D., et al. A Learning Health System for Pediatric Liver Transplant: The Starzl Network for Excellence in Pediatric Transplantation. *J Pediatr Gastroenterol Nutr.* March 1, 2021;72(3):417–424. doi:10.1097/MPG.0000000000002974.

priorities and experiences of patients and families who entrust their lives to this system is critical to understanding—and improving it.

Network members have reviewed the testimony and wish to add several areas of additional focus:

We appreciate the committee's focus on inequalities faced by marginalized populations and those mentioned in the hearing—African Americans and persons living in rural communities—were rightly emphasized. However, disparity in care delivery is an unfortunate reality for many other vulnerable populations and we welcome the opportunity to specifically discuss why children deserve special protection and priority in any efforts to improve the national system of organ allocation.

Among pediatric patients listed for liver transplant in the U.S. today, 1 in 10 infants and 1 in 20 children die while awaiting a suitable organ. This is an unacceptable reality. Particularly since in those children that do receive a liver transplant— either a deceased donor allocated through UNOS or a living donor—the vast majority survive and thrive well into adulthood.

And while improvements can surely be applied to the current system, we do strongly support the management of organ allocation by a single, nationally organized, non-profit institution. Should the U.S. organ allocation system be overseen by a forprofit entity, we are extremely concerned that disadvantaged populations such as children, which represent only 2% of the transplant wait list, would be further deprioritized and undervalued.

Saving the lives of children awaiting liver transplant requires that they have reliable access to offers of the rare organs that are right for them. Here, the Committees focus on decreasing organ discard rates presents another opportunity. To ensure that every child awaiting transplant has access to the best possible care, we believe it is critical that offers to vulnerable, under-represented populations—like children—are not bypassed in favor of expedited placement from organ procurement organizations (OPO) to adult transplant centers.

Having a well-coordinated, technologically efficient, and up-to-date national transplant system is critical for getting children to life-saving liver transplants. If OPTN functions are divided amongst multiple contractors, it is imperative that there is an oversight body to ensure that the work of all contractors is carefully aligned and collaborative. For the pediatric liver transplant community, having centralized data collection on ALL children awaiting transplant has been critical to identifying those at highest risk of waiting list death—and to designing policies that will prioritize and protect those at-risk children.

Among other technological initiatives, we urge the prioritization of an application programing interface (API) serving the integration, coordination, and centralization of streaming data among the community of stakeholders around the OPTN, including verified 3rd party IT support systems, custom interfaces, and electronic health record systems. Deeper, two-way integration of the OPTN data with verified stakeholder systems create a fertile environment for innovation that is both ancillary and complementary to the primary functions of the OPTN technology ecosystem.

Notably, modification of the current system is possible and recent policy changes have enabled modest improvements in access to care. With contemporary adaptations, more than 60% of children now receive livers that are "shared nationally;" meaning that the organ travels to the child who needs it most. Since this change, more timely transplants have occurred, and fewer children have died awaiting an acceptable organ offer.

Unfortunately, other policy initiatives, such as prioritizing the splitting of donor allografts so that a child and an adult can benefit from one liver, have not been implemented. A "split-first" liver allocation policy has proven efficacious in Europe resulting in increased access to transplant for kids while maintaining access for adults. Evidence suggests that outcomes are equivalent for both adult and pediatric split-liver recipients. The Network would welcome the opportunity to provide additional data and documentation on this topic and firmly believe legislation that would mandate improved organ utilization using split liver transplantation is a move that could efficiently improve wait-list outcomes for both adults and children.

We also recommend optimization of the policy review and implementation process. Currently, most policy changes from proposal to Board approval may take 18–24 months and then still await programming or implementation challenges. Efforts for improvement should focus on ensuring stakeholder engagement, public review, and expert input while still allowing for more rapid implementation of life saving policies.

Finally, to help children access the liver donors they need, OPOs must have the training and resources to work with families of pediatric donors, to appropriately manage pediatric donors, and to help deliver the "gift of life" from those children and families to transplant centers that can use them for children.

In the Starzl Network, our mission is to unite big data, technology, patient advocacy, and transplant thought leaders to deliver the best possible care and develop new, scalable solutions to pediatric transplantation's most challenging problems. We believe the OPTN, and the U.S. transplant system, can and should provide this same support to all organ transplant candidates.

Respectfully submitted on behalf of the Starzl Network,
George Mazariegos, Chair
James E Squires, Co-Chair

Tennessee Donor Services

566 Mainstream Drive
Nashville, TN 37203
(O) 615–564–3642
(F) 615–564–3911
Website: tds.dcids.org

I am writing to CORRECT THE RECORD as it pertains to Dr. Jayme Locke's testimony on August 3, 2022. She described 4 kidneys that, for various reasons, she declined to transplant. The subject of my response is the one noted to have had a "botched biopsy" pictured in image 4 of her written testimony (https://www.finance.senate.gov/imo/media/doc/Senate Testimony/8.2.22/Written%20Finalv2. pdf). She was seemingly unaware the kidney was successfully transplanted elsewhere. When we got word it was being declined for the specific reason, we were essentially 100% confident it was transplantable. Given the importance of every hour of being outside the body with no blood flow that Dr. Locke accurately described, we retrieved it from her hospital over a 3-hour drive away, while simultaneously attempting to reallocate it. Fortunately, another transplant center approximately 4 hours away accepted and successfully transplanted this kidney. As of August 5, 2022, the recipient was doing "great" according to that center and had a creatinine = 1.16, which signifies excellent kidney function,

3 months post-transplant. Since her testimony was based on specific anecdotes and not aggregate data, I felt it necessary to correct the one anecdote I knew to be wrong.

Dr. Locke and her colleagues at UAB need to be recognized for their superior kidney offer acceptance ratios (OARs). UAB has been a leader in kidney transplantation in that regard for decades. If every kidney transplant program in the U.S. emulated their offer acceptance behavior, morbidity and mortality from end-stage renal disease would be far less in this country. They are within 250 nautical miles of much of our donation service area, which means their patients are likely to heavily populate the match runs on many of our donors. As such, their OAR undoubtedly benefits our organ transplantation rate, which is a very important metric for us as an organ procurement organization. Again, their acceptance practice is laudable.

In addition to the kidney described in her testimony, which was clearly transplantable, we had another kidney declined earlier this year by them for the same reason. Unfortunately, it was declined too many hours after removal from the donor for us to reallocate it, and it was discarded. We retrieved it for surgical review and unequivocally concluded it was transplantable. This was a 37 year-old kidney donor with normal kidney function and a normal biopsy, so it would have likely gotten someone off dialysis for many years. So, despite being an exemplary program in most respects, even model programs like hers contribute to our tragically high kidney discard rate, which now is approximately 30%. We respectfully reached out to her asking her to re-examine their practice of assessing transplantability of biopsied kidneys and to clarify how we can do a biopsy that they don't deem a kidney non-transplantable. We want to help her help her waitlisted patients. They deserve for us to be on the same page.

While it is not appropriate to make system changes based on anecdotes, each of these anecdotes have many similar sister-anecdotes, which means we have a worsening problem. The ones detailed here and ones Dr. Locke eloquently testified to each equate to a life saved or lost, depending on whether the system functions optimally. They also illustrate the fact that all persons and steps in the process must function optimally; failure by any person/step can derail the entire endeavor and contributes to the problems of organ discard and wait-list mortality. Moreover, each failure robs the donor and their family of an important component of their legacy and/or emotional healing; the importance of this cannot be overstated.

I have been in the organ donation/transplantation profession for over 25 years and have seen first-hand the amazing work that has resulted from it. I have also witnessed the amazing progress made. Wait-list mortality, however, remains unacceptably and unnecessarily high. It is not overdramatic to say that each death represents a failure of our current system, processes, and society.

All in the system—CMS, UNOS/OPTN, OPOs, donor hospitals, transplant centers— are responsible for addressing failures, and all must be held accountable to serve our mission to candidates on the wait list and to donors and donor families. Meaningful accountability is lacking. We all, including and especially you, are in a position to improve it; so, thank you for your attention to this life-and-death matter.

If you have any questions regarding my thoughts or desire further information from me, please reach out anytime.

Sincerely,

Marty T. Sellers, M.D., MPH Organ recovery surgeon
Tennessee Donor Services Former transplant surgeon

University of Alabama at Birmingham University of Pennsylvania
University of Pittsburgh Piedmont Atlanta Hospital Emory University
Medical Advisor
Association of Organ Procurement Organizations

Transplant Families

24654 N. Lake Pleasant Pkwy #103–187
Peoria, AZ 85383

August 12, 2022

The Honorable Ron Wyden Chairman
U.S. Senate Committee on Finance
219 Dirksen Senate Office Building Washington, DC 20510
The Honorable Mike Crapo Ranking Member
U.S. Senate Committee on Finance
219 Dirksen Senate Office Building Washington, DC 20510

Dear Chairman Wyden and Ranking Member Crapo:

We are writing to you today as a coalition of community-based organizations with a vested interest in pediatric transplantation. Each of us has either watched our child slowly succumb to organ failure, not knowing if they would live or die, or we have supported someone who has been through this process. We, caregivers, have watched our childrens' transplant teams work extremely hard to list our children on the national organ waiting list, and, thereafter, they have provided around-the-clock care and a shoulder to cry on in our most helpless of hours. We have celebrated with our transplant teams when algorithm matching is successful, and our child is offered a second chance at life. We are especially thankful when a donor family makes a heartbreaking and selfless choice to allow that second chance at life for our loved ones. Many of these things were discussed in your hearing on August 3rd, 2022. We commend the Committee on their commitment to continuous improvement for a system that saves the lives of so many.

However, we couldn't help but notice that the most vulnerable recipients were left out of consideration. We are writing to you to consider pediatric patients in future proceedings regarding the Organ Procurement and Transplantation System (OPTN) and its contractor, United Network for Organ Sharing (UNOS).

We believe the current system needs improvement, as it is not representative of people who live with organ failure: patients and caregivers. Often the voices of one of the most marginalized groups of organ failure are underrepresented throughout the system: children. Time and time again, past policies created around organ procurement, such as multi-organ transplants, have harmed pediatric patients. In this example, multi-organ transplants take priority over those children waiting for kidney transplant.[131] Children need fair access to the national system, and all involved need specialized training to work with donor families who are losing a child and recipient families who receive the gift of life. We all agree the list is too long, and organ discard rates need to decrease, but not at the expense of children who may be passed over in favor of adult transplant centers.

A few items to consider are:

1) Incorporating the patient and family's voice in the OPTN's work is critical! There should be appropriate representation on Committees, in the discussion of policy priorities, and in considering patient-centered outcomes and metrics— these advocates need to have adequate training and support from the organization. They should not have to be employed by a hospital, OPO, or the like to be considered. Sometimes the best advocates that will give an objective point of view do not work within the transplant system.
2) There was important attention in the Committee's Report and in the hearing to that of minority groups, like African-Americans, which are at risk for limited access to transplant and poorer outcomes. We applaud the Committee for bringing attention to this and would like to add that races other than white often make up over half of all pediatric transplants, according to the SRTR donation and transplant analytics page.[132] Many of these are Hispanic families with no access to Spanish patient education.
3) Currently, there are just 2,100 children on the U.S. wait list for solid organ transplant—this is less than 2% of the total wait list (1 in 100 on the kidney wait list, 1 in 20 for liver, 1 in 10 for heart, 1 in 50 for lung). But every one of those children is on the organ transplant wait list because they have a risk of dying without transplant—and every one of them is likely to survive and thrive into adulthood IF they get a transplant.
    a) There was NO mention in the report, accompanying documents, or the hearing itself about children on the transplant wait list—another vulnerable population that is critical to prioritize and protect.
    b) In terms of the amount of patient years they have lived, children are underrepresented in policy-making but almost always see the full impact of policies, good or bad.
4) A well-coordinated national transplant system is imperative for these children. Because children are small, they have fewer options for suitable donors. Well-organized, efficient, regional, and national sharing of organs is thus critical for children and pediatric transplant centers to obtain the right organ for every child.
5) Ensuring that OPOs have the training and resources needed to approach families of pediatric donors—and to manage pediatric donors and connect them to transplant centers that can utilize them effectively for children—is an important need. There is little known about OPO performance specifically as relates to pediatric donors.
6) In considering OPO strategies for decreasing organ discard rates, it is imperative to ensure that potential offers to marginalized populations—like children— are not

---

[131] Organ Procurement and Transplant Network. [Ethical implications of multi-organ transplants]. *[https://optn.transplant.hrsa.gov/policies-bylaws/public-comment/ethical-implications-of-multi-organ-transplants/].* Accessed [August 2022].

[132] Scientific Registry of Transplant Recipients. [Donation and Transplantation Analytics]. *[https://www.srtr.org/tools/donation-and-transplantation-analytics/].* Accessed [August 2022].

skipped over in favor of expedited placement along well-trodden paths from OPOs to adult transplant centers. To save the lives of children on the transplant wait list, they need to have broad, trustworthy access to offers of organs that are right for them. This is specified in the "Maximin" principle as spelled out in the Ethical principles of pediatric organ updated November 2014 on the OPTN website.[133]

Finally, we would like to address a few line items based on the recommendations outlined in the Staff Memo on Organizational Failures of the United States Organ Procurement.[134]

- While we encourage competition to improve any system, specifically opening the contract to for-profit entities as the first line item concerns patients and families as this will most certainly drive costs up for organ transplant, pre- and post-care. As we have seen in other for-profit areas, these costs are always shifted to the consumer (or patient in this case), who already shoulders significant costs when it comes to life-saving transplants. We hope that the Committee will please take this into consideration.
- The second line item stating that policy can be enacted by several contractors is also concerning. Having centralized organ allocation (i.e., a "clearinghouse function") is almost necessary in order to keep seamless exchange to and from OPOs and transplant hospitals. In other countries that have separate organ allocation systems (that would mimic the several contractor's scenario), there aren't easy or automated ways to share life-saving resources. Our current data allocation system works well. It is the discards and transport that is one of the most concerning items, along with access to the wait list. We hope the solution that you are alluding to in item 4 is actually a centralized data store and allocation with potential contractors involved at another point besides decisioning and would like clarification between points 2 and 4.
- All of the other suggestions we strongly support and are willing to give specifics as to why.

Thank you for your compassion, time, and effort during these hearings. It is clear that the Committee shares a desire for positive change within our organ allocation system. We write to you in hopes that these changes will always include and consider those it affects the most: the donor and recipient patients and their families.

Sincerely, Melissa McQueen

Parent to heart transplant recipient Dylan (14, transplanted 8 months old) Executive Director/Founder Transplant Families

Member, OPTN/UNOS Board of Directors

Member, OPTN/UNOS IT Advisory Committee/Network Ops and Oversight Committee

Former Member, OPTN Data Advisory Committee Former Member, OPTN Pediatric Committee

---

133 Organ Procurement and Transplant Network. [Ethical implications of multi-organ transplants]. *[https://optn.transplant.hrsa.gov/policies-bylaws/public-comment/ethical-implications-of-multi-organ-transplants/].* Accessed [August 2022].

134 United States Senate Committee on Finance (August 3, 2022) Staff Memo on Organizational Failures of the United States Organ Procurement *[https://www.finance.senate.gov/imo/media/doc/UNOS%20Hearing%20Confidential%20Memo%20(FOR%20RELEASE).pdf].*

Families in Action Council Co-Chair, Advanced Cardiac Therapies Improving Outcomes Network (ACTION)

PARTNER Project Lead—PCORI project facilitated by Starzl Network and Transplant Families

Jennifer Lau

Parent to liver transplant recipient Nathan (10, transplanted 9 months old) Board Vice President, Transplant Families

Member, OPTN Pediatric Committee Co-Founder/President BARE Inc.

Chair, Patient and Family Engaged Partners of SPLIT (Society of Pediatric Liver Transplantation)

PARTNER Project Lead—PCORI project facilitated by Starzl Network and Transplant Families

PFV Member, Starzl Network

Stacy Hillenburg

Parent to pediatric heart transplant recipient (10 years old, 2 months old at transplant)

Board Secretary, Transplant Families

Jill L. Brown, MPA

Parent and Living Donor to kidney transplant recipient Kylee (12, transplanted at 3 years old)

Executive Director of NW Kidney Kids Board Treasurer, Transplant Families

Riki Graves, MHA

Parent to heart transplant recipient, Juliana (8, transplanted at 17 days old) Board Member, Transplant Families

Quality Initiatives Committee Member, Pediatric Heart Transplant Society

Families in Action Council Member, Advanced Cardiac Therapies Improving Outcomes Network (ACTION)

Joseph Hillenburg

Parent to pediatric heart transplant recipient (10 years old, 2 months old at transplant)

Strategy Advisor, Transplant Families

Member, Scientific Committee, Pediatric Heart Transplant Society

Member, Families in Action (FACT), Advanced Cardiac Therapies Improving Outcomes Network (ACTION)

Member, American Society of Transplantation Transplant Community Advisory Committee

Member, Donate Life America Volunteer Committee Former Member, OPTN/UNOS Board of Directors

Former Member, OPTN/UNOS IT Advisory Committee/Network Ops and Oversight Committee

Former Member, OPTN Patient Affairs Committee Former Member, OPTN Pediatric Committee

Ansara Piebenga
Parent to kidney/liver transplant recipient, Lauren (16, transplanted at 16 months old)
Board Member, Transplant Families
Member, Improving Renal Outcomes Collaborative (IROC)'s Community Engage- ment Workgroup
Ambassador and Volunteer, National Kidney Foundation

Sarah Vargas
Parent to pediatric two-time liver transplant recipient, Rosie (8, 9 months and 4 years of age)
Board Member, Transplant Families
PFV and Executive Steering Committee, Starzl Network

Erin Babin, LCSW
Parent to liver transplant recipient Elise (10, transplanted at 17 months)
Member, Patient and Family Engaged Partners of SPLIT (Society of Pediatric Liver Transplantation)

Anna Beeman
Parent to liver transplant recipient, Will (4, 6 months old at transplant) CEO of Liver Mommas and Families, Inc.

Christopher Beeman
Parent to liver transplant recipient, Will (4, 6 months old at transplant) Board Member, BARE, Inc.

Bonnie Bolin, RN, BSN
Mother to heart transplant recipient Raylan (2, transplanted at 3 months old) Advanced Cardiac Therapies Improving Outcomes Network (ACTION) Committee Member
Hospital Services Coordinator for Southwest Transplant Alliance

Jessica Callear
Parent to liver transplant recipient Hazel (6, transplanted 10 months old)
Member, Patient and Family Engaged Partners of SPLIT (Society of Pediatric Liver Transplantation)

Hilary Camille
Parent to heart transplant recipient Shiloh (11, heart transplant at 2 years old) Certified Grief and Trauma Coach
Advocate and Co-Administrator of Pediatric Heart Transplant Caregiver Group, representing nearly 2,000 caregivers nationwide

Amanda Morcheles Goldstein
Parent to pediatric kidney transplant recipient (Lily, transplanted in 2016, 11 years old)
Co-Chair of the Improving Renal Outcome Collaborative's (IROC) Community Engagement Workgroup

Serina Guerrero

Parent to heart transplant recipient Amaya (9, transplanted at 8 months old) Advocate and Co-Administrator of Pediatric Heart Transplant Caregiver Group, rep- resenting nearly 2,000 caregivers nationwide

Jasmine Hollingsworth

Parent to liver transplant recipient, Kai (14, 4 months old at transplant) Founder/Executive Director of Liver Mommas and Families, Inc.

Amanda Kammes

Parent to current liver wait-list child, William (12) Board Member BARE, Inc.

Sherrie Logan, BSc, BA

Parent to liver transplant recipient, Ashley (15, 2 years old at transplant)

Co-Founder of Ashley's Angels (Third party fundraising initiative in support of The Hospital for Sick Children)

Executive Committee Member Starzl Network

Member, Patient and Family Engaged Partners of SPLIT (Society of Pediatric Liver Transplantation)

Kimberly Matthews

Parent to liver transplant recipient, Isaac (18, transplanted at 5 months)

Member, Patient and Family Engaged Partners of SPLIT (Society of Pediatric Liver Transplantation)

Stephanie Mullett

Parent to pediatric liver transplant recipient (4, 10 months old at transplant) Program Administrator, Alagille Syndrome Alliance

CHOC Representative for PFV, Starzl Network

Brittany Munn

Parent to liver transplant recipient Caleb (8, transplanted at 6 months old) Board Member, BARE Inc.

Member, Patient and Family Engaged Partners of SPLIT (Society of Pediatric Liver Transplantation)

Jennifer Rodriguez

Parent of pediatric kidney transplant recipient Emily (3.5 years post-transplant) IROC Community Engagement Workgroup Member

Jordan Sarbaugh

Parent to liver transplant recipient Hudson (5, transplanted 9 months old) Co-Founder, VP BARE Inc.

Member, Patient and Family Engaged Partners of SPLIT (Society of Pediatric Liver Transplantation)

Krupa Shah
Parent of liver transplant recipient Jaisal (11, transplanted 15 months old) Member Parent and Family Voice, Starzl Network

Stephanie Skrede
Parent to liver transplant recipient Sophia (9, transplanted at 91⁄2 months old) Board Member, BARE Inc.

Vanessa Smith, Living Liver Donor
Parent to liver transplant recipient Rylie (15, transplanted at 10 months)
Member, Patient and Family Engaged Partners of SPLIT (Society of Pediatric Liver Transplantation)

Jennifer White
Parent to liver transplant recipient Joshua (24, transplanted 14 years old)
Co-Chair, Patient and Family Engaged Partners of SPLIT (Society of Pediatric Liver Transplantation)

Tawanna Williams, CPC
Parent to heart transplant recipient Avery Grace (6, 2 years old at transplant) Diversity, Equity, and Inclusion Consultant
Certified Professional Coach
National Board Member/Medical Advisory Council The Children's Heart Foundation
Parent and Advisory Board Member Additional Ventures

Cheryl Witty
Parent to pediatric kidney transplant recipient Kimberly (transplanted at 12 years old)
Co-Founder, Children's Transplant Initiative

Ross Witty
Parent and living kidney donor to daughter Kimberly (transplanted at 12 years old) President/CEO, Co-Founder, Children's Transplant Initiative

Leslie Wyers
Parent to TWO pediatric kidney transplant recipients (Logan, transplanted 10 years ago, and Kylie, transplanted 8 years ago)
Living Donor
Co-Chair of Improving Renal Outcome Collaborative's (IROC) Community Engagement Workgroup
President NephHope Foundation
Past UNOS Patient Affairs Committee member

Kathleen Yago
Parent to heart transplant recipient Hana (7, transplanted at 21 months old) Member, Families in Action (FACT), Advanced Cardiac Therapies Improving Outcomes Network (ACTION)

Family Advisory Council Member, Stanford Medicine Children's Health at Lucile Packard Children's Hospital

Susan Zohner
Parent to pediatric heart transplant recipient (10 years old, 4 months old at transplant)

Deborah Morrissey Pham
Parent to pediatric heart transplant recipient Madelyn (18, transplanted at 7 weeks old)

Madelyn Pham (18)
Pediatric heart transplant recipient at 7 weeks of age

Diana D. Kendall
Executive Director Transplants for Children

Rick Lofgren
President and CEO of the Children's Organ Transplant Association (COTA) Representing more than 2,000 pediatric transplant families across the country since 1986

Carolyn Salvador
Chief Executive Officer, Enduring Hearts

Diann Begley R.N., BSN
Program Administrator, Enduring Hearts

Lisa Yue
President and Founder
Children's Cardiomyopathy Foundation

Letter Submitted by a Transplant Surgeon

August 10, 2022
To whom it may concern;

I am a transplant surgeon at Thomas Jefferson University Hospital. I have worked in transplantation for slightly more than 22 years. I am a current OPTN/UNOS board member. My comments are based on my viewing of the entire hearing. I have not had the time to review the accompanying documents. I have gotten to know Brian Shepard during the time I have served on the UNOS board and have found him to be an effective leader who is unflappable and professional. Of course, he is not perfect and I am sure that in the 10 years that he has been the CEO of UNOS, there have been a few things that he wished he had done differently. All in all, his leadership has been highly effective and 41K transplants while the country is still struggling with a pandemic is testament to his focused leadership. I found the hearing to be disheartening as someone who has worked tirelessly in my profession. There was a gross over simplification of the problems faced and a is characterization of who are the heroes and who are the "villains." Seeing an individual, Brian Shepard who I know to be a force of good being vilified by several U.S. Senators, was mockery of good governance and the fact that it was bipartisan did nothing to lessen the blow. Fortunately, my State Senator, Senator Casey, stood out as being reserved in judgement. There were no real solutions proposed during this hearing. Dividing UNOS and OPTN leadership perhaps might improve things, but I humbly submit it would do little and on the whole the mission of UNOS and the OPTN are largely quite aligned.

I would hope the Senators consider the following: (1) There has been a profound push within the OPTN/UNOS leadership to encourage diversification of the committee membership to ensure that all voices are heard in making policy. Having a greater voice for patient and donor representatives, has been a significant part of this push. These moves have championed by UNOS leaders like Brian Shepard and Dr. Mathew Cooper. (2) Geographic disparity with regards to deceased donor kidney transplant access has been a great inequity within the U.S. and is in violation of the final rule from 2000. OPTN policies have been placed into effect to deal with this inequity which have caused strains on the transplant system. Dealing with this inequity does require greater deceased donor kidney travel and with travel comes risk. (3) Sensational stories of deceased donor kidneys being incorrectly surgically procured; incorrectly package leading to the organ being frozen; mishandled during transport; or even run over by likely a poor chain of custody for the organ are not the real story of the problems that plague the system. That does not mean that they do not need to be addressed, but these are not the real numbers behind kidney discards. (4) Deceased donor kidney discards are a real problem and I know the Senators recognize this. Many deceased donor kidneys do come with sizeable risks including donor derived disease which was discussed during the hearing.

I humbly submit my comments as a transplant surgeon and as citizen of this country. I found the approach of several Senators to be overly opinionated and devoid of balance that I expect of our country's leaders.

University of Pittsburgh Medical Center

U.S. Steel Tower Suite 6200
600 Grant Street
Pittsburgh, PA 15219

August 16, 2022
Hon. Ron Wyden Chairman
Hon. Mike Crapo Ranking Member
U.S. Senate
Committee on Finance

219 Dirksen Senate Office Building Washington, DC 20510–6200

Dear Chairman Wyden and Ranking Member Crapo:

UPMC appreciates the Committee's diligence in reviewing and spotlighting short- comings in the nation's organ procurement, allocation and transplantation systems.

Since 1981, UPMC Transplant Services has performed more than 20,000 organ transplant surgery procedures, including liver, kidney, pancreas, small bowel, liver/ small bowel, heart/lung, double lung, single lung and multiple-organ transplants. UPMC is home to some of the world's foremost transplant experts and has a long history of developing new anit-rejection therapies, allowing organ recipients to enjoy better health. Our program is also distinguished by its commitment to discussing living donation with each patient who will benefit. Our living-donor liver and kidney transplant programs have helped many patients receive the gift of life through living donation.

Executive Summary

As a leader in transplantation, we share many of the concerns raised by the Committee, and write today to include our perspectives with respect to additional opportunities not addressed during the hearing that United Network for Organ Sharing (UNOS) can implement to drive system innovation and improvement and that can ultimately reduce or eliminate wait-list mortality. First, UNOS' policies unnecessarily deny children the most optimal care by failing to fully endorse and support deceased donor liver transplant (DDLT) splitting, a practice common in other countries that has effectively reduced wait-list mortality elsewhere.[135] Second, UNOS' policies do nothing to improve adult and pediatric wait-list mortality by failing to promote and implement living donor liver transplant (LDLT) options. Third, UNOS has for years displayed a lack of sincere effort, and in some instances a total breakdown in communication, in responding to UPMC and other living donor allied groups in seeking to better educate the public about the benefits of living donor transplants.[136]

UNOS is slow to embrace these and other innovations in transplantation. In UPMC's experience, it is very difficult to raise pediatric voices within UNOS' committee structure, in particular, and even more challenging to implement policy change in general. UNOS' policy review process is lengthy and all too often years elapse between peer-reviewed recommendations and policy implementation, increasing mortality risk for adults and tragically, to even greater degrees, for children.[137] With respect to pending liver transplants alone, approximately 20 percent of adults die while waiting, and in some centers, up to 10 percent of children perish or get to sick for transplant while waiting for transplant therapies.

This mortality trend is unacceptable and could be substantially improved or eliminated with robust support for DDLT splitting, with substantial LDLT program implementation, and for other novel transplantation innovations. Currently at UPMC, LDLTs comprise 65 percent of

---

[135] For example, the United Kingdom's intent-to-split study policy resulted in [a] dramatic reduction of wait-list mortality and was accomplished with deceased donor liver transplant (DDLT) variant split grafts. Sixty-five percent of pediatric liver transplants were performed as split deceased donor grafts with excellent outcomes . . . [and] most significantly, pediatric waitlist mortality was eliminated during the last 4 years of the study period. Battula N.R., Platto, M., Anbarasab R., Perera M.T.P.R., Ong E., Roll G.R., et al. *Intention to split policy: A successful strategy in a combined pediatric and adult liver transplant center.* Ann Surg. 2017;265:1009– 15.

[136] *See* Addendum I, Index of Communications with UNOS on Educational Initiatives Since 2018.

[137] The U.S. transplant community does regularly assess the impact of policy change, although these assessments may take too much time and often do not distinguish between pediatric and adult outcomes, limiting their ability to drive efficient cycles of continuous improvement. Mazariegos G.V., Soltys K.A., Perito E.R.; Editorial, *Waitlist mortality in pediatric liver transplantation: The Goal is Zero.* Liver Transpl 2022;00:1–2.

our total number of liver transplants (contrasted with the national average of 6 percent), resulting in substantial increases in transplant rates and reductions in wait-list mortality.

Innovations in Pediatric Liver Allocation

Deceased donor livers remain a limited resource, in the U.S. and elsewhere. In the U.S., mortality of pediatric patients on liver transplant waiting lists persists despite improved care for patients and directed efforts to increase pediatric priority in liver allocation. Organ allocation systems, like those managed by UNOS in the U.S., play a primary role in determining wait time and likelihood of transplantation on the pediatric waiting list. As long as wait-list mortality persists, a need exists to use all available methods, especially technical variant grafts that should drive increased utilization of split-liver transplantation, which U.S. and international data now suggest equivalent outcomes for both adult and pediatric split recipients.[138] However, under UNOS oversight, voluntary splitting of livers to 2 recipients is rare in the U.S. and essentially only occurs when the organ is first allocated to a pediatric recipient.[139]

More generally, UNOS, in implementing the Institute of Medicine's recommendations on Congress' Final Rule[140] with respect to liver allocation in 2002, adopted the Model for End-Stage Liver Disease (MELD) and Pediatric End-Stage Liver Disease (PELD) scoring system, which UNOS recognized did not accurately reflect the true mortality risk of every pediatric patient on the waiting list. And so UNOS created standardized exceptions that were designed to elevate the priority score in those children who met certain criteria, and additional nonstandard case-by-case exceptions reviewed by UNOS Regional Review Boards.

By 2005, UPMC and others in the pediatric liver transplant community observed an increasing dependence on standard PELD exception requests for allocation.[141] Further examination of the nonstandard (case-by-case) exception requests found a five-fold increase,[142] with variation in approval rates from 65 percent (Region 5) to 100 percent (Region 6).[143] The case-by-case exceptions were associated with better outcomes and lower mortality in children, but UPMC was then and remains today concerned that such significant regional and racial variation in case-by-case or non-standard exception rates, with those of caucasian identity and private insurance being more likely to benefit,[144] creates an unfair imbalance in the system that UNOS should address in a more consistent manner, ideally in a uniform fashion rather than a provider-directed, case-by-case one, which would reduce both regional and racial disparity.

---

[138] Hsu E.K., Mazariegos G.V., *Global Lessons in Graft Type and Pediatric Liver Allocation: A Path Toward Improving Outcomes and Eliminating Wait-List Mortality,* Liver Transpl 23:86– 95 2017.

[139] *Id.* at 89.

[140] The Final Rule mandated that an objective wait list of patients be established. 63 Fed. Reg. 16296–16338 (1998).

[141] Shneider B.L., Suchy F.J., Emre S., National and regional analysis of exceptions to the Pedi- atric End-Stage Liver Disease scoring system (2003–2004), Liver Transpl 2006;12:40–45.

[142] Braun H.J., Perito, E.R., Dodge J.L., Rhee S., Roberts J.P., Nonstandard exception requests impact outcomes for pediatric liver transplant candidates, Am. J Transplant 2016;16:3181–3191.

[143] *Id*

[144] Hsu E.K., Shaffer M., Bradford M., Mayer-Hamblett N., Horslen S., *Heterogeneity and disparities in the use of exception scores in pediatric liver allocation.* Am. J. Transplant 2015;15:436– 444.

More broadly, UNOS' attempt at redistricting to resolve regional disparity concerns like those discussed supra have shown little significant impact upon pediatric allocation and transplantation rates.[145]

With the exception of the U.S., many other countries have prioritized liver allocation in a definitive manner without detriment to adult liver access. Revisiting splitting criteria is critical. UNOS policy 9.8.A allows for regional splitting when the adult is the index patient, but the policy has not resulted in a significant increase in split grafts benefitting children. This lack of change in split utilization in the U.S. suggests that pediatric prioritization will be essential to improve split application.[146] UNOS can and should repurpose resources and policies to prioritize pediatric access to life saving therapy, primarily by emphasizing the importance of split-graft utilization.

Innovations in Adult Liver and Kidney Allocation

UPMC believes that the Committee's investigation and hearing offer a critical opportunity to raise awareness to what we strongly believe is a key part of the solution to organ shortages, and, by extension, long patient wait lists: living donation. We hope this letter augments the Committee's work in acknowledging that certain diseases, like diabetes, chronic kidney disease and end-stage liver and renal dis eases are on the rise and will drive an even greater need for kidney and liver transplantation in the coming years.

It is our hope that UNOS establishes a substantial commitment to broader education and public awareness about living donation for kidney and liver transplantation, in addition to split-graft liver transplant procedures like those discussed supra.

So far, UNOS has not shown this level of interest or commitment. In fact, as UPMC has pressed UNOS for greater promotion of living donor options, including the publication and dissemination of materials and data to the public that make the case for living donation, UNOS has, for the most part, stood down.

Either because of ambivalence or because of bureaucratic red tape, UNOS' failure to move in the direction of advancing living donor transplantation forced UPMC to act on its own.[147] Understanding the great need for public awareness and acceptance of living donor liver transplantation, UPMC invested in and launched its own national awareness campaign in 2018 to educate the public about the option.[148] Our own results with LDLT clearly demonstrate the successes of educational campaigns to promote living donation and beneficial effects on patient outcomes. UPMC has partnered with other non-profit and transplant-related organizations to help continue to promote awareness and education of this life-saving procedure, and of the benefits of living donation overall. We believe UNOS can, and should, join us.

---

[145] Gentry S.E., Massie A.B., Cheek S.W., Lentine K.L., Chow E. H,. Wickliffe C.E., et al. *Addressing Geographic Disparities in liver transplantation through redistricting.* Am. J Transplant 2013; 13:2052–2058.

[146] *See supra* FN 3 and 1, respectively.

[147] A description of UPMC's efforts to coordinate with and convince UNOS of the benefits of novel transplant options since 2018, like living donation, is attached as Addendum I.

[148] *See generally https://www.upmc.com/services/transplant/liver/living-donor.*

Conclusion

As the Committee continues to examine possible structural alternatives to the current UNOS-governed organ procurement and allocation system, we strongly advocate that greater attention be given to LDLT, split liver and novel transplant procedures that can increase organ availability and reduce wait-list mortality. We are pleased to submit this response to the Committee's hearing and stand ready to further expand on our points and references described herein at your convenience. Thank you for your ongoing attention to this matter.

Sincerely,
Abhinav Humar, M.D.
Clinical Director of the Thomas E. Starzl Transplantation Institute
Chief, Division of Transplantation in the Department of Surgery at UPMC

George Mazariegos, M.D.
Chief Pediatric Transplantation, UPMC Children's Hospital of Pittsburgh
Professor of Surgery and Critical Care, University of Pittsburgh School of Medicine

Addendum I

Index of Communications with UNOS on Educational Initiatives Since 2018

Fall 2018. UPMC submitted topics for a co-branded consumer webinar to UNOS communications officials. UPMC met with UNOS designees and UPMC was advised to provide content for review before UNOS would commit to the webinar. UPMC developed content and submitted it but never received return acknowledgement from UNOS on topics including (1) current status of living donor liver transplantation in the U.S.; (2) shifting the paradigm toward living donor liver transplant; and (3) novel indications for living donor liver transplant.

Winter 2019. UPMC submitted copy to UNOS for a co-branded consumer-directed brochure on living donor liver options. UPMC met with UNOS officials and were advised that the project would be held pending a rebuild of the UNOS website. UPMC did not receive any further contact.

Summer 2019. UPMC, Donate Life America, American Liver Foundation and WedMD participated in an educational summit in Washington, DC to educate the public about the shortage of deceased-donor livers available for transplantation and living donation as an option to reduce wait-list deaths. Brian Shepherd represented UNOS on a panel of experts.

Summer 2020. UPMC submitted three patient stories and photographs for the newly rebuilt UNOS website. The patient stories were only temporarily posted publicly.

March 2022. UPMC convened a phone call with Brian Shepherd to introduce a new idea for updating the multi-listing brochure that all transplant centers are required to give waitlisted patients to include information about living donation. UNOS agreed this could be part of the brochure update but advised that it would be assigned to a work group of the UNOS Patient Committee and could take up to a year to complete because of the levels of review involved.

UPMC followed up in late May and received no response from UNOS. As an alternative, UPMC has been working with contacts at Donate Life America to reach members of the UNOS Patient Committee directly to facilitate approval and publication of the new information about living donation. Success of those efforts is to be determined.

Vanderbilt University Medical Center

1161 21st Avenue South D–4316 Medical Center North Nashville, TN 37232–2730
tel 615–322–2363
fax 615–343–5365
seth.karp@vumc.org

August 16, 2022
U.S. Senate
Committee on Finance
219 Dirksen Senate Office Building Washington, DC 20510

Dear Chairman Wyden, Ranking Member Crapo, Senator Grassley, and Members of the Senate Finance Committee:

As the largest heart transplant center, largest donor hospital and one of the largest overall transplant centers in the United States, Vanderbilt University Medical Center (VUMC) would like to express its gratitude to the Senate Finance Committee for holding an important and compelling oversight hearing on the Organ Procurement and Transplantation Network (OPTN). The hearing and related Committee investigation highlighted numerous failings of the current OPTN contractor, the United Network for Organ Sharing (UNOS), running this central component of the nation's transplant system.

Members of the Vanderbilt Transplant Center have served on the Board of Directors of OPTN/UNOS, have testified before Congress on related subject matter,[149] and held numerous national leadership positions in transplantation over a period of more than 30 years. Based on this experience, we strongly endorse the conclusions reached by the Committee in its investigative findings, namely that there is widespread and consequential failure by UNOS in managing the OPTN contract. These failings most certainly have led to patient harm and death, demanding prompt action by the Department of Health and Human Services (HHS) to ensure stewards of the U.S. transplant donation and allocation system immediately address deficiencies and improve service for prospective transplant patients.

Although the problems are widespread, we believe significant improvement can be made by addressing the following issues identified by the Committee:

(i) Lack of effective oversight of Organ Procurement Organizations (OPOs):

---

[149] Testimony of Seth Karp, M.D. before the U.S. House Committee on Oversight and Reform, "The Urgent Need to Reform the Organ Transplantation System to Secure More Organs for Waiting, Ailing, and Dying Patients", May 4, 2021. Online at *https://oversight.house.gov/legislation/hearings/the-urgent-need-to-reform-the-organ-transplantation-system-to-secure-more.*

Assessment: Many in the governance and leadership of UNOS are also leaders of OPOs. Although the Final Rule § 121.10 instructs the OPTN to design appropriate plans and procedures to review the performance of each member OPO, this is simply not occurring. In fact, multiple Board Members are actively involved in blocking oversight of OPO performance. Twenty years of high-quality research suggests the number of donors in the U.S. should be 2–3 times the number of actual donors, and that poor OPO performance is a principal cause of this gap between what is, and what could be, the number of organs available for transplant.

Recommendation: OPO performance oversight must be immediately removed from the purview of UNOS. We applaud the new CMS guidelines (CALC metric) for assessing OPO performance but stress the need for active enforcement by HHS to ensure the intended goal of improving OPO performance is being achieved. All stakeholders, including OPOs, transplant centers and the OPTN must be held to account when we fail patients.

(ii) Obsolete technology:

Assessment: As the hearing elucidated in great detail, UNOS technology is failing with respect to logistics, safety, usability, reliability and efficiency. As Members of the Committee described, UNOS lacks the core competency to improve the system.

Recommendation: A new contract should be issued after an open bidding process for the OPTN commences. HHS should take necessary steps to assure that HHS or another appropriate Federal oversight agency has permanent rights of use and further development in the current technology and software platforms used by UNOS, as well as those that may be developed in the future by any new organization retained to serve as the OPTN contractor.

(iii) UNOS is a bad faith actor:

Assessment: Although the majority of members of UNOS are motivated by a desire to serve the transplant community, the leadership of UNOS subverts this energy to serve the interests and objectives of UNOS, whether or not those interests ultimately will serve transplant candidates well. When UNOS senior leadership reports to Congress that only 10% of the UNOS budget is taxpayer funded and ignores the significant contributions by the Medicare program (and in some cases Medicaid) through payment of organ acquisition fees, it undermines the transplant community's trust of the OPTN. When UNOS lobbies HRSA to require anyone competing for the OPTN contract to have extensive experience in running the OPTN, it eliminates competition and perpetuates the same poor performance. When UNOS refuses to separate the Boards of UNOS and the OPTN, it ensures that the OPTN cannot separately hold UNOS to account for deficits in its operating performance, and thus prevents HHS from regulating the OPTN contractor effectively. When multiple members of the community are subject to reprisals for speaking out against UNOS policy, as detailed by Dr. Jayme Locke, an environment of fear and intimidation is created.

Recommendation: HHS and HRSA should immediately bid out the OPTN contract and prevent any current or recent board member of UNOS from taking on a leadership position in whatever organization may be awarded the contract. In addition, HHS and HRSA should assure that the boards of the OPTN and any new contractor retained to operate the OPTN are separate and distinct, and that a majority of members of the OPTN Board are independent from, and do not serve in the leadership or governance of, any organization selected to serve as the OPTN contractor.

In our view, these aims can only fully be achieved by HHS awarding a new contractor that is fully committed to improving upon the status quo. VUMC and the Vanderbilt Transplant Center stand ready to be a resource to policymakers as you seek additional oversight and accountability, and as you push for meaningful reforms of the OPTN.

Thank you for your commitment to this critical issue.

Sincerely,
Seth J. Karp, M.D.
Professor and Chair, Section of Surgical Sciences Surgeon-in-Chief,
Vanderbilt University Medical Center Director,
Vanderbilt Transplant Center

Chapter 2

Organ Transplants: Changes in Allocation Policies for Donated Livers and Lungs*

United States Government Accountability Office

Abbreviations

DSA	donation service area
HHS	Department of Health and Human Services
HRSA	Health Resources and Services Administration
MELD	Model for End-Stage Liver Disease
OPTN	Organ Procurement and Transplantation Network

Why GAO Did This Study

Organ transplantation is the leading form of treatment for patients with severe organ failure. OPTN, a nonprofit entity that was established in 1984 under the National Organ Transplant Act, manages the nation's organ allocation system. In 2019, 32,322 organs were transplanted from deceased donors in the United States. Nevertheless, as of July 2020, close to 110,000 individuals remained on waiting lists for donor organs.

Previously, donated livers and lungs were generally offered first to the sickest candidates in donation service areas. However, livers and lungs are now generally offered first to the sickest candidates based on distance.

GAO was asked to review the changes to the liver and lung allocation policies. This report describes (1) changes to the liver allocation policy, and (2) similarities and differences in the processes OPTN used to change the liver and lung allocation policies, and federal oversight of these processes, among other things.

GAO reviewed documents, including those related to the current liver and lung allocation policies, and the 2017 liver allocation policy; interviewed HHS officials and OPTN members;

* This is an edited, reformatted and augmented version of the United States Government Accountability Office Report to Congressional Requesters, Publication No. GAO-21-70, dated October 2020.

In: Organ Transplants: Procurement, Procedures and Allocation Policies
Editor: Nathalie B. Larson
ISBN: 979-8-89530-729-8

reviewed the National Organ Transplant Act and its implementing regulations; and conducted a literature review of studies published from January 2017 through April 2020 in peer-reviewed and other publications.

HHS and the United Network for Organ Sharing (the contractor serving as OPTN) provided technical comments on a draft of this report, which GAO incorporated as appropriate.

What GAO Found

The Organ Procurement and Transplantation Network (OPTN) develops allocation policies in the United States to determine which transplant candidates receive offers for organs, such as livers or lungs, that are donated from deceased donors. In July 2018, the Department of Health and Human Services (HHS), which oversees OPTN, directed it to change the liver allocation policy to be more consistent with federal regulations. The liver allocation policy changed in February 2020 from a system that, in general, offered donated livers first to the sickest candidates within the fixed boundaries of a donation service area or region to a system based on a candidate's level of illness and distance from the donor hospital. The current liver allocation policy offers livers first to the sickest candidates within 500 nautical miles of the donor hospital using a series of distance-based concentric circles, called acuity circles.

Timeline of Selected Events Related to Three Organ Allocation Policies

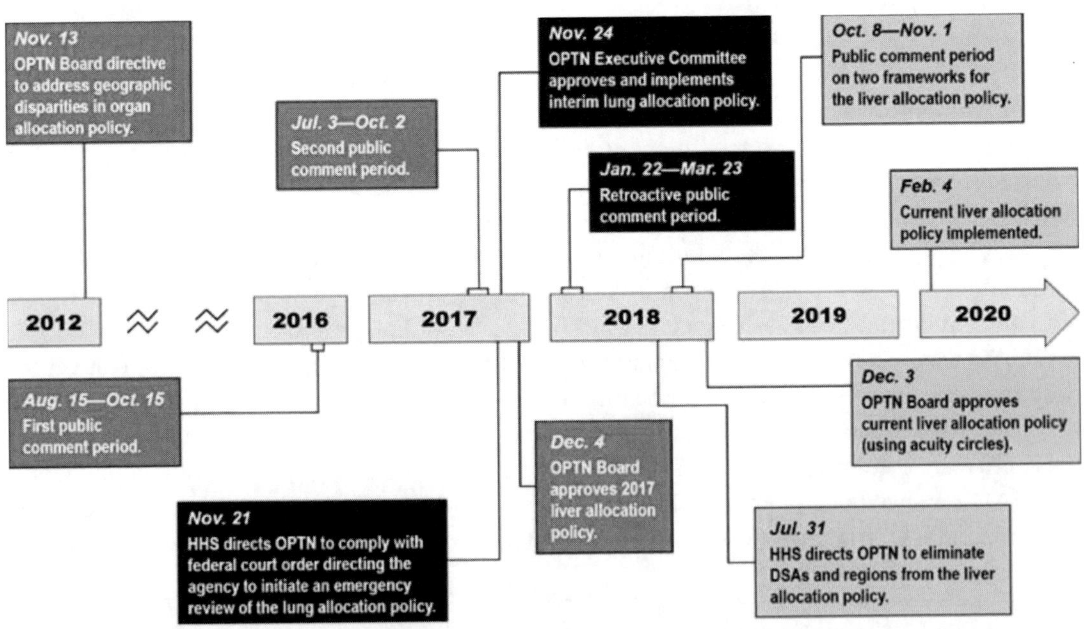

Legend: DSA=donation service area; HHS=Department of Health and Human Services; OPTN=Organ Procurement and Transplantation Network.

2017 liver allocation policy | Current lung allocation policy | Current liver allocation policy

Source: GAO. | GAO-21-70.

The processes used to develop the liver and lung allocation policies had various similarities and differences. For example, while the current liver allocation policy, the 2017 liver allocation policy, and the current lung allocation policy each had public comment periods, the length of these comment periods varied—25 days for the current liver allocation policy; two separate 62-day and 64-day periods for the 2017 liver allocation policy; and 61 days (retroactive) for the current lung allocation policy. In addition, the current lung allocation policy resulted in part from a federal district court order directing HHS to initiate emergency review of the policy. However, the 2017 liver allocation policy—that was approved but never implemented—resulted from a 2012 OPTN Board directive to reduce geographic disparities in organ allocation. HHS oversight of OPTN's processes were similar for all three allocation policies and included reviewing the proposed changes to the policies to ensure compliance with federal regulations, according to HHS officials.

October 16, 2020

The Honorable Roy Blunt Chairman
Subcommittee on Labor, Health and Human Services, Education, and Related Agencies
Committee on Appropriations United States Senate

The Honorable Jerry Moran Chairman
Subcommittee on Commerce, Justice, Science, and Related Agencies Committee on Appropriations
United States Senate

Organ transplantation is the leading form of treatment for patients with severe organ failure. In 2019, individuals received 32,322 organ transplants from deceased donors across the United States. However, as of July 2020, close to 110,000 individuals remained on a waiting list to receive an organ. On average, more than 20 people die each day waiting for an organ transplant.

Within the Department of Health and Human Services (HHS), the Health Resources and Services Administration (HRSA) oversees the Organ Procurement and Transplantation Network (OPTN), a nonprofit entity that was established in 1984 under the National Organ Transplant Act to manage the nation's organ allocation system.[150] OPTN develops national allocation policies that determine which patients receive organs from deceased donors, maintains the waiting lists of individuals seeking organ transplants, and tracks data on individuals awaiting and receiving donated organs in the United States, among other things.

OPTN implemented the current liver allocation policy in February 2020 and the current lung allocation policy in November 2017. Livers and lungs that are donated for transplants are now generally offered first to the sickest candidates based on distance from the donor hospital. Previously, donated livers were generally offered first to the sickest candidates within the fixed boundaries of donation service areas (DSA) and then within the boundaries of OPTN regions before being offered nationally. Donated lungs were generally offered first to the sickest candidates within the DSA and then in increasing increments of 500 nautical mile circles outside the donor hospital's DSA. You asked us to report on these changes, as well as federal oversight of OPTN's processes to change allocation policies and the effects of the changes to the lung allocation policy. Specifically, this report describes

---

[150] Pub. L. No. 98-507, § 201, 98 Stat. 2339, 2344 (1984) (codified, as amended, at 42U.S.C. § 274(b)).

1. how the liver allocation policy changed and the rationale for the changes;
2. similarities and differences in the processes OPTN used to change the liver and lung allocation policies, and HRSA's oversight of these processes; and
3. what is known about changes to outcomes and spending following the lung allocation policy changes made in 2017.

To examine how the liver allocation policy changed and the rationale for the changes, we reviewed OPTN and United Network for Organ Sharing documents, such as a December 2018 briefing paper from the OPTN Liver and Intestine Transplantation Committee (OPTN Liver Committee) that included proposals to revise the liver allocation policy.[151] We also reviewed federal agency documents, including a July 2018 letter from HRSA directing OPTN to review the liver allocation policy; and reports and analyses from the Scientific Registry of Transplant Recipients, including the modeling conducted to assess the potential effects of the proposals to revise the liver allocation policy.[152] In addition, we reviewed the National Organ Transplant Act, which established the framework for the U.S organ transplant system, and the OPTN Final Rule, which established the regulatory framework for the structure and operations of OPTN[153] We also interviewed HRSA and United Network for Organ Sharing officials and OPTN members, including OPTN Liver Committee members, to obtain information on the changes to the liver allocation policy.

To examine the similarities and differences in the processes OPTN used to change the liver and lung allocation policies, and HRSA's oversight of these processes, we reviewed information related to the current liver allocation policy and two other policies: a 2017 liver allocation policy approved by the OPTN board but never implemented (2017 liver allocation policy), and the current lung allocation policy, which was implemented in November 2017. Specifically, we reviewed Scientific Registry of Transplant Recipients reports and analyses, including the modeling conducted for the proposals to revise the liver allocation policy. We also reviewed the National Organ Transplant Act and the OPTN Final Rule. We examined federal agency documents pertaining to organ allocation, to the liver and lung allocation policies, and to HRSA's oversight of these policies, including a November 2017 letter from HRSA directing OPTN to comply with a court order to initiate an emergency review of the lung allocation policy. We also reviewed OPTN bylaws, policies, and other documents, including documents on the processes used to make changes to organ allocation policies and on HRSA's oversight processes, such as OPTN meeting notes and briefing papers. We also interviewed HRSA and United Network for Organ Sharing officials and OPTN members to obtain information on changes to the liver and lung allocation policies and HRSA's oversight of these changes.

To examine what is known about changes to outcomes and spending following the lung allocation policy changes made in 2017, we conducted a literature review of peer-reviewed and

---

151 The United Network for Organ Sharing—a private, nonprofit organization—serves as the OPTN through a contract with HRSA.

152 The Scientific Registry of Transplant Recipients conducts analyses of data on organ donors, and transplant candidates and recipients, as well as modeling for proposed organ allocation policies. The Chronic Disease Research Group, a division of the Hennepin Healthcare Research Institute in Minneapolis, Minnesota, has a contract with HRSA to administer the Scientific Registry of Transplant Recipients.

153 Pub. L. No. 98-507, 98 Stat. 2339 (1984) (codified, as amended, at 42 U.S.C. § 273 et seq.); and 63 Fed. Reg. 16,296 (Apr. 2, 1998).

trade publications since January 2017, examined OPTN monitoring reports, and interviewed federal officials and other stakeholders:

- *Literature review.* We identified peer-reviewed studies, and government, legislative, and trade articles published from January 2017 through April 2020 through a search of bibliographic databases, including ProQuest, Scopus, DIALOG, and EBSCO, using terms such as “organ,” “transplant,” “allocation,” “liver,” and “lung.” Of the 242 citations we identified, we obtained 89 full studies and articles for further review. Of those, we determined that one study included relevant information. We examined this study for information related to the effects of changes in the lung allocation policy on outcomes, such as the level of illness of lung transplant recipients, and spending. We also reviewed the methodology of the relevant study to confirm our understanding of the data and analyses.
- *OPTN monitoring reports.* We reviewed data from OPTN’s monitoring reports on changes to the lung allocation policy, including outcomes, such as the number of lung transplants, the distance to recover donor lungs for transplants, and 6-month post-transplant patient survival for lung transplant recipients before and after the lung allocation policy change in 2017.[154] We focused on the 2-year monitoring report that contains data from the 2-year period before the current lung allocation policy was implemented and the 2-year period after the policy was implemented.[155] We analyzed these data and obtained additional data from the United Network for Organ Sharing that was not included in the 2-year monitoring report, including data on lung transplant recipients by OPTN region.[156]
- *Federal agency and stakeholder interviews.* We interviewed federal agency officials from HRSA and the Centers for Medicare & Medicaid Services, and relevant stakeholders, including OPTN members, officials from the United Network for Organ Sharing, and officials from the Association of Organ Procurement Organizations, to identify available information related to the effect of the lung allocation policy changes on outcomes and spending.[157]

---

[154] OPTN’s monitoring reports were completed by the United Network for Organ Sharing’s Research Department for the OPTN Lung Transplantation Committee, which is responsible for developing national lung allocation policies, among other things. The OPTN Lung Transplantation Committee was called the OPTN Thoracic Transplantation Committee prior to July 1, 2020. We refer to both the current OPTN Lung Transplantation Committee and the OPTN Thoracic Transplantation Committee as the OPTN Lung Committee in this report. We defined outcomes to include data on lung transplants and lung transplant recipients.

[155] OPTN Thoracic Transplantation Committee, *Monitoring of the Lung Allocation Change, 2 Year Report: Removal of DSA as a Unit Of Allocation,* accessed June 18, 2020, https://optn.transplant.hrsa.gov/media/3661/item_25_thoracic_committee_20200212.pdf. OPTN has issued six monitoring reports since the current lung allocation policy was implemented in November 2017.

[156] We reviewed the methodology of OPTN’s 2-year monitoring report, compared the additional data we received with figures in the report, and interviewed United Network for Organ Sharing officials to confirm our understanding of the data and analyses.

[157] The Association of Organ Procurement Organizations is a national nonprofit organization that represents the 58 organ procurement organizations in the United States, which are the nonprofit organizations responsible for recovering organs from deceased donors for transplantation and transporting these organs to those awaiting transplantation.

We conducted this performance audit from October 2019 to October 2020 in accordance with generally accepted government auditing standards.

Those standards require that we plan and perform the audit to obtain sufficient, appropriate evidence to provide a reasonable basis for our findings and conclusions based on our audit objectives. We believe that the evidence obtained provides a reasonable basis for our findings and conclusions based on our audit objectives.

Background

The National Organ Transplant Act, enacted in 1984, established the framework for the U.S organ transplant system; and the OPTN Final Rule, issued in April 1998 and implemented in March 2000, established the regulatory framework for the structure and operations of OPTN.[158] The OPTN Final Rule requires OPTN to develop policies for the equitable allocation of organs to candidates who need transplants.[159] Such allocation policies must, among other things,

- be based on sound medical judgment;
- seek to achieve the best use of donated organs;
- be designed to promote the efficient management of organ placement;
- not be based on the candidate's place of residence or place of listing (i.e., where the candidate does not necessarily reside), except as otherwise required; and
- include appropriate procedures to promote and review compliance.[160]

As part of its responsibilities to oversee OPTN, HRSA awarded the United Network for Organ Sharing the initial contract to manage OPTN in 1986. The United Network for Organ Sharing has rebid on and been awarded the contract to continue to manage the national transplant network through eight terms of operation since that date.

The Scientific Registry of Transplant Recipients is an organization that conducts modeling for allocation policy proposals, including for livers and lungs, to inform OPTN's organ allocation policymaking. In addition, as called for by the National Organ Transplant Act, the Scientific Registry of Transplant Recipients analyzes data collected from OPTN on organ donors, and transplant candidates and recipients. The Chronic Disease Research Group, a division of the Hennepin Healthcare Research Institute, has a contract with HRSA to administer the Scientific Registry of Transplant Recipients.

---

[158] Pub. L. No. 98-507, 98 Stat. 2339 (1984) (codified, as amended, at 42 U.S.C. § 273 et seq.); and 63 Fed. Reg. 16,296 (Apr. 2, 1998).

[159] OPTN is responsible for developing equitable allocation policy for organs from deceased donors. In addition to organs donated by deceased donors, some organs are donated by living donors. The OPTN policies discussed in our report are for organs from deceased donors.

[160] See 42 C.F.R. § 121.8(a) (2019).

OPTN's Role and Responsibilities

Through its members, board of directors, and committees, OPTN develops and implements the policies that govern the distribution of organs from deceased donors and other issues related to transplantation.[161] OPTN's functions include:

- maintaining a list of patients (candidates) waiting for transplants;
- operating a system for matching donated organs with candidates on the list;
- establishing a national system for allocating organs in accordance with medical criteria;
- collecting and analyzing data on organs donated and transplanted, including monitoring reports on the implementation of policy changes; and
- conducting work, such as promoting knowledge of effective donation practices, to increase the supply of donated organs.[162]

The OPTN Liver Committee and the OPTN Lung Committee are responsible for developing evidence-based policies aimed at reducing the burden of liver, and heart and lung disease, respectively, in transplant patients, among other responsibilities.[163] OPTN's processes for making changes to organ allocation policies include an impetus for policy change, evidence gathering and proposal development, public comment periods, review and revision of proposals, OPTN Board approvals, and implementation.

Organ Allocation

Historically, OPTN's policies allocated organs to candidates based on 58 local DSAs and 11 OPTN regions. While these administrative boundaries are no longer used for allocating donated livers and lungs, they continue to serve other purposes. For example, DSAs continue to define the boundaries of organ procurement organizations that conduct other activities, including activities to promote organ donation, and OPTN regions are used to coordinate regional activities for the transplant community.

---

[161] OPTN's members include transplant hospitals participating in Medicare or Medicaid and all organ procurement organizations in the country. Members may also include other organizations, institutions, and individuals interested in organ donation or transplantation, such as organ donors, recipients, and their families. Membership generally means that their institution meets OPTN requirements and that they play an active role in forming the policies that govern the transplant community.

[162] See 42 U.S.C. § 274(b)(2). Monitoring reports compare certain outcomes before implementation of changes to an organ allocation policy to those same outcomes after implementation of the revised policy. Outcomes include the number of candidates on the waiting list and number of transplants, and patient survival probabilities.

[163] Goals of the work of the OPTN Liver and Lung Committees also include increasing liver and thoracic organ utilization, improving access to liver and thoracic transplantation, and improving the health outcomes of liver and thoracic transplant recipients. In addition to the organ-specific OPTN committees, the OPTN Board of Directors' Executive Committee continues the work of the board between meetings of the full board, including addressing emergency actions for allocation policies and approving the committees' allocation policy proposals for public comment distribution. OPTN also forms ad hoc committees for specific purposes, such as the Ad Hoc Geography Committee that was formed to develop principles for the appropriate consideration of geography in organ allocation policies.

- *DSAs.* DSAs are geographic areas established by the Centers for Medicare & Medicaid Services, which are served by one designated organ procurement organization, one or more transplant programs, and one or more donor hospitals. DSAs, which differ in size, define the boundaries in which organ procurement organizations recover organs from eligible donors. (See fig. 1.)

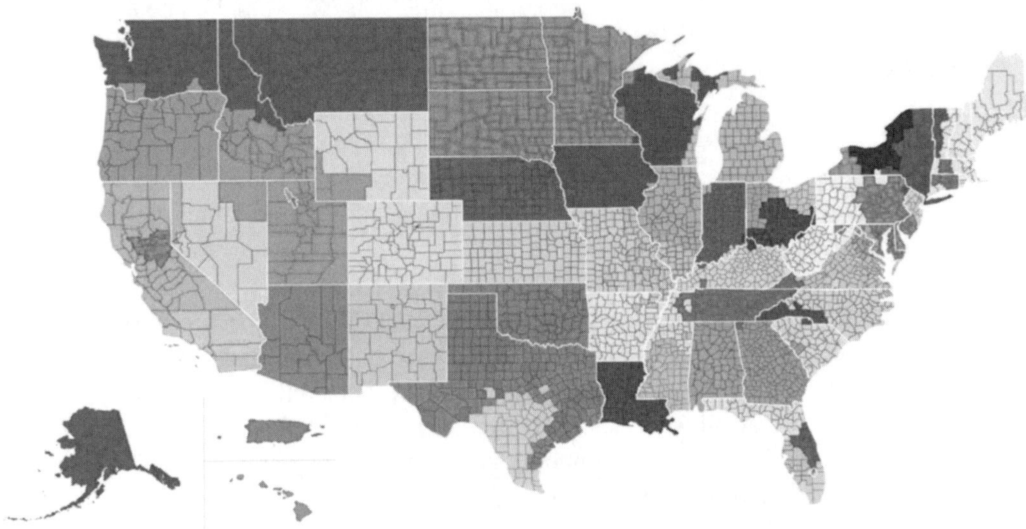

Source: United Network for Organ Sharing. | GAO-21-70.

Figure 1. United States Map of the 58 Donation Service Areas, as of August 2020.

- *OPTN regions.* OPTN regions are administrative boundaries used to facilitate OPTN governance activities, such as collecting public comments and establishing board and committee representation. Each of the 11 OPTN regions is a collection of states. (See fig. 2.)

Many factors, including a candidate's compatibility with the donor organ, are used to allocate organs to transplant candidates. Specifically, once an organ becomes available, those transplant candidates who are incompatible with the donor because of certain factors, such as blood type, height, and weight, are automatically screened out. For the remaining candidates on the waiting list for that type of organ, OPTN uses a computer program that determines the order in which candidates will be offered the organ, according to the national organ allocation policies.

Factors that weigh into the computer program's ordering include geography, proper organ size, and organ-specific factors.[164] Candidates waiting for a liver or lung transplant are given a score—for example, a Model for End-Stage Liver Disease (MELD) score for livers and a Lung

---

[164] The amount of time an organ spends being preserved after recovery from the donor, referred to as cold ischemic time, can affect transplant outcomes. In organ allocation policies, cold ischemic time is a factor when considering the optimal distance between the donor hospital and transplant hospital.

Allocation Score for lungs. The higher the score, the greater the medical need and urgency for a transplant.

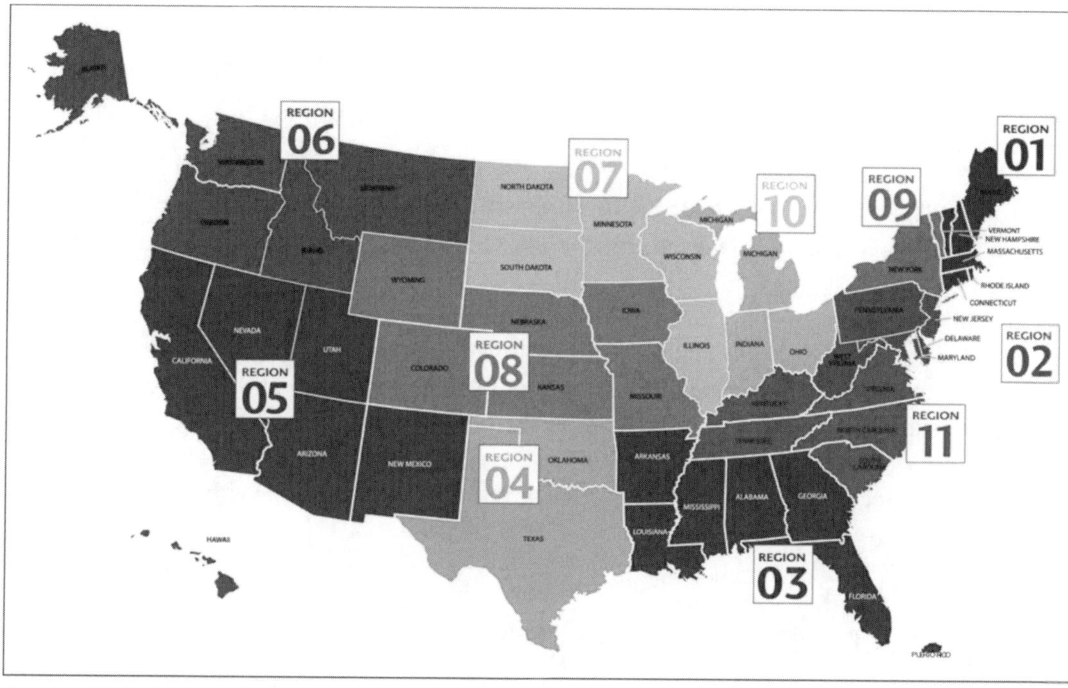

Source: United Network for Organ Sharing. | GAO-21-70.

Figure 2. United States Map of the 11 Organ Procurement and Transplantation Network (OPTN) Regions, as of August 2020.

- MELD scores range from 6 (less ill) to 40 (severely ill) and are used for liver transplant candidates age 12 and older.[165] Each candidate for a liver receives a MELD score based on how urgently a liver transplant is needed within the next 3 months. Those liver candidates who have acute (sudden and severe onset) liver failure and a life expectancy of hours to a few days without a transplant, called status 1A, are given higher priority than the candidates with the highest MELD score. Similarly, very sick, chronically ill candidates (registered on the waiting list and younger than 18 years old), called status 1B, also have higher priority. Status 1A and 1B candidates together represent less than 1 percent of liver transplant candidates.
- Lung Allocation Scores range from 0 (less ill) to 100 (severely ill) and are used for lung transplant candidates age 12 and older.[166] Lung Allocation Scores are used, along

---

[165] The MELD score is calculated by a formula using three routine lab test results: 1) bilirubin, which measures how effectively the liver excretes bile; 2) INR (prothrombin time), which measures the liver's ability to make blood clotting factors; and 3) creatinine, which measures kidney function (impaired kidney function is often associated with severe liver disease). Pediatric liver candidates are prioritized according to the Pediatric End-Stage Liver Disease scoring system based on lab values, growth failure, and whether the child is less than 1 year old. The liver allocation policy uses this scoring system for candidates younger than age 12.

[166] Each candidate for a lung receives a Lung Allocation Score based on lab values, such as creatinine (high creatinine levels reflect impaired kidney function, sometimes associated with severe lung disease); test results, including pulmonary artery pressure (the pressure the heart generates to pump blood through the lungs, which may be high

with other factors, to determine priority for receiving a lung transplant when a donor lung becomes available. Pediatric lung candidates younger than 12 years old are classified as Priority 1 or Priority 2, based on their medical condition.

Those that meet criteria reflecting a more urgent status are listed as Priority 1; all other candidates in this age range are Priority 2.

Liver Allocation Policy Changed to Include Distance after HHS Directed OPTN to Create a Policy Consistent with Federal Regulations

The liver allocation policy changed from a system that, in general, offered deceased donor livers first to the candidates with the highest level of illness within the deceased donor's DSA and OPTN region before offering them outside the region, to a system that allocates livers based on a candidate's level of illness and distance from the donor hospital.[167] OPTN made this change after it developed but did not implement the 2017 liver allocation policy, and after HHS, in July 2018, further directed OPTN to develop a policy that was consistent with the OPTN Final Rule.[168]

Liver Allocation Policy from June 2013 – February 2020

Under the previous liver allocation policy, which was in effect from 2013 to 2020 (2013-2020 liver allocation policy), generally, the sickest transplant candidates within a liver donor's DSA and OPTN region, were offered a liver first. Specifically, status 1A candidates (those with acute liver failure) within the deceased donor's DSA and OPTN region were offered the liver first, followed by status 1B candidates (very sick, chronically ill candidates 18 years and younger) within the same areas. Livers were then generally offered to candidates with a MELD score greater than or equal to 35 within the DSA and then OPTN region, and then to candidates within the DSA and OPTN region with MELD scores from 15 to 34, before being offered nationally.[169] (See fig. 3.)

---

in some people with serious lung disease); and disease diagnosis (success following a lung transplant varies among people with different lung diseases.

167 While we are describing the allocation procedures for liver allocation policies at a general level, there may be some variances based on particular donor characteristics, such as by age groups.

168 See app. I for a timeline of selected events related to organ allocation policies, including the liver and lung allocation policies.

169 For candidates with MELD scores from 40 (the highest MELD score) to 35, candidates within a DSA ranked above regional candidates at each MELD score. For example, candidates with a MELD score of 40 within the DSA and then OPTN region were offered the liver followed by candidates with a MELD score of 39 within the DSA and then OPTN region.

PREVIOUS LIVER ALLOCATION POLICY

SEVERITY OF ILLNESS

Order in which livers are offered:	*Illness category*[a]	*Geographic unit of allocation* Organs donated to candidates in descending order of illness in the:
1 2	Status 1A Status 1B	DSA and OPTN region
3	≥ 35 MELD score	DSA and OPTN region (DSA candidates ranked above regional candidates at each MELD score)
4	29-34 MELD score	DSA
5	Liver-intestine candidates[b]	Nation
6	15-28 MELD score	DSA
7	15-34 MELD score	OPTN region
8 9 10	Status 1A Status 1B ≥15 MELD score	Nation
11	<15 MELD score	DSA
12	<15 MELD score	OPTN region
13	<15 MELD score	Nation

(Rows 1–7: Less to more severe; Rows 8–13: Less to more severe)

Legend: DSA=donation service area; MELD=Model for End-Stage Liver Disease; OPTN=Organ Procurement and Transplantation Network

Source: GAO. | GAO-21-70.

Note: We are describing the previous liver allocation policy at a general level for adult deceased donors, and there may be some variances based on particular donor characteristics, such as by age groups.

[a]The illness category is the assigned status or score assignment for a liver transplant candidate that reflects the probability of death within a 3-month period, including assignments of MELD scores, and status 1A, status 1B, or liver-intestine candidates. MELD scores range from 6 (less ill) to 40 (severely ill) and are used for liver transplant candidates age 12 and older. The higher the score, the greater the medical need and urgency for a transplant. Status 1A liver candidates are those who have acute (sudden and severe onset) liver failure and a life expectancy of hours to a few days without a transplant. Status 1B candidates are very sick, chronically ill candidates age 18 and younger. In addition to MELD scores, the previous liver allocation policy used the Pediatric End-Stage Liver Disease scoring system for pediatric liver candidates (younger than age 12), which prioritizes pediatric candidates based on lab values, growth failure, and whether the child is less than 1 year old.

[b]Liver-intestine candidates are adult and pediatric liver candidates who are also registered and active on the waiting list for an intestine transplant.

Figure 3. Sequence of Offers for Livers from Deceased Donors under Previous Liver Allocation Policy, June 2013 – February 2020.

2017 Liver Allocation Policy

On December 1, 2017, HHS received a critical comment from a liver transplant candidate, asking HHS to require that livers from deceased donors be allocated to candidates based on medical priority and not on "arbitrary geographical boundaries" (i.e., DSAs and OPTN regions).[170] The comment stated that the liver allocation policy in effect at that time offered an available liver to candidates within the local DSA first, even if there were candidates with a higher medical priority (i.e., a higher MELD score) within a closer distance of the donor but in a different DSA or OPTN region. Also, in December 2017, the OPTN Board approved the 2017 liver allocation policy, which expanded the first unit of distribution to include candidates within the same OPTN region as a liver donor and those within 150 nautical miles of the donor hospital, but in a different OPTN region.[171] OPTN planned to implement the 2017 liver allocation policy in December 2018, but this policy was never put into effect.

On May 30, 2018, HHS received a second critical comment from a group of liver transplant candidates regarding the use of DSAs and OPTN regions in the 2013-2020 liver allocation policy, as well as in the 2017 liver allocation policy. Following the second critical comment, in June 2018, HRSA requested OPTN's views on whether aspects of the 2017 liver allocation policy, including the use of DSAs and OPTN regions as units of allocation, alone or in combination with a nautical mile circle distance from donor hospitals, were consistent with the requirements of the National Organ Transplant Act and the OPTN Final Rule.

In its June 2018 response to HRSA, OPTN stated that the 2017 liver allocation policy did not include an over-reliance on DSAs as the primary unit of liver distribution, but also stated that DSAs and OPTN regions were not good proxies for geographic distance between donors and transplant candidates. Specifically, OPTN stated that the most medically urgent patients under the 2017 liver allocation policy would be prioritized regardless of whether they were located within or outside of the DSA of the donor. However, OPTN also stated that the disparate sizes, shapes, and populations of DSAs and OPTN regions resulted in an inconsistent application for all candidates and committed to adopt a liver allocation policy without DSAs or OPTN regions by December 2018.

On July 31, 2018, HRSA stated that OPTN had not justified and could not justify the use of DSAs and OPTN regions in the 2013-2020 liver allocation policy and the 2017 liver allocation policy, under the OPTN Final Rule.[172] HRSA directed OPTN to approve another liver allocation policy by December 2018 that eliminated DSAs and OPTN regions, and was consistent with the OPTN Final Rule. The July 2018 letter directed OPTN to revise the liver allocation policy to eliminate the use of DSAs and OPTN regions, without "directing any particular policy outcome or allocation scheme." HRSA officials told us the agency left it to OPTN to determine how to eliminate the use of DSAs and OPTN regions.

---

170 Any interested individual or entity may submit to the Secretary of Health and Human Services critical comments related to the manner in which OPTN is carrying out its duties. See 42 U.S.C. § 274(c) and 42 C.F.R. § 121.4(d) (2019).

171 OPTN uses nautical miles, as opposed to statutory miles, because if an organ had to travel over any significant distance, it would be flown, which requires use of the units for aviation (i.e., nautical miles), according to United Network for Organ Sharing officials. A nautical mile is approximately 1.15 statutory miles.

172 HRSA also found that the use of DSAs and OPTN regions in all other organ allocation policies had not been, and could not be, justified under the OPTN Final Rule.

Liver Allocation Policy Options

Following HRSA's July 2018 directive to develop a liver allocation policy that eliminated the use of DSAs and OPTN regions, the OPTN Liver Committee subsequently developed and distributed for public comment two options: one called the broader 2-circle framework and another called the acuity circles framework. Each framework eliminated the use of DSAs and OPTN regions, but each allocated livers based on different distances from the donor hospital, and based on different ways to group transplant recipients' severity of illness.

- The broader 2-circle framework would allocate livers first to candidates with the highest medical urgency within 500 nautical miles of the donor hospital, then to candidates with a MELD score of 29 or higher within 250 nautical miles of donor hospitals, and then to candidates with a MELD score of 15 to 28 within 150, 250, or 500 nautical miles of donor hospitals before offering them nationally to candidates with the highest medical urgency.
- The acuity circles framework would also allocate livers first to candidates with the highest medical urgency within 500 nautical miles of the donor hospital, then to candidates in a series of concentric circles of different distances (150, 250, and 500 nautical miles) from the donor hospital in bands of MELD scores that got progressively lower (i.e., 37 and higher, 33-36, 29-32, 15-28), before offering the livers nationally to candidates with the highest medical urgency.

Figure 4 illustrates how the broader 2-circle framework would offer donated livers to transplant candidates, and figure 5 illustrates how the acuity circles framework would offer donated livers to transplant candidates.

The Scientific Registry of Transplant Recipients conducted modeling for the OPTN Liver Committee of which candidates would receive transplants under the two liver allocation policy options. It found that both frameworks reduced the variance in the median MELD scores for transplant recipients at the time of the transplant across DSAs—that is, they both prioritized candidates based on MELD scores with less regard for their geographic location, which would result in improving equity in access to transplants. However, the modeling for the acuity circles framework showed greater reductions in the variance in the median MELD scores than the broader

2-circles framework, and therefore showed greater prioritization of more medically urgent candidates.[173]2 In addition, both frameworks showed greater distances to recover livers than the 2013-2020 liver allocation policy, but the acuity circles framework showed transport metrics (e.g., number of flights to recover livers and transport time) that were higher than the broader 2-circle framework. Specifically, the acuity circles framework showed that 71.4 percent to 74 percent of livers would be flown, and 58.4 percent to 60.8 percent would be flown using the broader 2-circle framework.

[173] The median MELD score is calculated from transplant recipients' MELD scores at the time of the transplant from all liver transplant programs within a DSA. There was variance in the median MELD scores across the 58 DSAs, which resulted in candidates having to achieve higher MELD scores in order to receive an offer in some DSAs than candidates with lower MELD scores in other DSAs.

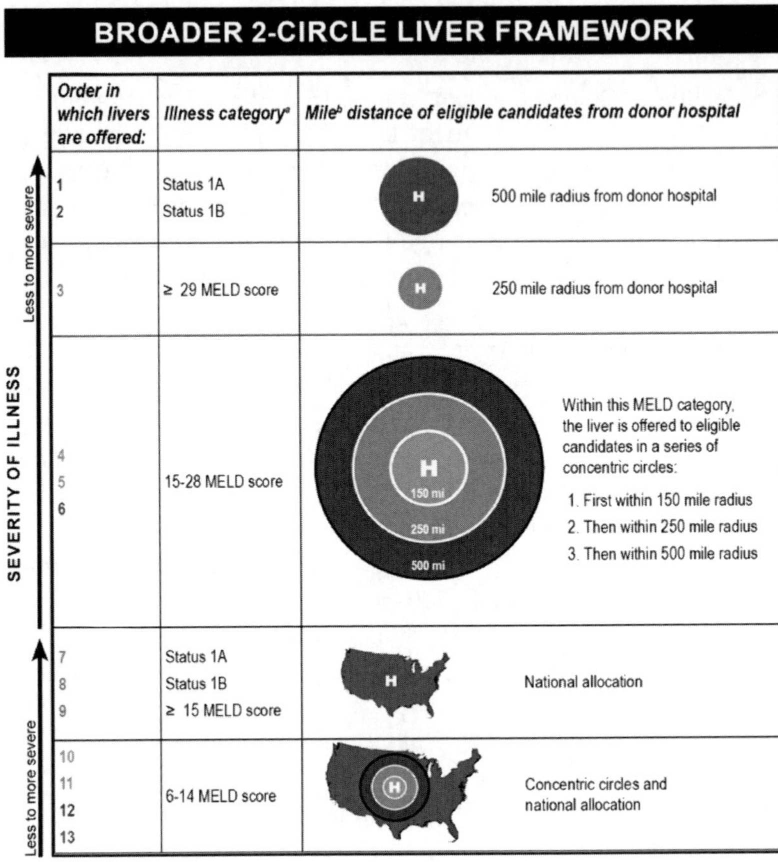

Source: GAO. | GAO-21-70.

Note: We are describing the broader 2-circle liver framework at a general level for adult deceased donors, and there may be some variances based on particular donor characteristics, such as by age groups.

[a]The illness category is the assigned status or score assignment for a liver transplant candidate that reflects the probability of death within a 3-month period, including assignments of Model for End- Stage Liver Disease (MELD) scores, and status 1A, status 1B, or liver-intestine candidates. MELD scores range from 6 (less ill) to 40 (severely ill) and are used for liver transplant candidates age 12 and older. The higher the score, the greater the medical need and urgency for a transplant. Status 1A liver candidates are those who have acute (sudden and severe onset) liver failure and a life expectancy of hours to a few days without a transplant. Status 1B candidates are highly urgent candidates age 18 and younger. In addition to MELD scores, the broader 2-circle liver framework used the Pediatric End-Stage Liver Disease scoring system for pediatric liver candidates (younger than age 12), which prioritizes pediatric candidates based on lab values, growth failure, and whether the child is less than 1 year old.

[b]Mile refers to nautical mile, which the Organ Procurement and Transplantation Network uses because if an organ had to travel over any significant distance, it would be flown, requiring the use of the units for aviation (i.e., nautical miles), according to United Network for Organ Sharing officials. A nautical mile is approximately 1.15 statutory miles.

Figure 4. Sequence of Offers for Livers from Deceased Donors under Broader 2- Circle Liver Allocation Framework.

ACUITY CIRCLES LIVER FRAMEWORK

SEVERITY OF ILLNESS (Less to more severe)

Order in which livers are offered:	*Illness category[a]*	*Mile[b] distance of eligible candidates from donor hospital*
1 2	Status 1A Status 1B	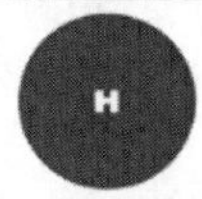 H — 500 mile radius from donor hospital
3 4 5	≥ 37 MELD score	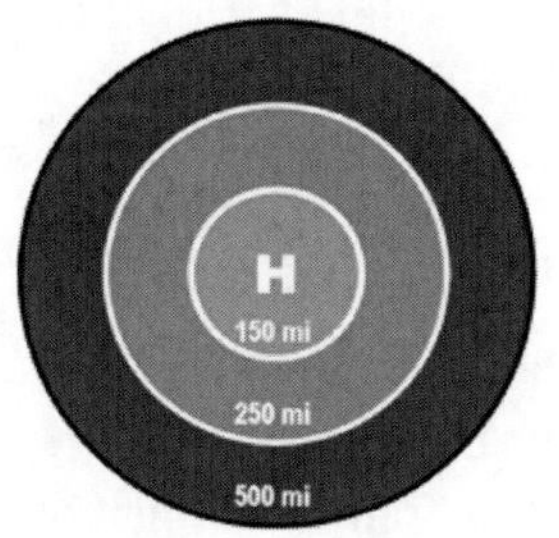 H; 150 mi; 250 mi; 500 mi — Within this MELD category, the liver is offered to eligible candidates in a series of concentric circles: 1. First within 150 mile radius 2. Then within 250 mile radius 3. Then within 500 mile radius
6 7 8	33-36 MELD score	
9 10 11	29-32 MELD score	
12 13 14	15-28 MELD score	
15 16 17	Status 1A Status 1B 15-40 MELD score	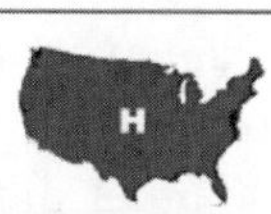 H — National allocation
18 19 20 21	6-14 MELD score	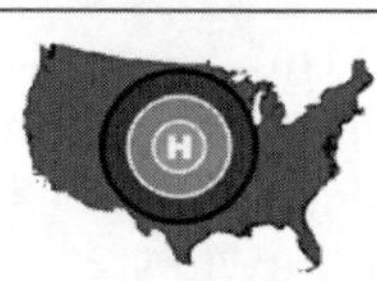 H — Concentric circles and national allocation

Source: GAO. | GAO-21-70.

Note: We are describing the acuity circles liver framework at a general level for adult deceased donors, and there may be some variances based on particular donor characteristics, such as by age groups.

[a]The illness category is the assigned status or score assignment for a liver transplant candidate that reflects the probability of death within a 3-month period, including assignments of Model for End- Stage Liver Disease (MELD) scores, and status 1A, status 1B, or liver-intestine candidates. MELD scores range from 6 (less ill) to 40 (severely ill) and are used for liver transplant candidates age 12 and older. The higher the score, the greater the medical need and urgency for a transplant. Status 1A liver candidates are those who have acute (sudden and severe onset) liver failure and a life expectancy of hours to a few days without a transplant. Status 1B candidates are highly urgent candidates age 18 and younger. In addition to MELD scores, the acuity circles liver framework used the Pediatric End-Stage Liver Disease scoring system for pediatric liver candidates (younger than age 12), which prioritizes pediatric candidates based on lab values, growth failure, and whether the child is less than 1 year old.

[b]Mile refers to nautical mile, which the Organ Procurement and Transplantation Network uses because if an organ had to travel over any significant distance, it would be flown, requiring the use of the units for aviation (i.e., nautical miles), according to United Network for Organ Sharing officials. A nautical mile is approximately 1.15 statutory miles.

Figure 5. Sequence of Offers for Livers from Deceased Donors under Acuity Circles Liver Allocation Framework.

Examples of Sequence of Liver Offers with Broader 2-Circle and Acuity Circles Frameworks

Examples of the order in which livers from deceased donors would be offered to transplant candidates for the two policy options for three hypothetical liver transplant candidates are shown below. These examples of sequences are for liver donations that did not occur after cardiac death and donors that are younger than 70 years old.

Candidate A – Status 1A (highest medical urgency); 550 nautical miles from donor hospital

Candidate B – MELD score = 38 (less ill than candidate A, but severely ill); 300 nautical miles from donor hospital Candidate C – MELD score = 30 (less ill than candidates A and B); 100 nautical miles from donor hospital

How the broader 2-circle framework and acuity circles framework would affect these three candidates:

- Among the three candidates, Candidate C is closest to the donor, but has the least severe illness. Under the broader 2-circle framework, Candidate C would be offered the liver first, because this framework prioritizes patients within 250 nautical miles if they have a MELD score of 29 or higher.
- Candidate B is farther from the donor than Candidate C, but has a more severe illness. Under the acuity circles framework, Candidate B would be offered the liver first, because this framework prioritizes patients with a MELD score of 37 or greater if they are within 150, 250, or 500 miles of the donor.
- Candidate A is the farthest from the donor, but has the most severe illness. Candidate A would not be offered the liver first under either of the frameworks, due to the combination of the other candidates' distance from the donor and severity of illness. Both frameworks give top priority to status 1A candidates if they are within 500 miles of the donor, but Candidate A is outside of this range.

Source: GAO. | GAO-21-70.

In November 2018, the OPTN Liver Committee voted to recommend the broader 2-circle framework to the OPTN Board for approval, with 11 members in favor of the broader 2-circle framework and 9 members in favor of the acuity circles framework. Based on the modeling for both frameworks, the majority of the committee determined the broader 2- circle framework had the optimal balance of broader distribution and distance to meet the requirements of the OPTN Final Rule, according to an OPTN Liver Committee report.[174]

Current Liver Allocation Policy

After reviewing both frameworks, at its December 2018 board meeting the OPTN Board voted 24 in favor and 14 in opposition on an amendment to adopt the acuity circles framework, rather than the broader 2-circle framework recommended by the OPTN Liver Committee. The acuity

[174] OPTN Liver and Intestine Transplantation Committee, Liver and Intestine Distribution Using Distance from Donor Hospital, accessed June 18, 2020, https://optn.transplant.hrsa.gov/media/2766/liver_boardreport_ 201812.pdf.

circles framework allocates livers first to the sickest candidates within 500 nautical miles of the donor hospital and then in a series of concentric circles of different distances (150, 250, and 500 nautical miles) from the donor hospital. The OPTN Board stated that it selected the acuity circles framework for the liver allocation policy because this framework allocated livers to candidates with the greatest need (i.e., sicker patients) while distributing livers as broadly as possible, according to a report by the OPTN Board.[175]

The current liver allocation policy (using acuity circles) was briefly implemented for a little over a week in May 2019, but HRSA directed OPTN to revert back to the 2013-2020 liver allocation policy in response to a federal district court order imposing a stay on implementation of the liver allocation policy.[176] OPTN ultimately implemented the current liver allocation policy on February 4, 2020. For a timeline of selected events related to organ allocation policies, including the liver and lung allocation policies, see appendix I.

Processes for Changing Liver and Lung Allocation Policies Had Similarities and Differences; HRSA's Oversight Processes Were Similar

OPTN used similar processes to develop three organ allocation policies that we reviewed—the current liver allocation policy, the 2017 liver allocation policy that was never implemented, and the current lung allocation policy, which was implemented in November 2017. There were also differences, including the impetus for making changes to the policies and the public comment periods, among other things. In addition, HRSA officials told us that the agency's oversight of OPTN's processes to make changes to organ allocation policies is the same for all policies and includes reviewing organ allocation policy proposals to ensure compliance with the National Organ Transplant Act and the OPTN Final Rule. Table 1 provides an overview of OPTN's policy development process steps for the three policies.

Table 1. Organ procurement and transplantation network's (OPTN) policy development process steps for three organ allocation policies

OPTN policy process step	Current liver allocation policy	2017 liver allocation policy (not implemented)	Current lung allocation policy
Impetus	HHS directive following receipt of critical comment[a]	OPTN Board directive to address geographic disparities	Federal district court order and HHS directive following receipt of critical comment[b]
Evidence gathering and proposal development	OPTN Liver Committee reviewed Scientific Registry of Transplant Recipients models and evidence	OPTN Liver Committee conducted a survey, held two public forums, and reviewed Scientific Registry of	OPTN Lung Committee reviewed existing OPTN data and literature

[175] OPTN, Executive Summary of OPTN Approval of Policies to Eliminate the Use of DSAs and Regions in Liver Allocation, accessed June 18, 2020, https://optn.transplant.hrsa.gov/MEDIA/2779/BOARD_EXECUTIVE SUMMARY_LIVER_20 1812.PDF.

[176] This order was issued during the course of an April 2019 lawsuit filed in the U.S. District Court for the Northern District of Georgia, in which four liver transplant candidates and 14 transplant centers alleged, among other things, that HHS failed to follow legally required procedures in developing the current liver allocation policy (using acuity circles) and instead deferred authority to the United Network for Organ Sharing. Callahan v. Azar, No. 19-cv-01783 (N.D. Ga. Apr. 22, 2019). As of July 2020, this litigation was still ongoing.

Table 1. (Continued)

OPTN policy process step	Current liver allocation policy	2017 liver allocation policy (not implemented)	Current lung allocation policy
	collected and modeled in prior policy discussions	Transplant Recipients models	
Public comment	One 25-day public comment period (10/8/18 - 11/1/18)	Two public comment periods, one 62 days (8/15/16 - 10/15/16) and the next 64 days (7/31/17 - 10/2/17)	Retroactive 61-day public comment period after the policy became effective (1/22/18 - 3/23/18)
Review/revision of proposals	OPTN Liver Committee met 20 times over a 6-month period after receiving HHS directive	OPTN Liver Committee reviewed and revised the proposal over several years after considering the findings of public forums and the first public comment period	OPTN Executive Committee reviewed and revised the proposal over 4 days because this was an emergency action
Board approval	Proposal approved on 12/3/2018	Proposal approved on 12/4/2017	Interim policy adopted by the OPTN Executive Committee on 11/24/17 and approved by the OPTN Board as permanent policy on 6/12/18
Implementation	Implemented on 5/14/19, reverted back to previous policy on 5/23/19 in response to a federal district court order, and implemented again on 2/4/20[c]	Never implemented	Implemented on 11/24/17

Source: GAO. | GAO-21-70.

[a] Any interested individual or entity may submit to the Secretary of Health and Human Services critical comments related to the manner in which OPTN is carrying out its duties. See 42 U.S.C. § 274(c) and 42 C.F.R. § 121.4(d) (2019).

[b] This order was issued during the course of a November 2017 lawsuit filed in the U.S. District Court for the Southern District of New York, in which a lung transplant candidate requested the court require the Department of Health and Human Services (HHS) to allocate donor lungs based on medical priority, rather than donation service areas. Holman v. Hargan, No. 17-cv-09041 (S.D.N.Y. Nov. 19, 2017).

[c] This order was issued during the course of an April 2019 lawsuit filed in the U.S. District Court for the Northern District of Georgia, in which four liver transplant candidates and 14 transplant centers alleged, among other things, that HHS failed to follow legally required procedures in developing the current liver allocation policy (using acuity circles) and instead deferred authority to the United Network for Organ Sharing. Callahan v. Azar, No. 19-cv-01783 (N.D. Ga. Apr. 22, 2019).

The following are descriptions of the similarities and differences in OPTN's standard policy approval processes used to develop the current liver allocation policy, the 2017 liver allocation policy, and the current lung allocation policy.[177]

- *Impetus for the policy change.* The impetus for the changes resulting in each allocation policy varied. Specifically, the impetus for the changes resulting in the current liver

[177] OPTN's bylaws outline a policy approval process for developing organ allocation policies, which includes the main steps of 1) identifying issues (impetus), 2) creating a policy proposal (evidence gathering and proposal development), 3) distributing the proposal to the public for review and comment (public comment periods), 4) responding to comments and developing a final policy proposal (review and revision of proposals), 5) sending the final proposal to the OPTN Board for a vote (Board approval), 6) providing notice to the transplant community of the approved changes to OPTN policy and taking the necessary steps to implement the changes (implementation), and 7) periodically evaluating the policy's impact and effectiveness (oversight).

allocation policy was an HHS directive following the agency's receipt of a critical comment regarding the use of DSAs and OPTN Regions in the 2013-2020 liver allocation policy and the 2017 liver allocation policy. The impetus for the changes resulting in the current lung allocation policy was two-fold. First, a federal district court ordered HHS to initiate an emergency review of the lung allocation policy.[178] Second, HRSA directed OPTN to initiate an emergency review of the lung allocation policy in accordance with the court order and as a first step in responding to a critical comment asking HHS to require OPTN to set aside portions of the lung allocation policy that utilize DSAs. The impetus for the changes that resulted in the 2017 liver allocation policy was a November 2012 OPTN Board directive to address geographic disparities.[179]

- *Evidence gathering and proposal development.* The evidence reviewed to develop each of these organ allocation policies varied. For example, the OPTN Liver Committee reviewed Scientific Registry of Transplant Recipients modeling of allocation policy proposals for the development of both the current liver allocation policy and the 2017 liver allocation policy prior to submitting these policies to the OPTN Board for approval. In addition, OPTN Liver Committee members presented 32 webinars over a 5-month period to the transplant community as part of the proposal development for the current liver allocation policy, according to OPTN members.[180] For the 2017 liver allocation policy, the OPTN Liver Committee also conducted a survey and held two public forums to gather input regarding drawing new boundaries for liver allocation. For the current lung allocation policy, the OPTN Lung Committee reviewed existing OPTN data and literature prior to OPTN Executive Committee approval of an interim lung allocation policy and reviewed Scientific Registry of Transplant Recipients modeling after the interim policy was implemented in November 2017. According to HRSA officials, the evidence gathering and proposal development process was different for the current lung allocation policy because the process was part of an emergency review.
- *Public comment periods.* The timing of the public comment periods differed for each of the policy proposals prior to OPTN Board approval. There was a public comment period for the current liver allocation policy over 25 days from October 8, 2018, through November 1, 2018, whereas the 2017 liver allocation policy had two public comment periods, each 62 days or more (August 15, 2016 to October 15, 2016, and July 31, 2017 to October 2, 2017), prior to OPTN Board approval. The comment period for the current lung allocation policy differed in that it occurred after the policy was implemented in November 2017, which is permissible under an emergency action.[181]

---

[178] This order was issued during the course of a November 2017 lawsuit filed in the U.S. District Court for the Southern District of New York, in which a lung transplant candidate requested the court require HHS to allocate donor lungs based on medical priority, rather than DSAs. Holman v. Hargan, No. 17-cv-09041 (S.D.N.Y. Nov. 19, 2017).

[179] OPTN Liver and Intestinal Organ Transplantation Committee, *Redesigning Liver Distribution to Reduce Variation in Access to Liver Transplantation*, accessed February 3, 2020, https://optn.transplant.hrsa.gov/MEDIA/1269/LIVER_CONCEPTS_2014.PDF.

[180] While developing the current liver allocation policy, the OPTN Liver Committee was able to utilize and build on modeling and analyses performed for the 2017 liver allocation policy.

[181] OPTN's bylaws designate policy proposals that meet at least one of the following criteria as emergency actions that may be adopted by the OPTN Board prior to public comment: 1) a proposal that is necessitated by a pending statutory or regulatory change; 2) a proposal that is required due to an emergent public health issue or patient

OPTN provided for a 61-day retroactive comment period on the current lung allocation policy from January 22, 2018, to March 23, 2018, after the policy became effective in November 2017.

- *Review and revision of proposals.* The time frames for reviews and revisions of policy proposals differed across the three allocation policies. For the current liver allocation policy, the full OPTN Liver Committee met 20 times over a 6-month period to revise the policy proposal. For the 2017 liver allocation policy, the OPTN Liver Committee reviewed and revised the proposal over a 5-year time frame after considering the findings of two public forums in September 2014 and June 2015 and following the first of two public comment periods described earlier. OPTN members told us that the committee held the public forums to solicit feedback from experts and revised the proposal for the 2017 liver allocation policy by incorporating ideas from these forums. For the current lung allocation policy, the OPTN Executive Committee reviewed and revised the proposal over 4 days.
- *OPTN Board approvals.* The current liver allocation policy and 2017 liver allocation policy approvals were similar in that the OPTN Board approved both as permanent policy. The OPTN Executive Committee approved the current lung allocation policy in November 2017 on an interim basis and then, after a public comment period from January 22, 2018, to March 23, 2018, the OPTN Board approved it as permanent policy in June 2018.
- *Implementation.* Implementation differed across the three policies. For example, the current liver allocation policy was initially implemented in May 2019, but reverted back to the 2013-2020 liver allocation policy 9 days later in response to a federal district court order imposing a stay on implementation. The current liver allocation policy was implemented again in February 2020. Conversely, the 2017 liver allocation policy was approved by the OPTN Board but was never implemented. The current lung allocation policy was implemented immediately after it was approved.

HRSA's oversight of OPTN's processes to make changes to organ allocation policies is the same for all allocation policies, according to HRSA officials and OPTN members. As ex officio, nonvoting members of the OPTN Board and all OPTN committees, HRSA officials participate in OPTN committee meetings. This participation entails reviewing organ allocation policy proposals to ensure compliance with the National Organ Transplant Act and the OPTN Final Rule, OPTN briefing papers on policy proposals, summaries of committee meetings, and modeling results, according to HRSA officials and OPTN members. OPTN members also told us that OPTN has frequent, collaborative interactions with HRSA officials (e.g., meetings and phone calls) regarding OPTN's changes to organ allocation policies, as well as other activities.

Figure 6 shows a timeline of selected events related to the current liver allocation policy, the current lung allocation policy, and the 2017 liver allocation policy, including public comment periods for the three policies.

---

safety factors; or 3) a proposal that is necessitated by a new medical device or technology that affects organ allocation. Such policy proposals must be distributed for public comment no more than six months after OPTN Board approval.

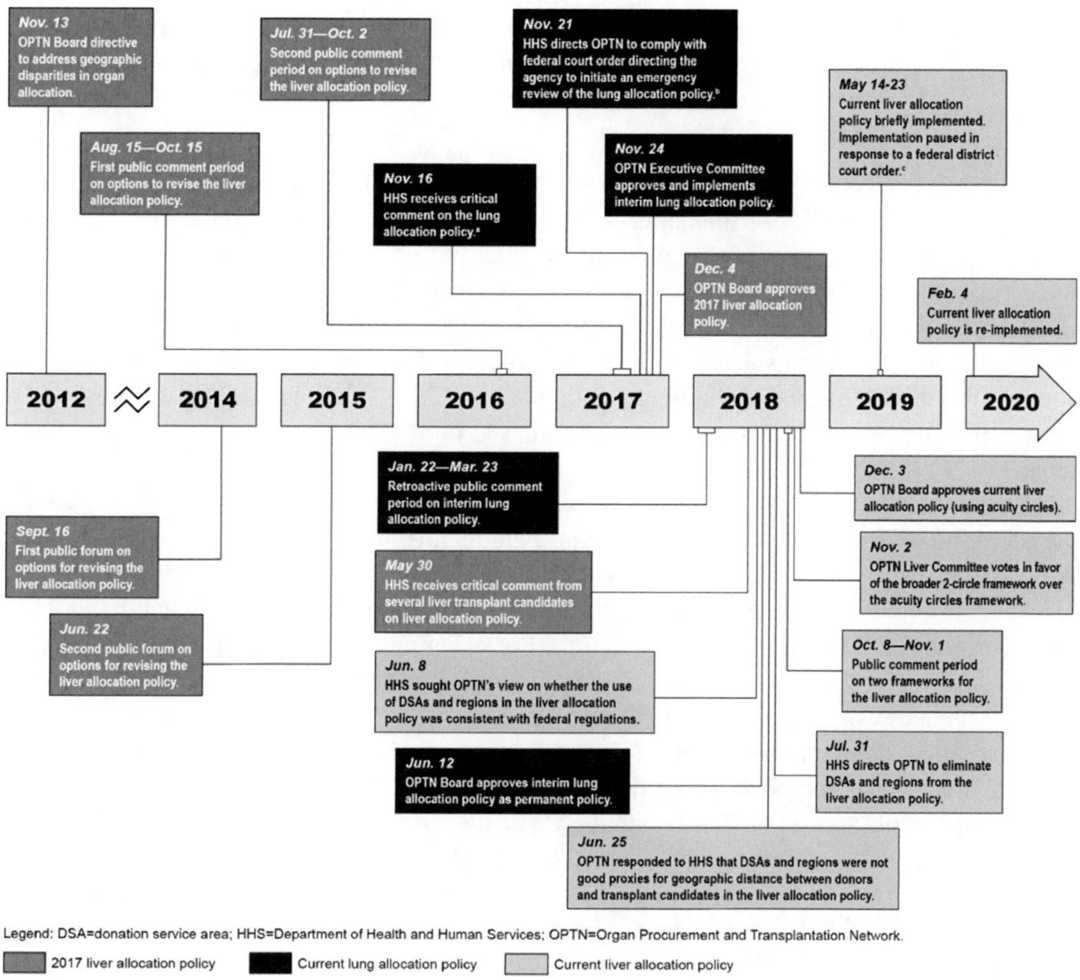

Source: GAO. | GAO-21-70.

[a]Any interested individual or entity may submit to the Secretary of Health and Human Services critical comments related to the manner in which OPTN is carrying out its duties. See 42 U.S.C. § 274(c) and 42 C.F.R. § 121.4(d) (2019).

[b]This order was issued during the course of a November 2017 lawsuit filed in the U.S. District Court for the Southern District of New York, in which a lung transplant candidate requested the court require HHS to allocate donor lungs based on medical priority, rather than DSAs. Holman v. Hargan, No. 17- cv-09041 (S.D.N.Y. Nov. 19, 2017).

[c]This order was issued during the course of an April 2019 lawsuit filed in the U.S. District Court for the Northern District of Georgia, in which four liver transplant candidates and 14 transplant centers alleged, among other things, that HHS failed to follow legally required procedures in developing the current liver allocation policy (using acuity circles) and instead deferred authority to the United Network for Organ Sharing. Callahan v. Azar, No. 19-cv-01783 (N.D. Ga. Apr. 22, 2019).

Figure 6. Timeline of Selected Events Related to the Current Liver Allocation Policy, Current Lung Allocation Policy, and 2017 Liver Allocation Policy.

OPTN Reported that Lung Transplants to Sicker Patients and Distance Increased after Changes in Allocation Policy; Little Is Known about Changes in Spending

OPTN's 2-year monitoring report following changes to the lung allocation policy found an increase nationally in sicker patients receiving lung transplants and an increase in the distance between recovering a lung from the donor hospital and the transplant center, among other selected outcomes; however, the report did not examine changes in spending.[182] HRSA officials said that the lung allocation policy was changed to provide more equitable allocation of lungs, specifically to provide transplants to sicker candidates and to provide greater access across the country through a broader distribution of available lungs. HRSA officials told us they therefore believe the current policy has met these goals based on the data from the 2-year monitoring report.

Specifically, the monitoring report found that the average Lung Allocation Score—which measures the severity of illness—for lung transplant recipients increased nationally from 47.25 in the two years preceding implementation of the current lung allocation policy to 49.79 in the two years following implementation of the current policy, a statistically significant increase.[183] However, this varied by the 11 OPTN regions. For example, the monitoring report found that nine of the regions had an increase in the average Lung Allocation Score for transplant recipients while two regions had a decrease.[184] (See fig. 7.)

In addition, the monitoring report showed increases in the distance to recover donor lungs from the donor hospital to the transplant center. Nationally, the median distance between the donor hospital and transplant center had a statistically significant increase, from 109 nautical miles in the 2 years preceding implementation of the current lung allocation policy to 166 nautical miles in the 2 years following implementation of the current policy. Consistent with this change, the number of transplants within 50 nautical miles decreased. According to the monitoring report, the number of transplants varied for other distance groups (e.g., 50-100 nautical mile group and 200-250 nautical mile group). Figure 8 shows that the number of lung transplants increased nationally in the distance groups from 50 nautical miles to 250 nautical miles and over 500 nautical miles pre- and post-policy changes, but decreased in the other distance groups. Officials from the United Network for Organ Sharing told us that because DSAs (many of which are smaller than 250 nautical miles) were removed as units of allocation from the lung allocation policy and the first geographic unit of distribution was changed to 250 nautical miles, lungs were more uniformly distributed within 250 nautical miles of the donor hospital in the 2-year period following implementation of the current lung allocation policy.

---

[182] See app. II for additional data from OPTN's 2-year monitoring report following changes in the lung allocation policy.

[183] Lung Allocation Scores are a measure of the level of illness of a lung transplant candidate or recipient. These scores range from 0 to 100, and a higher score represents a clinically sicker transplant candidate or recipient. The current lung allocation policy went into effect on November 24, 2017, at 8 p.m. Eastern Time. The 2 years preceding implementation of the current lung allocation policy for these analyses was November 26, 2015 through November 24, 2017. The 2 years following implementation of the current lung allocation policy was November 25, 2017 through November 24, 2019.

[184] It is not known whether any of the changes in the average lung allocation scores by OPTN region are statistically significant because comparisons of each of the 11 OPTN regions for the 2-year periods before and after the changes to the lung allocation policy were not performed or requested for the monitoring report, according to officials from the United Network for Organ Sharing.

They added that a large number of lung transplants between 0-50 nautical miles is expected due in part to the fact that a lung may be donated at the same hospital, or a hospital very close to, where it is transplanted, based on the general distribution of organ recovery and transplant hospitals across the country.

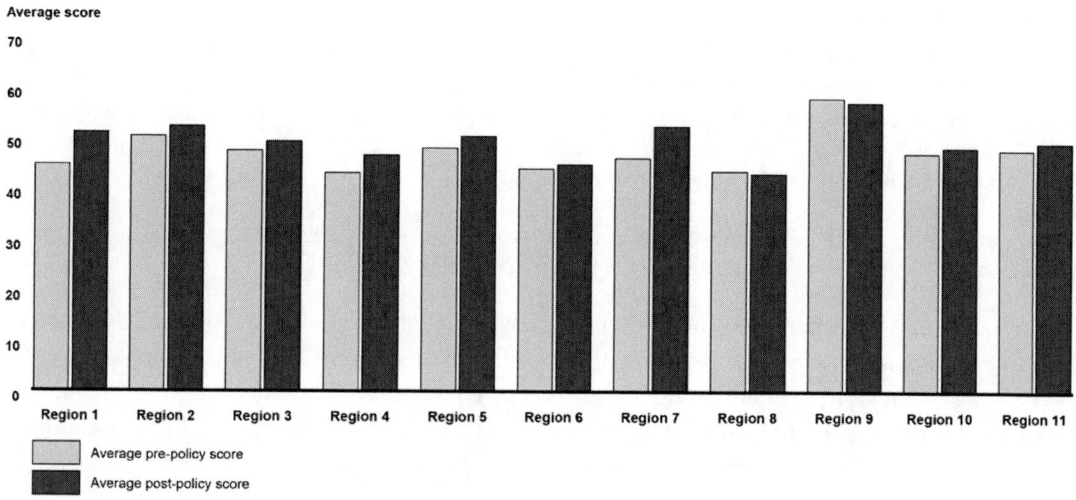

Source: Organ Procurement and Transportation Network (OPTN). | GAO-21-70.

Notes: The current lung allocation policy went into effect on November 24, 2017, at 8 p.m. Eastern Time. The pre-policy score refers to the average Lung Allocation Score for lung transplant recipients in the 2 years preceding implementation of the current lung allocation policy, which was November 26, 2015, through November 24, 2017. The post-policy score refers to the average Lung Allocation Score for lung transplant recipients in the 2 years following implementation of the current lung allocation policy, which was November 25, 2017, through November 24, 2019. Lung allocation scores are a measure of the level of illness of a lung transplant recipient. These scores range from 0 to 100, and a higher score represents a clinically sicker transplant recipient.

Figure 7. Average Lung Allocation Scores for Lung Transplant Recipients by OPTN Regions Pre- and Post-Policy Changes.

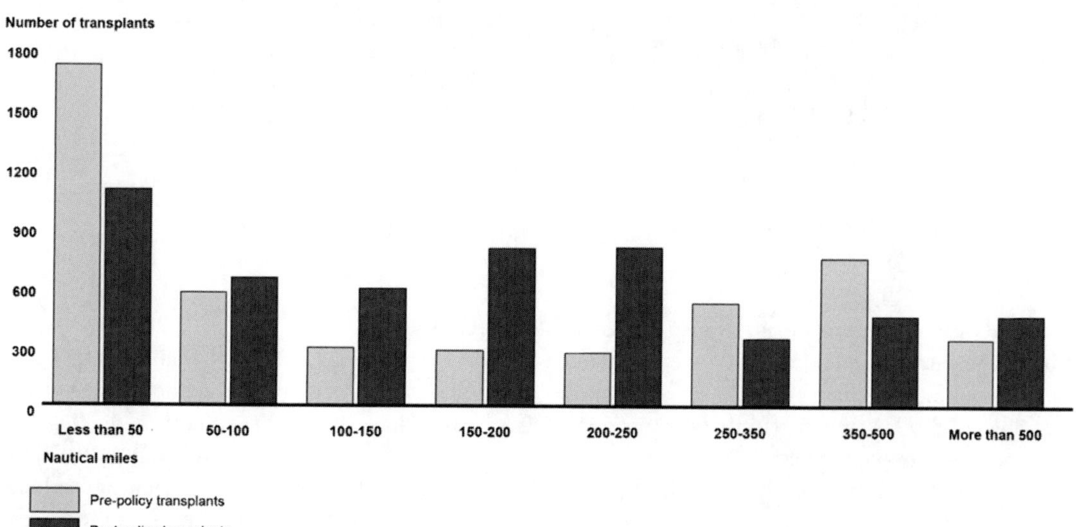

Source: Organ Procurement and Transportation Network (OPTN). | GAO-21-70.

Figure 8. (Continued).

Notes: The current lung allocation policy went into effect on November 24, 2017, at 8 p.m. Eastern Time.
Pre-policy transplants refer to the number of lung transplants in the 2 years preceding implementation of the current lung allocation policy, which was November 26, 2015, through November 24, 2017. Post-policy transplants refer to the number of lung transplants in the 2 years following implementation of the current lung allocation policy, which was November 25, 2017, through November 24, 2019.
Each of the distance groups includes their upper limit but not their lower limit (unless the lower limit is 0), according to the United Network for Organ Sharing, which conducted these analyses for OPTN. For example, a distance of exactly 50 nautical miles would be in the 0-50 nautical mile group, a distance of 50.1 would be in the 50-100 nautical mile group, and a distance of 100 nautical miles would be included in the 50-100 nautical mile group.

Figure 8. Number of Lung Transplants Nationally Pre- and Post-Policy Changes, by Distance Groups from Donor Hospital to Transplant Recipients in Nautical Miles.

The monitoring report also showed that for lung transplants performed within 250 nautical miles of the donor hospital (the first unit of allocation in the current lung allocation policy), the percentage of lungs transplanted outside of the DSA where the lung was recovered increased from a total of 19 percent before the policy change to a total of 62 percent after the policy change. The percentage of lungs transplanted nationally increased from 7 percent to 26 percent. (See fig. 9.)

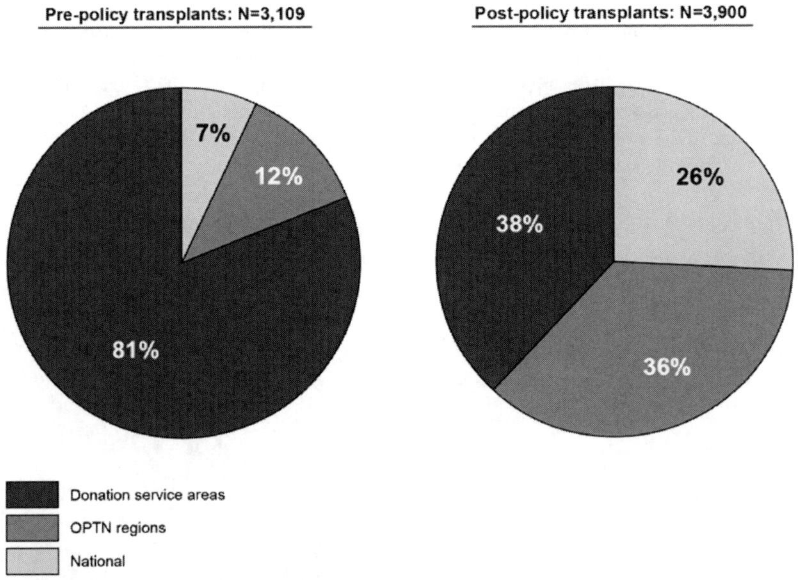

Source: Organ Procurement and Transportation Network (OPTN). | GAO-21-70.
Notes: The current lung allocation policy went into effect on November 24, 2017, at 8 p.m. Eastern Time.
Pre-policy transplants refer to the percentages of lung transplants within 250 nautical miles of the donor hospital (the first unit of allocation in the current lung allocation policy) in the 2 years preceding implementation of the current lung allocation policy, which was November 26, 2015, through November 24, 2017. Post-policy transplants refer to the percentages of lung transplants within 250 nautical miles of the donor hospital in the 2 years following implementation of the current lung allocation policy, which was November 25, 2017, through November 24. 2019.

Figure 9. Percentage Distribution of Lung Transplants within 250 Nautical Miles Pre- and Post-Policy November 2017 Changes.

Other selected outcomes from the monitoring report showed that the number of lung transplants nationally increased from 4,709 in the 2 years preceding implementation of the current lung allocation policy to 5,147 in the 2 years following implementation of the current policy. In addition, the utilization rate (the rate at which lungs are transplanted from all deceased donors) was consistent, with little change before and after the policy changes at just over 22 percent. Further, the discard rate (the number of lungs that were discarded out of the total number of lungs recovered for the purpose of transplant) increased nationally from 5.5 percent before the policy changes to 6.5 percent after the changes. However, when excluding lung transplants using certain types of lungs with unclear or initially insufficient function—perfused lungs and lungs from donations after circulatory death—the discard rate remained stable.[185]

The monitoring report also examined outcomes for 6-month post- transplant survival nationally for recipients of lung-alone transplants and found that there was not a statistically significant difference in the 6- month survival for lung transplant recipients before and after the lung allocation policy changes.[186] Lung transplant recipients had a 93.5 percent 6-month patient survival estimate in the 2-year period preceding implementation of the current lung allocation policy and 93.2 percent in the period following implementation of the current policy.

Little is known about changes in spending following the change to the current lung allocation policy.[187] Of the 89 studies and other publications we reviewed, we identified one 2019 peer-reviewed personal viewpoint article that reported data on costs from January 1, 2017, to June 4, 2018, from one lung transplant program. This article compared information on the costs to recover donor lungs for 77 lung transplants prior to the implementation of the current lung allocation policy in November 2017 with the costs for 50 transplants in the first 6 months after implementation.[188] This article reported that the median cost to recover a lung for transplantation increased from $34,000 to $70,203 for this transplant program. According to the article, this increase was to be expected given the decline in local lung transplants and higher transportation costs to procure lungs from greater distances. However, this information from one lung transplant program cannot be generalized to all lung transplant programs.

---

[185] Perfused lungs and lungs from donations after circulatory death are defined as lungs with unclear or initially insufficient function, and are sometimes referred to as marginal lungs. Lung transplants using perfused lungs and lungs from donations after circulatory death have increased in utilization since the lung allocation policy change, according to OPTN's 2-year monitoring report.

[186] Lung-alone transplants are transplants that are not in combination with another organ, such as a heart. The current lung allocation policy went into effect on November 24, 2017, at 8 p.m. Eastern Time. The 2-year period preceding implementation of the current lung allocation policy included recipients (age 12 and older) that received a lung-alone transplant from November 26, 2015, through November 24, 2017, and the period following implementation of the current lung allocation policy included recipients from November 25, 2017, through January 1, 2019. For this analysis, the period following implementation of the current lung allocation policy was limited to lung transplant recipients before January 1, 2019, to allow sufficient time to complete follow up, according to the OPTN 2-year monitoring report.

[187] We conducted a literature review of studies published from January 2017 through April 2020 in peer-reviewed journals and other publications.

[188] Organ costs included the organ acquisition charge from the organ procurement organization, cost of transportation by land or air, and administrative overhead charge by the local organ procurement organization when it had to coordinate organ import for organs procured from a distant organ procurement organization located in a different DSA. These costs do not include costs for lung transplants.

Agency and Third Party Comments

We provided a draft of this report to HHS for review and comment. HHS provided technical comments, which we incorporated as appropriate. In addition, we provided a draft report to the United Network for Organ Sharing for review and comment, and incorporated its technical comments, as appropriate.

As agreed with your offices, unless you publicly announce the contents of this report earlier, we plan no further distribution until 30 days from the report date. At that time, we will send copies of this report to the Secretary of Health and Human Services, appropriate congressional committees, and other interested parties. In addition, the report will be available at no charge on the GAO Web site at http://www.gao.gov.

If you or your staff have any questions about this report, please contact me at (202) 512-7114 or cosgrovej@gao.gov. Contact points for our Offices of Congressional Relations and Public Affairs are on the last page of this report. GAO staff who made major contributions to this report are listed in appendix III.

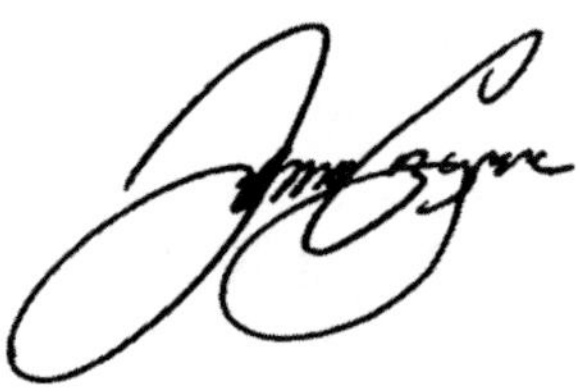

James Cosgrove Director, Health Care

Appendix I: Timeline of Selected Actions Related to Organ Allocation Policies

This appendix presents information on selected actions related to organ allocation policies, including actions specific to changes in organ allocation policies for livers and lungs. The actions in table 2 are in chronological order and range from October 19, 1984, to February 4, 2020.

Table 2. Timeline of selected actions related to organ allocation policies

Action date	Action
10/19/84	The National Organ Transplant Act (NOTA) was enacted, which • prohibited the selling of human organs; • established the Organ Procurement and Transplantation Network (OPTN) to ensure fair and equitable allocation of donated organs; • established the Scientific Registry of Transplant Recipients to conduct an ongoing evaluation of the scientific and clinical status of organ transplantation; and • provided for grants for the establishment, initial operation, and expansion of organ procurement organizations.
9/30/86	The U.S. Department of Health and Human Services (HHS) awarded the first contract for the establishment and operation of OPTN to the United Network for Organ Sharing.
4/2/98	HHS issued the OPTN Final Rule, which established the regulatory framework for the structure and operations of OPTN.

Action date	Action
3/16/00	HHS implemented the OPTN Final Rule, which requires OPTN to develop policies for the equitable allocation of organs. Such allocation policies must, among other things, • be based on sound medical judgment; • seek to achieve the best use of donated organs; • be designed to promote the efficient management of organ placement; • not be based on the candidate's place of residence or place of listing, except as otherwise required; and • include appropriate procedures to promote and review compliance.
11/13/12	The OPTN Board of Directors (OPTN Board) approved a resolution stating that the existing geographic disparity in allocation of organs for transplant was unacceptably high, and directed the organ-specific committees to define the measurement of fairness and any constraints for each organ system by 6/30/13.
6/18/13	The OPTN Board implemented a revised liver allocation policy to broaden regional and national access for highly urgent liver candidates with a Model for End-Stage Liver Disease (MELD) score of 35 or higher, but allocation continued to be based primarily on donation service areas (DSA) and OPTN regions.
6/5/17-6/6/17	The OPTN Board approved the establishment of a National Liver Review Board to replace individual review boards in each of the 11 OPTN regions. The National Liver Review Board is a body established to promote consistency in assigning exception points to allocation scores of liver transplant candidates with special medical conditions.
7/31/17-10/2/17	The OPTN Liver Committee sought public comments on a proposed change to the liver allocation policy, which would enhance liver distribution.
10/10/17	The OPTN Liver Committee reviewed public comments collected from 7/31/17-10/2/17 on its proposal to revise the liver allocation policy and voted to advance a modified proposal to the OPTN Board.
11/16/17	HHS received a critical comment from a lung transplant candidate asking HHS to require OPTN to set aside the portions of the lung allocation policy that utilize DSAs.
11/19/17	The lung transplant candidate who submitted a critical comment to HHS on 11/16/17 filed a lawsuit in the U.S. District Court for the Southern District of New York, requesting the court require HHS to allocate donor lungs based on medical priority rather than DSAs. (Holman v. Hargan)
11/20/17	The district court ordered HHS to initiate an emergency review of the lung allocation policy and submit a report by 11/28/17 to address "whether and to what extent the policy will be changed and a timetable for the implementation of any change(s)." (Holman v. Hargan)
11/21/17	HHS' Health Resources and Services Administration (HRSA) sent a letter to the OPTN President directing OPTN to comply with the court order to initiate an emergency review of the lung allocation policy and as a first step in responding to the 11/16/17 critical comment.
11/24/17	The OPTN Executive Committee reported to HRSA its conclusion that the lung allocation policy could be modified to replace DSAs as the first level of distribution with a 250 nautical mile circle around the donor hospital in order to be consistent with the OPTN Final Rule.
11/24/17	OPTN implemented and adopted the interim lung allocation policy changes effective at 8 p.m. Eastern Time on 11/24/17, with an expiration date of 11/24/18.
12/1/17	HHS received a critical comment from a liver transplant candidate asking HHS to require that livers from deceased donors be allocated to candidates based on medical priority and not on arbitrary geographical boundaries.
12/4/17-12/5/17	The OPTN Board approved a revised liver allocation policy (2017 liver allocation policy) that included DSAs and OPTN regions, but expanded the first unit of distribution to include candidates within the same DSA as a liver donor and those within 150 nautical miles of the donor hospital but in a different DSA. This liver allocation policy was never implemented.
12/4/17-12/5/17	OPTN announced the formation of the Ad Hoc Geography Committee to develop principles for the appropriate consideration of geography in organ allocation policies.
1/22/18-3/23/18	The interim lung allocation policy approved by the OPTN Executive Committee and adopted nationwide on 11/24/17 was distributed for public comment after the policy became effective.
5/30/18	HHS received a second critical comment from several liver transplant candidates, asserting that the use of DSAs and OPTN Regions in liver allocation policies was inconsistent with the OPTN Final Rule.
6/8/18	HRSA sent OPTN a letter seeking its views on the 5/30/18 critical comment challenging the liver allocation policy and whether the 2017 liver allocation policy was consistent with the National Organ Transplant Act and the OPTN Final Rule.

Table 2. (Continued)

Action date	Action
6/12/18	The OPTN Board approved the interim lung allocation policy, which was implemented on 11/24/17, as permanent policy.
6/13/18-11/15/18	Following the critical comment HHS received on 5/30/18 and HRSA's 6/8/18 letter to OPTN to review the 2017 liver allocation policy, the full OPTN Liver Committee held 20 meetings from 6/13/18-11/15/18 to consider whether the use of DSAs and OPTN regions in the liver allocation policy was consistent with the National Organ Transplant Act and the OPTN Final Rule, and subsequently developed a proposal for a revised liver allocation policy that eliminated the use of DSAs and OPTN regions.
6/25/18	OPTN submitted to HRSA its opinion that DSAs are not a good proxy for geographic distance between donors and transplant candidates because of the disparate sizes and shapes of the DSAs, and OPTN noted similar problems with OPTN Regions. OPTN committed to adopting a revised liver allocation policy that eliminated DSAs and OPTN regions by December 2018.
7/13/18	The liver transplant candidates who submitted a critical comment to HHS on 5/30/18 filed a lawsuit in the U.S. District Court for the Southern District of New York, challenging the use of DSAs and OPTN regions as units of allocation in the liver allocation policy and contending that the then-current liver allocation policy and the 2017 liver allocation policy were inconsistent with the OPTN Final Rule. (Cruz v. Azar)
7/31/18	To address the 5/30/18 critical comment on the liver allocation policy and respond to OPTN's 6/25/18 opinion that DSAs are not a good proxy for geographic distance between donors and transplant candidates, HRSA sent a letter to OPTN directing it to adopt a liver allocation policy that eliminated the use of DSAs and OPTN Regions and was compliant with the OPTN Final Rule. HRSA also directed OPTN to submit a report outlining OPTN's plans to eliminate DSAs and OPTN regions from all other organ allocation policies.
8/13/18	OPTN responded to HRSA's 7/31/18 letter with its proposed plans to eliminate DSAs and OPTN regions from all organ-specific allocation policies.
10/8/18-11/1/18	OPTN circulated a liver allocation policy proposal for public comment that solicited input on the acuity circles and broader 2-circle frameworks. All comments were posted to the OPTN website and available to the public throughout the public comment period from 10/8/18-11/1/18. During this period, officials from the United Network for Organ Sharing, a government contractor that serves as OPTN, and OPTN Liver Committee leadership periodically shared updates with OPTN Liver Committee members on participation and themes observed from the comments submitted up to that date.
11/2/18	The OPTN Liver Committee met to discuss public comments collected from 10/8/18-11/1/18 and voted to recommend the broader 2-circle framework rather than the acuity circles framework as part of a revised liver policy with 11 members in favor of the broader 2-circle framework and 9 members in favor of the acuity circles framework.
12/3/18-12/4/18	The OPTN Board approved the revised liver allocation policy with the acuity circles framework, instead of the broader 2-circle framework that was presented earlier in the meeting by the OPTN Liver Committee. The OPTN Board voted 24 in favor and 14 in opposition of an amendment adopting the acuity circles framework. The OPTN Board voted on a few more amendments, and then voted on the policy package as a whole once all amendments were considered and voted upon. The final vote on the policy package as a whole (which included the acuity circles framework) was 30 in favor, 7 opposed, and 2 abstain.
12/3/18-12/4/18	The OPTN Board adopted the continuous distribution allocation framework as best suited for future policies for the geographic distribution of organs. The continuous distribution allocation framework distributes organs to candidates using a statistical formula that combines important clinical factors with proximity to the donor location so that candidates receive organs based on their relative distribution score. There is no absolute geographic boundary in this allocation framework.
2/13/19	HHS received a new critical comment from 10 liver transplant centers, asking that HHS set aside the revised liver allocation policy (using acuity circles) and work to expeditiously develop a new liver allocation policy.
3/14/19	HRSA requested that OPTN provide its views on issues raised in the 2/13/19 critical comment.
3/18/19-4/8/20	The OPTN Liver Committee's Acuity Circles Subcommittee held 7 meetings from 3/18/19-4/8/20 that focused on issues related to the revised liver allocation policy (using acuity circles) approved by the OPTN Board in Dec. 2018, including challenges associated with implementation, MELD at transplant calculations, local organ recovery guidance, and conducting a local organ recovery survey.

Action date	Action
3/26/19	OPTN responded to HRSA's 3/14/19 letter concerning the 2/13/19 critical comment and found that the revised liver allocation policy (using acuity circles) adopted on 12/3/18 complied with the OPTN Final Rule.
4/22/19	Four liver transplant candidates and 14 transplant centers filed a lawsuit in the U.S. District Court for the Northern District of Georgia, alleging that HHS failed to follow legally required procedures in developing the revised liver allocation policy (using acuity circles) and instead deferred authority to the United Network for Organ Sharing. (Callahan v. Azar)
4/22/19	The plaintiffs filed a request for a temporary restraining order of the revised liver allocation policy (using acuity circles). (Callahan v. Azar)
4/23/19	HRSA responded to the 2/13/19 critical comment explaining that after careful review and correspondence about the revised liver allocation policy (using acuity circles), it determined that no further HHS actions were warranted.
5/13/19	The district court denied the plaintiffs' request for a temporary restraining order. (Callahan v. Azar)
5/14/19	The revised liver allocation policy (using acuity circles) was briefly implemented following the district court's denial of plaintiff's request for a temporary restraining order. (Callahan v. Azar)
5/14/19	The plaintiffs filed an appeal to the U.S. Court of Appeals for the 11th Circuit, requesting review of the district court's denial of the plaintiffs' request for a temporary restraining order. (Callahan v. Azar)
5/15/19	The district court imposed a stay on implementation of the revised liver allocation policy (using acuity circles) pending the appeal to the 11th Circuit. (Callahan v. Azar)
5/23/19	The previous liver allocation policy (using DSAs) was reinstated and went into effect pending the 11th Circuit's review of the plaintiffs' appeal. (Callahan v. Azar)
8/16/19	The parties agreed to delay implementation of the revised liver allocation policy (using acuity circles) until at least 14 days after the earliest of (1) the district court issuing an order lifting its 5/15/19 stay, (2) the 11th Circuit issuing a mandate in the appeal, or (3) the 11th Circuit issuing an order dissolving the stay pending the appeal. (Callahan v. Azar)
9/25/19	The 11th Circuit affirmed in part and remanded in part the district court's denial of plaintiffs' request for a temporary restraining order. (Callahan v. Azar)
12/3/19	The parties agreed to delay implementation of the revised liver allocation policy (using acuity circles). (Callahan v. Azar)
12/11/19	The plaintiffs renewed their request for a temporary restraining order of the revised liver allocation policy (using acuity circles). (Callahan v. Azar)
1/16/20	The district court denied plaintiffs' renewed request for a temporary restraining order. (Callahan v. Azar)
2/4/20	The revised liver allocation policy (using acuity circles) was reimplemented.

Source: GAO. | GAO-21-70.

Note: Any interested individual or entity may submit to the Secretary of Health and Human Services critical comments related to the manner in which OPTN is carrying out its duties. See 42 U.S.C. § 274(c) and 42 C.F.R. § 121.4(d) (2019).

Appendix II: Data on Outcomes from 2-Year Monitoring Report following Changes to Lung Allocation Policy

This appendix presents data from the Organ Procurement and Transplantation Network's (OPTN) monitoring report following the changes in the current lung allocation policy that went into effect on November 24, 2017, at 8 p.m. Eastern Time. This monitoring report examined changes in health outcomes in the 2-year period before the policy changes and the 2-year period after the policy changes.[189] Table 3 shows outcomes related to candidates on the waiting list, transplant recipients, and the percent of donor lungs used for transplants before and after the

[189] OPTN Thoracic Transplantation Committee, *Monitoring of the Lung Allocation Change, 2 Year Report: Removal of DSA as a Unit Of Allocation,* accessed June 18, 2020, https://optn.transplant.hrsa.gov/media/3661/item_25_thoracic_committee_20200212.pdf.

policy changes, by OPTN region.[190] Table 4 shows the number of lung transplant recipients nationally by groups of Lung Allocation Scores before and after the policy changes.[191]

Table 3. Outcomes following changes to the lung allocation policy by OPTN region

Pre-policy changes period: 11/26/15 - 11/24/17
Post-policy changes period: 11/25/17 - 11/24/19

Candidates on the waiting list						Transplant recipients			Use of deceased donor lungs for transplants	
Outcomes			Number of candidates added	Average Lung Allocation Score at listing for candidates added[a]	Median Lung Allocation Score at listing for candidates added	Number of transplants	Average Lung Allocation Score at time of transplant	Median Lung Allocation Score at time of transplant	Utilization rate[b] (%)	Discard rate[c] (%)
OPTN region	1	Pre	202	41.50	36.86	208	44.78	38.77	22.93	2.75
		Post	195	43.46	36.55	164	51.10	43.71	18.48	6.64
	2	Pre	995	44.01	37.90	746	50.38	42.19	20.57	14.59
		Post	1,061	45.50	38.30	862	52.33	43.41	22.62	14.76
	3	Pre	566	43.45	37.66	479	47.53	40.12	19.70	6.11
		Post	606	44.77	37.86	522	49.35	40.42	20.55	6.64
	4	Pre	665	41.60	37.72	588	43.17	38.82	25.34	2.53
		Post	658	44.04	38.40	554	46.65	40.07	24.34	3.72
	5	Pre	928	43.15	38.34	770	48.06	42.14	24.66	2.47
		Post	1,028	44.77	38.88	808	50.38	42.87	22.62	2.84
	6	Pre	113	39.22	35.95	106	44.03	40.42	16.24	1.59
		Post	152	39.69	35.58	109	44.89	39.31	16.50	2.30
	7	Pre	454	42.97	37.24	376	46.14	38.58	24.63	5.51
		Post	480	45.56	40.06	367	52.43	44.80	21.94	6.86
	8	Pre	327	20.73	32.24	276	43.56	37.25	25.09	1.82
		Post	351	34.37	34.96	333	43.08	37.22	24.48	5.13
	9	Pre	206	45.97	41.86	139	57.92	48.55	13.06	8.68
		Post	449	46.33	41.33	294	57.06	50.66	16.92	4.66
	10	Pre	706	43.89	36.50	596	47.11	39.0	24.22	4.55
		Post	781	44.24	37.57	634	48.27	40.02	26.22	7.77
	11	Pre	462	44.17	39.38	425	47.76	42.27	23.72	6.32
		Post	563	44.95	39.90	500	49.19	42.61	23.74	5.97

Source: Organ Procurement and Transplantation Network (OPTN). | GAO-21-70.

Notes: The current lung allocation policy went into effect on November 24, 2017, at 8 p.m. Eastern Time. There are 11 OPTN regions in the United States, which include two or more states.

[a] Lung Allocation Scores indicate the level of illness for a lung transplant candidate or recipient, and range from 0 to 100. A higher score represents a clinically sicker candidate or recipient.

[b] The utilization rate is the rate at which lungs are transplanted from all deceased donors.

[c] The discard rate is the number of lungs that were discarded out of the total number of lungs recovered for the purpose of transplant.

[c]The discard rate is the number of lungs that were discarded out of the total number of lungs recovered for the purpose of transplant.

---

[190] There are 11 OPTN regions in the United States; each region includes two or more states.

[191] Lung Allocation Scores are a measure of the level of illness of a lung transplant candidate or recipient. These scores range from 0 to 100, and a higher score represents a clinically sicker transplant candidate or recipient.

Table 4. Number of lung transplants by lung allocation score groups, nationally

Pre-policy changes period: 11/26/15 - 11/24/17
Post-policy changes period: 11/25/17 - 11/24/19

Lung Allocation Score groupsb									
Policy period	Total number of lung transplantsa	<20	20 - 30	30 - 35	35 - 40	40 - 50	50 - 60	60 - 70	70 and higher
Pre	4,709	3	2	1,186	1,136	1,122	409	157	694
Post	5,147	0	2	1,124	1,111	1,208	500	273	929

Source: Organ Procurement and Transplantation Network. | GAO-21-70.

Notes: The current lung allocation policy went into effect on November 24, 2017, at 8 p.m. Eastern Time.

[a] These numbers represent lung transplant recipients who did not receive a lung transplant in combination with another organ, such as a heart.

[b] Lung Allocation Scores indicate the level of illness for a lung transplant candidate or recipient, and range from 0 to 100. A higher score represents a clinically sicker candidate or recipient.

Chapter 3

Federal Support for Organ Transplantation: Frequently Asked Questions*

Jared S. Sussman
Marco A. Villagrana
Evelyne P. Baumrucker
Sylvia L. Bryan
Vanessa C. Forsberg
Elayne J. Heisler
Nathan James
Abigail F. Kolker
and Bryce H. P. Mendez

Summary

Organ transplantation is a complex medical procedure, often requiring coordination among multiple entities, medical teams, and medical facilities. It is also unique in that it requires the use of an organ procured from one individual that is then implanted into another individual. The federal government supports organ procurement and transplantation in various ways. For example, the federal government has established a uniform system for allocating organs in the United States and set coverage requirements and payment for organ acquisition and transplantation. In some cases, the federal government directly provides organ transplantation services. This report focuses on federal coverage, financing, and the provision of organ transplantation by federal agencies and health programs, as well as the federal role in private health insurance coverage of such.

There is not a standard federal support or coverage for organ transplantation services. Each federal department, agency, program, and private health insurance plan has its own unique policies. Even within a program such as Medicaid, there are baseline federal requirements with flexibilities for states to determine what organ transplantation-related services and which subpopulations are covered, resulting in variability across state Medicaid programs.

---

* This is an edited, reformatted and augmented version of Congressional Research Service Publication No. R48257, dated November 8, 2024.

In: Organ Transplants: Procurement, Procedures and Allocation Policies
Editor: Nathalie B. Larson
ISBN: 979-8-89530-729-8

This report provides an overview of organ transplantation, defines key terms, addresses the role of key federal agencies in coverage and payment for organ transplantation, including a discussion of the federal role in regulating private health insurance with regard to organ transplantation.

Introduction

Organ transplantation is a complex medical procedure, often requiring coordination among multiple entities, medical teams, and medical facilities. It is also unique in that it requires the use of an organ procured from one individual that is then implanted into another individual. In addition, organ transplantation involves a complex set of policies, processes, and payments with implications for fairness in the allocation of organs, quality, and patient safety related to procurement, acquisition, and transplantation. All of these complexities are underscored by the fact that the supply of organs is not sufficient to meet the demand.

The federal government supports organ procurement and transplantation in various ways. It has established a system for allocating organs; set coverage requirements and payment for organ acquisition and transplantation; and, in some cases, directly provided organ transplantation, among other activities.

This report provides an overview of organ transplantation, describes key concepts, and addresses the role of selected federal agencies in coverage and payment for organ transplantation, including through a discussion of the federal role in regulating private health insurance with regard to organ transplantation.

What Is an Organ?

There exists both a biological definition of organs and a functional definition for the purpose of transplantation established by statute and regulatory action. These two definitions share some commonalities, but they are not mutually inclusive of each other. Some organs defined by statutes would not be considered organs in a biological sense; inversely, some biologically defined organs are not defined as such in statute or regulation.

Biologically, organs are defined as "a part of the body, composed of more than one tissue, that forms a structural unit responsible for a particular function (or functions)."[192] Examples of organs include the heart, which serves a distinct function of pumping blood through the body; the skin, which protects against germs and regulates body temperate; or the eye, which enables sight.

Statutorily, the National Organ Transplant Act of 1984 (NOTA; P.L. 98-507) defines an organ to mean the kidney, liver, heart, lung, pancreas, and any other human organ specified by the Secretary of Health and Human Services (HHS) by regulation.[193] These organs are generally ones for which there is an established or developing medical procedure to facilitate transplantation. At the time that NOTA was enacted, kidney transplantation was already an accepted medical practice, while heart and liver transplantation was transitioning from

---

[192] Harvey Marcovitch, ed., *Black's Medical Dictionary*, 43rd ed. (A&C Black, 2018).

[193] 42 U.S.C. §274b(d)(2).

experimental to accepted medical practice.[194] The Secretary has expanded the definition through regulation to also include intestine and vascularized composite allografts.[195] *Table 1* describes each organ as defined for this purpose.

What Is Involved in Organ Donation?

Organ donation involves the surgical removal of an organ from an individual, either living or deceased, to be transplanted into another individual experiencing organ failure. This process raises a number of legal and ethical questions.[196] The legality of organ donation and brain death were addressed at the state level with the adoption of the Uniform Anatomical Gift Act (UAGA; 1968) and the Uniform Determination of Death Act (1981), respectively. These acts were uniform bills created by the Uniform Law Commission intended for adoption throughout the states.[197] Every state and Washington, DC, have adopted some version of these two laws. These two acts created a legal basis by which both living and deceased individuals could donate organs.

The majority of organs are donated by deceased donors. However, certain organs, such as whole kidneys and portions of other organs, can be donated while living. In 2023, there were 23,295 individual organ donors.[198] Of those, 16,336 (70.1%) were deceased and 6,959 (29.9%) were living donors.[199] Each deceased donor generally donates multiple organs. In 2023, 54,054 organs in total were recovered from deceased donors.[200]

Table 1. Organs for transplantation

Organ	Description
Kidney	One of a pair. The kidneys separate fluid and certain solids from the blood.
Liver	The liver is divided into four lobes. It serves a role in many metabolic processes.
Heart	The heart maintains circulation of blood through the body.
Lung	One of a pair. Primarily acts as a respiratory organ so that blood can absorb oxygen.
Pancreas	Functions in digestion and production of certain hormones responsible for regulating blood sugar levels.
Intestine	Divided into small and large intestine. It takes the form of one continuous tube. Serves primarily in digestion.
Vascularized Composite Allografts	A minimally manipulated body part containing multiple tissue types. Common examples include a face or hand for transplantation.

Source: 42 U.S.C. §274b(d)(2); 42 C.F.R. §121.2; and Harvey Marcovitch, ed., Black's Medical Dictionary, 43rd ed. (A&C Black, 2018).

---

[194] U. S. Congress, Senate Health, Education, Labor, and Pensions Committee, *Organ Transplant and Procurement Act of 1984*, 98th Cong., 2nd sess., April 6, 1984, S. Rpt. 98-382, p. 3.

[195] 42 C.F.R. §121.2. Blood vessels considered integral to an organ used in transplantation also are included in the definition of an organ.

[196] For ethical considerations of organ recovery, see Organ Procurement & Transplantation Network (OPTN), *Ethics of Deceased Organ Donor Recovery*, December 2016, https://optn.transplant.hrsa.gov/professionals/by-topic/ethical-considerations/ethics-of-deceased-organ-donor-recovery/.

[197] The Uniform Law Commission provides states with nonpartisan legislation to address issues that affect all states. For more information, see https://www.uniformlaws.org/home.

[198] Based on OPTN data as of August 5, 2024. For more information, see OPTN, "National Data," https://optn.transplant.hrsa.gov/data/view-data-reports/national-data/#.

[199] Ibid.

[200] Ibid.

Deceased Organ Donation[201]

Under the typical scenario, when an individual experiences a potentially life-threatening medical event, the individual is transported to a hospital where a medical team provides life-saving care. Organ donation is not considered as an option until the individual is declared functionally brain dead. At that point, the body will be supported by artificial means, such as a ventilator. The purpose of artificial life support is to provide the necessary time to obtain authorization for donation from either a state or national registry of donors or from the individual's family, match the donor with potential transplant recipients, and recover the organs.

If the deceased individual had voluntarily opted in to donation via their state or national registry while alive, that is considered sufficient consent for donation, thus eliminating the need to obtain authorization for donation. If there were no indication that the individual opted in to donate, the organ recovery team would discuss options with the individual's family, which could include authorization for donation.

Organ retrieval is a time-sensitive process due to the limited viability of an organ after death. Therefore, the individual is kept on artificial life support while his or her information is entered into a national computer system to identify a transplant candidate that is a good match. Factors used for organ matching include

- Blood type,
- Tissue type,
- Organ size,
- Donor height and weight,
- Urgency for the transplant candidate,
- Length of time on the organ waitlist,
- Age of both donor and transplant candidate, and
- Geographic distance between donor and transplant candidate.[202]

Once a match is made and accepted by the transplant team, the donor's organs are recovered by a surgical team. The surgical team is not the same as the medical team that was responsible for providing care to the donor. The recovered organ(s) are then transported in a manner that is most expeditious depending on the distance involved (e.g., ambulance, helicopter, airplane) to the transplant hospital where the transplant candidate will receive surgery.

Living Organ Donation[203]

Only certain organs can be donated by a living donor. Specifically, a living donor can donate one of their kidneys or a portion of their liver, lung, pancreas, or intestine. The majority of

---

[201] This section is largely adapted from information available on the OPTN website landing page for deceased donation. For more information, see OPTN, "Deceased Donation," https://optn.transplant.hrsa.gov/patients/about-donation/ deceased-donation/.

[202] The OPTN maintains a series of detailed policies for matching each type of organ. For more information, see OPTN, *OPTN Policies*, September 3, 2024, https://optn.transplant.hrsa. gov/media/eavh5bf3/optn_policies.pdf.

[203] This section is largely adapted from information available on the OPTN website landing page for living donation. For more information, see OPTN, "Living Donation," https://optn. transplant.hrsa.gov/patients/about-donation/living- donation/living-donation/.

living donations are for kidneys—6,293 of 6,959 total organs (90.4%) recovered in 2023.[204] Living donors must meet certain criteria, such as being an adult in good health, understanding the risks involved, and not being coerced into donation.

Generally, living donors choose the recipient of their organ. This is referred to as *directed donation*. The majority of living donors donate organs to someone they know. In 2023, 72.8% of living donors donated to a relative, partner, or unrelated person who they knew.

Directed donation is possible only when the donor and the individual they choose to receive the organ are a match. In other words, the blood type, tissue type, size of organ, and other factors must match. In the case of living kidney donation, individuals who wish to direct a donation to someone but are not a match can use a process referred to as *paired donation*. Paired donation is when one incompatible donor/recipient pair is matched with another incompatible donor/recipient pair. Paired exchanges can become rather complex, as multiple donor/recipient pairs can form a chain that results in all recipients getting a kidney transplantation from a compatible donor. In 2023, 19.1% of living donors were involved in paired donation.

Finally, there are individuals who donate an organ anonymously. These individuals do not know who will receive the organ, and the donors are not known to the recipient. In 2023, 7.3% of living organ donations were made anonymously.

How Are Candidates for Organ Transplantation Identified and Organs Distributed?

Organ transplantation is one of the only medical procedures that uses a part of another person's body. As a result, the ability to get a transplant is limited by the supply of available organs. The nation has managed this by establishing a system by which potential transplant patients enter a waitlist that takes into account many factors in order to match them with an available organ.

Generally, an individual experiencing organ failure who has exhausted all other forms of treatment would be evaluated by a transplant team at a transplant hospital to determine if he or she is a good candidate for an organ transplantation. The federal government does not require transplant hospitals to use specific criteria when determining whether patients would be suitable candidates for transplantation, nor does it require transplant hospitals to have a specific selection process. Listing decisions are complex and involve both medical criteria (e.g., urgent need) and nonmedical criteria (e.g., life expectancy, adherence to medical advice, incarceration status, etc.).[205]

Once an individual is listed as a candidate on the waitlist, he or she remains on the waitlist until an organ becomes available that is suitable for the specific patient. This timeline can differ depending on the specific organ in need and other matching criteria. However, candidates can expect to wait for an extended period of time due to the limited supply of available organs. Of

[204] Based on OPTN data as of August 5, 2024. For more information see, OPTN, "National Data," https://optn.transplant.hrsa.gov/data/view-data-reports/national-data/#.

[205] OPTN, *General Considerations in Assessment for Transplant Candidacy*, 2021, https://optn.transplant.hrsa.gov/professionals/by-topic/ethical-considerations/general-considerations-in-assessment-for-transplant-candidacy/.

the approximately 104,000 candidates currently on the waitlist, nearly 64% have waited for over one year and 11% have waited five or more years.[206]

When an organ becomes available, the candidate is alerted and has to take immediate action to prepare for transplantation surgery.[207]

What Type of Posttransplant Care Do Organ Recipients Need?

Immediate posttransplant care resembles the type of care an individual would get following any similar surgical procedure. Rehabilitation, wound care, and pain management may be among the immediate care needs after the transplant procedure.[208] In addition, transplant recipients need to take certain medications to prevent rejection.[209] These medications are immunosuppressants, intended to prevent the recipient's own immune system from rejecting the transplanted organ.

Coverage and Payment for Organ Transplantation Services by Key Federal Agencies, Departments, and Programs

Several federal agencies and departments provide organ transplantation services directly or arrange to provide them and pay for them. For example, the Indian Health Service (IHS) funds hospitals and health care facilities; some are IHS-owned and operated, and others are tribally owned and operated. Medicare does not provide organ transplantation services directly but does have an oversight role and pays for such services. The following sections address coverage and payment for organ transplantation services by key federal agencies, departments, and federal health coverage programs. The content is organized alphabetically by federal department, agency, or program.

Bureau of Prisons

The Bureau of Prisons (BOP) within the Department of Justice (DOJ) operates the federal prison system, which includes 122 facilities in 35 states. BOP was established in 1930 to house federal prisoners, professionalize the prison service, and ensure consistent and centralized administration of the federal prison system.[210] BOP must confine any offender convicted and sentenced to a term of imprisonment in a federal court. As of the end of FY2023, there were

---

206 Based on OPTN data as of August 5, 2024. For more information see OPTN, "National Data," https://optn.transplant.hrsa.gov/data/view-data-reports/national-data/#.

207 For more information on this process, see United Network for Organ Sharing (UNOS), Transplant Living, "Receiving 'the Call,'" https://transplantliving.org/before-the-trans plant/waiting-for-your-transplant/receiving-the-call/.

208 OPTN Patient Affairs Committee, UNOS, *What Every Patient Needs to Know*, p. 31, https://unos.org/wp-content/uploads/Brochure-113-What-every-patient-needs-to-know.pdf.

209 According to UNOS, "Rejection is when the organ recipient's immune system recognizes the donor organ as foreign and attempts to eliminate it." UNOS, Transplant Living, "Preventing Rejection," https://transplantliving.org/after-the- transplant/preventing-rejection/.

210 U.S. Department of Justice (DOJ), Bureau of Prisons (BOP), *About the Bureau of Prisons*, June 2015, p. 1.

approximately 158,400 prisoners under BOP's jurisdiction, making BOP one of the largest correctional systems in the country.[211] BOP provides medically necessary health care treatment to all prisoners housed in BOP-operated facilities.[212] By statute, BOP is required to "provide for the safekeeping, care, and subsistence of all persons charged with or convicted of offenses against the United States, or held as witnesses or otherwise."[213]

Most medical treatment is provided through in-prison health care clinics operated by BOP. Most clinics have examination rooms, treatment rooms, dental clinics, radiology and laboratory areas, a pharmacy, and administrative offices.[214] When services for acute care cannot be provided at a facility, BOP transports prisoners to a community health care facility or provider (e.g., a hospital). Generally, each BOP facility maintains its own contract with community health care facilities or providers and sets the rate to be paid for providing medical treatment to inmates.[215] BOP transfers prisoners with acute or chronic long-term care needs that cannot be managed through in-prison clinics to one of its Federal Medical Centers (FMCs).[216]

Does BOP Provide for Individuals to Donate Organs?

Federal prisoners are allowed to donate organs, but only to immediate family members (i.e., parents, siblings, and biological children), and can receive an organ donation when BOP deems a transplant to be medically necessary. Federal prisoners are not allowed to list themselves as posthumous organ donors.

Prisoners who chose to donate an organ to an immediate family member must sign a consent form for the donation that indicates that

- the prisoner understands the possible risks of the operation,
- the prisoner agrees to the donation of his or her own free will, and
- the federal government will not be held responsible for any complications or financial obligations.[217]

BOP's patient care policy states that hospitalizations or fees associated with prisoners donating an organ to someone else will not be at the federal government's expense. This encompasses all costs associated with guarding the prisoner at off-site facilities, including any costs associated with the U.S. Marshals Service transporting the prisoner.[218] BOP handles the logistics associated with surgery for organ donation (e.g., arranging for transportation and hospitalization, conducting compatibility testing).[219]

---

[211] DOJ, BOP, "Statistics," https://www.bop.gov/about/statistics/population_statistics.jsp (data on the federal prison population was accessed on April 11, 2024).
[212] DOJ, BOP, FY2025 Performance Budget, Congressional Submission, Salaries and Expenses, p. 25.
[213] 18 U.S.C. §4042(a).
[214] U.S. Government Accountability Office (GAO), Bureau of Prisons: Better Planning and Evaluation Needed to Understand and Control Rising Inmate Health Care Costs, GAO-17-379, June 2017, p. 8.
[215] Ibid., p. 11.
[216] Federal Medical Centers (FMCs) are BOP facilities with the mission of providing care to prisoners with serious or chronic medical problems. Examples of services provided at FMCs include dialysis for inmates with chronic renal failure, oncology treatment (i.e., chemotherapy and radiation therapy), inpatient and forensic mental health, surgery (i.e., limited orthopedic and general surgery procedures), prosthetics and orthotics, long-term ventilator-dependent management, dementia care, and end-of-life care. Ibid., pp. 13, 64-65.
[217] DOJ, BOP, *Patient Care*, Program Statement 6031.04, p. 45.
[218] Ibid.
[219] Ibid.

Does BOP Provide for Organ Transplants?

Federal prisoners can receive donated organs if BOP determines an organ transplant is medically necessary. When a prison's clinical director (CD) determines it is medically necessary to evaluate a prisoner's suitability for an organ transplant, the CD will request an organ transplant workup from a medical specialist to be performed at the prison.[220] If the specialist concludes the prisoner may be a potential candidate for organ transplantation and the CD recommends that further evaluation is medically appropriate, the prisoner will be evaluated at an appropriate community health care facility, such as a transplant center, in the vicinity of the prison or at an FMC.[221] If the transplant center or FMC deems the prisoner suitable for a transplant, the CD compiles all the prisoner's pertinent records and forwards them to BOP's medical director (MD) for consideration.[222] If the MD determines an organ transplant is medically indicated, the prisoner will be approved for surgery at an appropriate transplant center in accordance with BOP policy, transplant center regulations, and state and federal laws.[223]

If a prisoner receives an organ transplant because it is deemed medically necessary, BOP will cover the direct costs of the procedure for both the prisoner and the organ donor.[224]

Does BOP Provide for Posttransplant Care?

As noted above, a prisoner is responsible for all costs associated with hospitalization if the prisoner is donating an organ to someone else. BOP covers costs for prisoners who receive a donated organ because a transplant is deemed medically necessary.

Does BOP Provide for Immunosuppressive Drugs Posttransplant?

BOP's patient care policy does not address immunosuppressive drugs for prisoners who receive an organ transplant. BOP also does not have clinical guidance regarding prescribing these drugs after an organ transplant. However, immunosuppressive drugs that are prescribed for transplant patients—such as tacrolimus, cyclosporine, mycophenolate mofetil, and azathioprine—are listed on BOP's formulary.[225]

Department of Defense

The Department of Defense (DOD) administers a statutory health benefit through the Military Health System (MHS).[226] The MHS offers health care benefits and services through its TRICARE program to approximately 9.6 million beneficiaries, comprising members and retirees of the uniformed services and their family members.[227] TRICARE offers a range of

---

220 Ibid, p. 45.
221 Ibid, p. 46.
222 Ibid.
223 Ibid.
224 Ibid.
225 DOJ, BOP, *Winter 2022 National Formulary Part 2*, https://www.bop.gov/resources/pdfs/2022_winter_formulary_part_2.pdf.
226 10 U.S.C. Chapter 55: Medical and Dental Care.
227 Military Health System (MHS), "Patients by Beneficiary Category," accessed April 17, 2024, https://health.mil/Military-Health-Topics/MHS-Toolkits/Media-Resources/Media-Center/Patient-Population-Statistics/Patients-by-Beneficiary-Category. The term uniformed services includes the Armed Forces (Army, Navy, Air Force, Space Force, Marine Corps, and Coast Guard), the Commissioned Corps of the Public Health

health care services, including organ transplant services, in military hospitals and clinics (also known as military treatment facilities, or MTFs) and through participating civilian health care providers. With the exception of active-duty servicemembers, beneficiaries are subject to certain cost-sharing requirements based on beneficiary category, health plan or benefit program, and the sponsor's initial enlistment or appointment date to military service.[228]

Does DOD Provide for Individuals to Donate Organs?

DOD policy stipulates that TRICARE beneficiaries are "without coercion ... afforded the opportunity and provided a convenient mechanism to donate organs and tissues."[229] TRICARE beneficiaries may declare their intent to donate their organs after death or serve as a living organ donor. Federal regulation authorizes TRICARE to cover certain organ donation costs when the donor or recipient is a TRICARE beneficiary.[230]

Intent to Donate After Death. Generally, DOD recognizes the "first person consent" or "donor designation" principle, which places an individual's desire to donate organs after death above the desire of the next of kin or designated power of attorney.[231] An individual with the capacity to provide informed consent may designate "an election to donate [their] organs" for transplantation or for the purposes of research and education.[232] DOD policies allow for TRICARE beneficiaries to declare their organ donor status at the time of DOD identification card issuance.[233] This policy also requires DOD to record an individual's organ donor status in the Defense Enrollment Eligibility System.[234]

Servicemembers as Living Organ Donors. All TRICARE beneficiaries may choose to be living organ donors. DOD policies outline specific requirements for a servicemember intending to serve as a living donor if the donation (1) requires an "absence from duty for more than one day" or (2) may potentially impact the servicemember's fitness for duty or deployability.[235] These requirements include

---

Service, and the Commissioned Corps of the National Oceanic and Atmospheric Administration. For additional information about the MHS, see CRS In Focus IF10530, Defense Primer: Military Health System.

[228] For more on TRICARE's cost-sharing features, see CRS Report R45399, *Military Medical Care: Frequently Asked Questions* ("Question 7. What are the Different TRICARE Plans?"). A *sponsor* refers to a servicemember or retired servicemember. For more on sponsors and family members, see TRICARE, "Plans and Eligibility," https://www.tricare. mil/Plans/Eligibility.

[229] Department of Defense (DOD) Instruction 6465.03, *Anatomic Gifts and Tissue Donation*, June 8, 2016, p. 3, https://www.esd.whs.mil/Portals/54/Documents/DD/issuances/dodi/646503p. pdf.

[230] 32 C.F.R. §199.4(e)(5)(i)(A)(3).

[231] DOD Instruction 6465.03, *Anatomic Gifts and Tissue Donation*, June 8, 2016, p. 6.

[232] Ibid. For more on informed consent, see U.S. Department of Health and Human Services (HHS), "Office for Human Research Protections," https://www.hhs.gov/ohrp/regulations-and-policy/guidance/faq/informed-consent/ index.html.

[233] Ibid; and Defense Health Agency (DHA) Procedural Instruction 6465.01, *Anatomic Gifts and Tissue Donation*, February 17, 2023, p. 12, https://www.health.mil/Reference-Center/DHA-Publications/2023/02/17/DHA-PI-6465-01.

[234] DHA Procedural Instruction 6465.01, *Anatomic Gifts and Tissue Donation*, February 17, 2023, p. 12, https://www.health.mil/Reference-Center/DHA-Publications/2023/02/17/DHA-PI-6465-01. The Defense Enrollment Eligibility Reporting System (DEERS) is a "database of information on uniformed services members (sponsors), U.S.- sponsored foreign military, DoD and uniformed services civilians, other personnel as directed by the DoD, and their family members." For more on DEERS, see milConnect, "About DEERS," https://milco nnect.dmdc.osd.mil/ milconnect/public/faq/DEERS-About_DEERS.

[235] DOD Instruction 6465.03, *Anatomic Gifts and Tissue Donation*, June 8, 2016, pp. 6-9; and DHA Procedural Instruction 6465.01, *Anatomic Gifts and Tissue Donation*, February 17, 2023, pp. 12-20.

- a servicemember's written request to be a living donor;
- written counseling and endorsement by the servicemember's chain of command;
- a medical examination by the servicemember's primary care manager;[236] and
- a statement from the transplant facility's attending physician that verifies the recipient's diagnosis, prognosis, and that no other donor is available.[237]

The surgeon general of the respective military service is the approval authority for servicemember requests to be a living organ donor.[238]

Does DOD Provide for Organ Transplants?

Federal regulation requires DOD to cover "services or supplies in connection with an organ transplant procedure, provided such transplant procedure is in accordance with accepted professional medical standards and is not considered unproven."[239] In addition to the transplant procedure, covered services and supplies can include

- evaluation of a potential candidate's suitability for an organ transplant,
- pre- and posttransplant inpatient hospital and outpatient services,
- pre- and postoperative services of the transplant team,
- blood and blood products,
- Food and Drug Administration (FDA)-approved immunosuppression medications,
- care to treat or mitigate complications of the transplant procedure,
- periodic evaluation and follow-up assessments,
- donor acquisition services and organ transportation, and
- maintenance of the viability of the donor organ.[240]

TRICARE policies stipulate that beneficiaries who require a medically necessary organ transplant obtain a preauthorization.[241] TRICARE covers organ transplant procedures performed only in TRICARE- or Medicare-certified transplantation centers.[242] Beneficiaries also may be subject to certain cost-sharing requirements for an organ transplant procedure and related services or supplies.[243] DOD policy requires the MHS to participate in the Organ

---

[236] DHA Procedural Instruction 6465.01 requires the medical examination to include completion of Defense Department (DD) Form 2807-1, *Report of Medical History*; DD Form 2808, *Report of Medical Examination*; and appropriate diagnostic testing.

[237] For more on the requirements of servicemembers intending to be a living organ donor, see DHA Procedural Instruction 6465.01, *Anatomic Gifts and Tissue Donation*, February 17, 2023, p. 35.

[238] DHA Procedural Instruction 6465.01, *Anatomic Gifts and Tissue Donation*, February 17, 2023, p. 10.

[239] 32 C.F.R. §199.4(e)(5)(i).

[240] 32 C.F.R. §199.4(e)(5) and CRS analysis of Chapter 4 of the *TRICARE Policy Manual 6010.60-M*, April 2015 (Change 125), https://manuals.health.mil/pages/ManualToc.aspx? Manual=TP15&Change=107. While outside the purview of this report, these regulatory and policy authorities also allow DOD to cover stem cell transplantation under certain conditions.

[241] Chapter 1, Section 6.1 of the *TRICARE Policy Manual 6010.60-M*, updated June 12, 2023, https://manuals.health.mil/pages/DisplayManualHtmlFile/2024-03-18/AsOf/TP15/C1S6_1.html.

[242] 2 C.F.R. §199.6(b)(4)(ii) and Chapter 11, §7.1 of the *TRICARE Policy Manual 6010.60-M*, April 2015 (Change 125), https://manuals.health.mil/pages/DisplayManualHtmlFile/2024-03-18/AsOf/TP15/C11S7_1.html.

[243] For more on TRICARE cost-sharing requirements, see TRICARE, "TRICARE Costs and Fees 2024," March 2024, https://tricare.mil/-/media/Files/TRICARE/Publications/FactSheets/TRICARE_Costs_Fees_FS_FINAL_032624.pdf.

Procurement and Transplantation Network (OPTN); as such, organ transplant procedures may be performed in certain MTFs with appropriate capabilities.[244]

Does DOD Provide for Posttransplant Care?

Federal regulation requires DOD to cover posttransplant care when the organ transplant procedure is "in accordance with accepted professional medical standards and is not considered unproven."[245] Posttransplant care may include related inpatient hospital services, outpatient services, and pharmacy services. For posttransplant care of living donors who are not TRICARE beneficiaries, federal regulation and TRICARE policy limit the coverage of costs to services and supplies "directly related to the transplant procedure itself and do not include medical care costs related to the treatment of the donor, including complications."[246]

Does DOD Provide for Immunosuppressive Drugs Posttransplant?

Federal regulation requires DOD to cover FDA-approved immunosuppressive drugs when the organ transplant procedure is "in accordance with accepted professional medical standards and is not considered unproven."[247] The regulation also authorizes TRICARE coverage of these drugs for "off-label uses when determined to be medically necessary for the treatment of the condition for which it is administered, according to accepted standards of medical practice."[248]

U.S. Immigration and Customs Enforcement Noncitizen Detention

Within the Department of Homeland Security (DHS), Immigration and Customs Enforcement's (ICE's) mission "is to protect America from the cross-border crime and illegal immigration that threaten national security and public safety."[249] ICE's Enforcement and Removal Operations component is responsible for immigration enforcement in the interior of the United States, including managing and overseeing the immigrant detention system.[250]

ICE detention standards were originally developed in 2000 and have been updated several times. Rather than there being one set of standards, there are currently various sets of standards that incorporate different laws and regulations and vary in terms of scope and rigor. Although there are different sets of standards, all facilities housing noncitizen detainees generally must comply with one of the sets of ICE detention standards, including health care standards.[251]

---

[244] DOD Instruction 6465.03, *Anatomic Gifts and Tissue Donation*, June 8, 2016, pp. 6-9; and DHA Procedural Instruction 6465.01, *Anatomic Gifts and Tissue Donation*, February 17, 2023, pp. 12-20.

[245] 32 C.F.R. §199.4(e)(5)(i).

[246] 32 C.F.R. §199.4(e)(5)(i)(A)(4); and Chapter 4, §24.9, of the *TRICARE Policy Manual 6010.60-M*, April 2015 (Change 125), https://manuals.health.mil/pages/DisplayManualHtmlFile/2024-03-18/AsOf/TP15/C4S24_9.html.

[247] 32 C.F.R. §199.4(e)(5)(i).

[248] 32 C.F.R. §199.4(e)(5)(i)(A)(1)(v).

[249] Department of Homeland Security (DHS), "Immigration and Customs Enforcement" (ICE), https://www.dhs.gov/topic/immigration-and-customs-enforcement.

[250] The law provides ICE with broad authority to detain noncitizens while awaiting a determination of whether they should be removed from the United States and mandates that certain categories of noncitizens are subject to mandatory detention (e.g., when the noncitizen is removable on account of certain criminal or terrorist activity). See 8 U.S.C. §§1225, 1226, 1226a, 1231, and 1357.

[251] For more information, see CRS In Focus IF12623, Medical Care Standards in Immigrant Detention Facilities.

Contracts or agreements between ICE and detention facilities specify which set of standards facilities are required to follow.[252]

Two sets of detention standards are applied at facilities that house the majority of the adult detained population: the 2011 Performance-Based National Detention Standards (PBNDS) and the 2000/2019 National Detention Standards (NDS).[253] The 2011 PBNDS and 2019 NDS provide identical guidance on certain standards. Multiple DHS Office of Inspector General (OIG) and Government Accountability Office reports indicate inadequate compliance with these standards in many ICE detention facilities.[254] For more information, see CRS In Focus IF12623, *Medical Care Standards in Immigrant Detention Facilities*.

Does ICE Provide for Organ Donation or Transplantation?

The PBNDS addresses detainees' ability to donate organs. It states that detainees may donate organs to immediate family members; the donation shall be at the detainees' expense, involving no government funds; and the government is not responsible for any associated medical complications.[255] The PBNDs does not reference detainees' ability to receive organ transplantations. The NDS does not address organ donation or transplantation.[256] CRS contacted ICE for more specifics and had not heard back by the date of publication.

---

[252] ICE owns and operates some of its own facilities, and it has arrangements through contracts with private companies that operate immigration detention facilities. In addition, immigrant detention facilities owned by state or local governments or private entities operate through intergovernmental agreements. (GAO, *ICE Should Enhance Its Use of Facility Oversight Data and Management of Detainee Complaints*, GAO-20-596, August 2020, pp. 6-7; hereinafter, GAO-20-596.)

[253] The 2011 Performance-Based National Detention Standards (PBNDS) was revised in 2016 to meet detention standards consistent with federal legal and regulatory requirements, as well as prior ICE policies and policy statements. The 2011 PBNDS is an updated version of the 2008 PBNDS; some facilities have contracts agreeing to adhere to the 2008 version (GAO-20-596). The 2019 National Detention Standards (NDS) is a modified version of the 2000 NDS. The data provided by GAO do not distinguish between the facilities using 2000 and 2019 NDS (GAO-20-596).

[254] For example, see DHS, Office of the Inspector General (OIG), Concerns About ICE Detainee Treatment and Care at Detention Facilities, OIG-18-32, December 11, 2017; DHS OIG, ICE Does Not Fully Use Contracting Tools to Hold Detention Facility Contractors Accountable for Failing to Meet Performance Standards, OIG-19-18, January 29, 2018; DHS OIG, Management Alert—Issues Requiring Action at the Adelanto ICE Processing Center in Adelanto, California, OIG-18-87, September 27, 2018; DHS OIG, Concerns About ICE Detainee Treatment and Care at Four Detention Facilities, OIG-19-57, June 3, 2019; DHS OIG, Capping Report: Observations of Unannounced Inspections of ICE Facilities in 2019, OIG-20-45, July 1, 2020; GAO, Immigrant Detention: Additional Actions Needed to Strengthen Management and Oversight of Detainee Medical Care, GAO-16-321, February 2016; GAO, Immigrant Detention: Care of Pregnant Women in DHS Facilities, GAO-20-330, March 2020; GAO, Immigrant Detention: ICE Should Enhance Its Use of Facility Oversight Data and Management of Detainee Complaints, GAO-20-956, August 2020. DHS OIG, Medical Processes and Communication Protocols Need Improvement at Irwin County Detention Center, OIG-22-14, January 3, 2022; GAO, Immigrant Detention: ICE Needs to Strengthen Oversight of Informed Consent for Medical Care, GAO-23-105196, October 2022; GAO, Immigration Detention: ICE Can Improve Oversight and Management, GAO-23-106350, January 2023; and DHS OIG, ICE and CBP Deaths in Custody During FY2021, OIG-23-12, February 1, 2023.

[255] ICE, "4.7 Terminal Illness, Advance Directives and Death," D. Organ Donation by Detainees," in *Performance-Based National Detention Standards 2011,* revised 2016, p. 341, https://www.ice.gov/doclib/detention-standards/2011/ 4-7.pdf. Note that while the section on "organ donation by detainees" is included in the chapter on "Terminal Illness, Advance Directives and Death," the guidelines do not specify that only dying or terminally ill detainees may donate organs to immediate family members.

[256] ICE, "4.3 Medical Care" and "4.6 Terminal Illness and Death," in *National Detention Standards for Non-Dedicated Facilities*, revised 2019, https://www.ice.gov/detain/ detention-management/2019.

Indian Health Service

American Indians and Alaska Natives who are members of federally recognized tribes are eligible to receive health care through IHS within HHS. IHS provides health care directly or provides funds for Indian tribes or tribal organizations to operate health care facilities.[257] It provides limited services free of charge to approximately 2.8 million eligible American Indians and Alaska Natives in 37 states.[258] IHS is organized into 12 geographic areas, which cover one or more states. Areas are then subdivided into service units that may consist of multiple facilities. Service units may cover a number of small reservations, or a larger reservation may be covered by multiple service units.

Not all individuals who are eligible to receive services will use IHS, and not all individuals who self-identify as American Indian and Alaska Native are eligible for IHS.[259] American Indians and Alaska Natives experience high rates of chronic conditions that may lead to organ failure (e.g., liver disease). Despite this, these individuals account for less than 1% of patients on the organ transplant waiting list. In 2020, 30% of American Indian/Alaska Native patients waiting for a transplant received one, compared with 49% of White patients that year.[260]

IHS does not have a standard medical benefit that includes or excludes certain services. The agency generally focuses on primary and preventive services through a network of nearly 700 facilities, which include hospitals (43), health centers (383), and small health stations (101). Other facility types include school health centers, youth regional treatment centers, and Alaska village clinics.[261] In general, IHS has limited funding and some facilities serve small populations. Most IHS hospitals are small and do not directly provide transplant services. IHS will pay for some services, potentially including transplant services, outside its system in non-IHS or non- tribally-owned or operated facilities (i.e., community health care facilities), through its Purchased/Referred Care (PRC) system as will be discussed further below.[262]

Does IHS Provide for Individuals to Donate Organs?

IHS's facilities are small and do not provide transplantation services directly. As such, IHS facilities would not retrieve organs for donation from IHS beneficiaries, nor would IHS facilitate the donation of organs that would be received by an IHS beneficiary. As discussed in the question below, IHS may pay for transplant services provided to IHS beneficiaries outside

---

[257] The Indian Health Service (IHS) also provides grants to Urban Indian Organizations (UIOs) that operate smaller health facilities in urban areas. These facilities vary in terms of the services available; some provide comprehensive services, whereas others provide information and referral services. UIOs do not provide inpatient services. As such, they would not be directly providing transplant services. Outside of the grants they receive, UIOs generally are not eligible to receive funds from the overall IHS budget; this includes purchased/referred care, which is the source of payment for IHS system transplant services. For more information on the IHS system and UIOs, see CRS Report R43330, *The Indian Health Service (IHS): An Overview*.

[258] HHS, IHS, *Fiscal Year 2025 Indian Health Service Justification of Estimates*, Justification of Estimates for Appropriations Committees (ihs.gov) https://www.ihs.gov/sites/budget formulation/themes/responsive2017/display_objects/documents/FY-2025-IHS-CJ030 824.pdf, see CJ.2.

[259] For discussion of issues related to measuring the American Indian and Alaska Native population, see Appendix A in CRS Report R43330, *The Indian Health Service (IHS): An Overview*.

[260] HHS, Office of Minority Health, "Organ Donation and American Indians/Alaska Natives," https://minorityhealth.hhs.gov/omh/browse.aspx?lvl=4&lvlid=42.

[261] HHS, IHS, *Fiscal Year 2024 Indian Health Service Justification of Estimates*, https://www. ihs.gov/sites/budgetformulation/themes/responsive2017/display_objects/documents/FY-2025-IHS-CJ030824.pdf, pp. 41-42.

[262] HHS, IHS, "Purchased/Referred Care," https://www.ihs.gov/prc/. In FY2024, the program received an appropriation of approximately $996.8 million in P.L. 118-42.

of IHS health facilities through the PRC program.[263] PRC information is not specific enough to determine whether IHS would pay for organ donation. IHS policy requires that a procedure be "medically necessary" but does not define that term.[264] Providing an organ to another individual would not be "medically necessary" for the donor; as such, it is unlikely that IHS funds would be available to pay for donor services.

Does IHS Provide for Organ Transplants?

IHS's facilities are small and do not provide transplantation services directly. IHS, however, may pay for transplant services provided to IHS beneficiaries outside of IHS health facilities through the PRC program.[265] IHS's PRC funds may be used to pay for an individual's transplant, subject to PRC program requirements. Only a subset of IHS beneficiaries are eligible for PRC, because eligibility is restricted to individuals who live in certain geographic areas.[266] PRC funds are authorized only for services in instances when the PRC-eligible individual does not have an alternate source of coverage or payment (e.g., Medicaid). In instances where the IHS beneficiary has alternate sources of coverage or payment, the program or plan rules of the alternate source apply.

For individuals without alternate sources, PRC referrals may be authorized and PRC funds would pay for services, to the extent that funds are available, based on medical priority rankings. These priorities range from Medical Priority Level I (emergency care services necessary to save life, limb, or senses, which are almost always paid) to Medical Priority Level V (excluded services, including those considered elective or experimental, which are not paid).[267] PRC programs are managed locally, and these local programs determine what priority level will be paid and may add or remove services within specific priority levels. In FY2022, 90% of IHS-operated PRC programs were able to pay for services beyond Medical Priority Level II services.[268] IHS's budget for PRC is limited, and funds may not be available toward the end of any given fiscal year. IHS reports that it denied or deferred 119,938 services for eligible IHS beneficiaries in FY2022 because of these funding limitations.[269]

Transplant services generally are considered Medical Priority Level IV (chronic tertiary care services). These treatments are not considered essential to treat an initial or emergent diagnosis, have less of an impact on mortality or morbidity, and are high cost. Transplant PRC referrals are subject to additional authorization than are PRC requests at higher priority levels. Specifically, for a transplant to be authorized, the service unit level PRC committee must concur

---

[263] Ibid.

[264] HHS, IHS, "Can PRC Pay for Your Referral Medical Care? Find Out in 3 Stages," https://www.ihs.gov/sites/prc/themes/responsive2017/display_objects/documents/PRC-ProcessHandout.pdf.

[265] HHS, IHS, "Purchased/Referred Care," https://www.ihs.gov/prc/.

[266] These are called *purchased/referred care delivery areas*. Each individual PRC program has its own purchased/referred care delivery area and in statute, some areas comprise entire states (e.g., Arizona under 25 U.S.C.§1678). The Purchased/Referred Care program was previously named the Contract Health Services program. In statute, these areas are referred to by the prior program name (i.e., *contract health service delivery areas*).

[267] For more information, see HHS, IHS, "Purchased/Referred Care: Requirements: Priorities of Care," https://www.ihs.gov/prc/eligibility/requirements-priorities-of-care/, see "Indian Health Service Medical Priority Levels" Word document.

[268] HHS, IHS, *Fiscal Year 2025 Indian Health Service Justification of Estimates*, Justification of Estimates for Appropriations Committees, https://www.ihs.gov/sites/budgetformulation/themes/responsive2017/display_objects/documents/FY-2025-IHS-CJ030824.pdf. See CJ-97.

[269] Ibid.

with the referral. The area level Chief Medical Officer or a designee also must monitor and, depending on cost, concur with the referral.[270]

Does IHS Provide Posttransplant Care?

IHS policies do not explicitly address posttransplant care. To the extent that a facility has the appropriate services that someone who has donated an organ or received a transplant requires, IHS would provide these services. In addition, to the extent that such services meet PRC medical priority levels (discussed above), PRC funds could be used to provide these services.

Does IHS Provide Immunosuppressive Drugs Posttransplant?

IHS does provide pharmaceutical benefits, and most facilities offer such services. IHS uses a National Core Formulary, which individual facilities can supplement with additional drugs, depending on facility needs. The formulary provides limited access to immunosuppressive drugs, based on CRS's search of the formulary as of April 2024. Some facilities may offer additional types of pharmaceuticals as part of supplementing the core formulary; in such cases, a facility could be providing immunosuppressive drugs.[271] As with other IHS services, pharmaceuticals are provided to eligible American Indians and Alaska Natives free of charge.

Department of Veterans Affairs

The Veterans Health Administration (VHA) of the Department of Veterans Affairs (VA) operates the nation's largest public integrated direct health care delivery system.[272] VHA's primary mission is to provide health care services to eligible veterans.[273] VHA provides care to approximately 6.4 million unique veteran patients on an annual basis.[274] VHA generally provides care directly through over 1,300 sites of care, including hospitals, clinics, and health care facilities.[275]

VHA is primarily a direct provider of care. It directly operates associated facilities and employs clinicians.[276] This model differs from the predominant health care financing and delivery model in the United States, in which there is a payer for health care services (e.g., Medicare, private health insurance plan), a provider (e.g., hospital, physician), and a recipient of care (patient). VHA is not a health insurance financing program that provides reimbursement to providers for all or a portion of a patient's health care costs.

---

[270] HHS, IHS, "Purchased/Referred Care—Requirements: Priorities of Care," https://www. ihs.gov/prc/ eligibility/requirements-priorities-of-care/, see "Indian Health Service Medical Priorities Levels," https://www.ihs.gov/prc/ eligibility/requirements-priorities-of-care/ (linked Word document).

[271] HHS, IHS, "National Core Formulary," https://www.ihs.gov/nptc/formularysearch/.

[272] Department of Veterans Affairs, *FY2025 Congressional Submission, Medical Programs*, vol. 2 of 4, March 2024, p. VHA-362.

[273] 38 U.S.C. §7301.

[274] Ibid., p. VHA-41.

[275] Department of Veterans Affairs, *FY2025 Congressional Submission, Medical Programs*, vol. 2 of 4, March 2024, p. VHA-17.

[276] The Veterans Health Administration (VHA) does pay for care in the community (i.e., non-Veterans Affairs [VA] providers) under certain circumstances. The VA Maintaining Internal Systems and Strengthening Integrated Outside Networks Act of 2018 (VA MISSION Act; P.L. 115-182) established the Veterans Community Care Program (VCCP), which requires VHA to provide for care in the community to all enrolled veterans who meet specified criteria.

VA has established, through regulation, a medical benefits package to standardize care provided to patients enrolled in the system.[277] The medical benefits package includes, among other things, inpatient care, outpatient care, and prescription drugs.[278]

VHA also provides health care to dependents, spouses, and caregivers of veterans who meet certain eligibility criteria through the Civilian Health and Medical Program of the Department of Veterans Affairs (CHAMPVA).[279] Unlike the provision of health care for veterans, which follows the standard medical benefits package, CHAMPVA is required to provide benefits similar to DOD's TRICARE Standard plan.[280] Furthermore, CHAMPVA is primarily a health insurance program in which enrollees receive care from private sector health care providers and CHAMPVA pays for a portion of the cost of care; this is in contrast to the provision of health care for veterans, which is generally provided by VA clinicians.

Does VA Have Protocols in Place for Individuals to Donate Organs?

VA has protocols in place to allow patients to donate organs upon death and for living donors to donate organs to patients in need.

VA policy requires that each VA medical center enter into an agreement with the local Organ Procurement Organization (OPO) to identify potential donors and to facilitate the donation-after- death process.[281] VA has established protocols for procession of donation after death, which includes conforming policy with specific state UAGAs and notifying OPOs of all hospital deaths, among other activities.

Subject to the availability of appropriations, the Secretary of Veterans Affairs is required to furnish any care or services that may be required in connection with a living donation for an eligible veteran's transplant procedure to any live donor, regardless of whether the donor is a veteran themselves.[282] The Secretary can furnish such services at a VA or non-VA facility.[283]

VA will provide the following for live donors pertaining to solid organ donation.[284]

- Any examinations, tests, and studies necessary to qualify a prospective live donor to donate.
- The surgical procedure to remove a solid organ or part of a solid organ.
- All hospital care, medical services, and other services that are necessary and appropriate to live donor follow-up for a period not less than that which the OPTN prescribes or recommends or for a period of two years, whichever is greater.

Under certain circumstances, VA will also reimburse living donors for the cost of travel for hospital care or medical services as well as for temporary lodging.[285]

---

[277] 38 C.F.R. §17.38.

[278] For more information on VA health care in general, see CRS Report R42747, *Health Care for Veterans: Answers to Frequently Asked Questions*.

[279] For more information on the Civilian Health and Medical Program of the Department of Veterans Affairs (CHAMPVA), see CRS Report RS22483, *Health Care for Dependents and Survivors of Veterans*.

[280] 38 U.S.C. §1781(b).

[281] VA, VHA, "Solid Organ, Tissue, and Eye Donation," VHA Directive 1101.3, August 23, 2021.

[282] 38 U.S.C. §1788.

[283] 38 C.F.R. §17.395(e).

[284] 38 C.F.R. §17.395(c).

[285] 38 C.F.R. §17.395(d).

Does VA Provide Organ Transplants?

VA operates a national transplant program for veterans enrolled in the VA health care system. As shown in *Figure 1*, VA operates its own transplant centers, which generally focus on a specific organ or organs for transplantation. Veterans generally travel to the nearest VA transplant center to receive transplant care. The veterans' care team at their VA medical center makes a referral to the VA transplant center when medically appropriate.[286]

Under the Veterans Community Care Program (VCCP), veterans can receive organ transplant care at a non-VA transplant center if the procedure is medically necessary and the veteran's primary care provider provides a medically compelling reason for the veteran to travel to a different OPTN region than where the veteran resides.[287] This differs from other types of care authorized under the VCCP, which can be authorized based on specified eligibility criteria or access standards.[288]

VA also pays for transplant services for certain spouses, dependents, and caregivers of veterans through the CHAMPVA program.[289] CHAMPVA beneficiaries generally do not need prior authorization (i.e., advanced approval) to receive care paid for by CHAMPVA. However, beneficiaries do require prior authorization for organ transplant care.

Does VA Provide Posttransplant Care?

VA provides enrolled veterans all medically necessary inpatient and outpatient care as part of the medical benefits package.[290] This includes any posttransplant care. VA generally does not pay for nonmedical expenses; however, under certain circumstances, it will reimburse veterans for certain travel costs.[291]

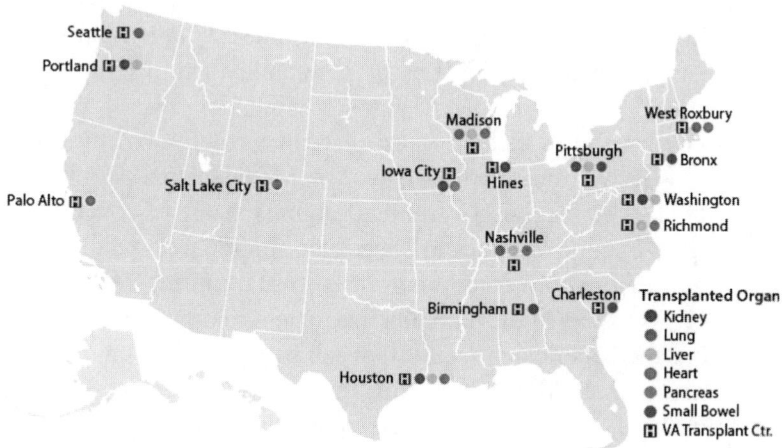

Source: Adapted by CRS from VA, https://www.va.gov/health/services/transplant/ (accessed on 02/07/2023).

Figure 1. VATransplant Centers.

---

[286] VA, VHA, "Solid Organ and Bone Marrow Transplantation," VHA Directive 2012-018(1), July 9, 2012.
[287] 38 C.F.R. §17.4020(d).
[288] For more information on the VCCP, see CRS Report R42747, Health Care for Veterans: Answers to Frequently Asked Questions.
[289] CHAMPVA, CHAMPVA Program Guide, p. 57, https://www.va.gov/COMMUNITY CARE/ docs/pubfiles/programguides/CHAMPVA-Guide.pdf.
[290] 38 C.F.R. 17.38(a)(1).
[291] 38 C.F.R. Part 70.

VA provides CHAMPVA beneficiaries postoperative services as well as any costs associated with complications of a transplant procedure.[292] CHAMPVA does not cover posttransplant nonmedical expenses, such as out-of-hospital living expenses.

Does VA Provide Immunosuppressive Drugs Posttransplant?

VA provides all medically necessary medications to enrolled veterans as required by the standard medical benefit package.[293] Veterans are generally required to pay copayments for medication.

However, copayments are not required if the organ transplant is related to a service-connected disability, among other potential reasons.[294]

CHAMPVA beneficiaries also are provided appropriate and FDA-approved immunosuppression therapy.[295] Beneficiaries are required to pay a specified cost sharing for pharmacy services unless they utilize the CHAMPVA *meds by mail* program. Under this program, beneficiaries pay no cost sharing for pharmacy services.[296]

Coverage of Organ Transplantation Services

Medicaid

Medicaid, authorized in Social Security Act (SSA) Title XIX, is a federal-state program that jointly finances primary and acute medical services, as well as long-term services and supports, to a diverse low-income population, including eligible children, pregnant women, adults, individuals with disabilities, and people aged 65 and older.[297] Participation in Medicaid is voluntary for states; all states, the District of Columbia, and U.S. territories choose to participate.

In general, states must follow federal rules to receive federal matching funds, but states have the flexibility to design their own versions of Medicaid within the federal statute's framework. For example, the federal government requires states to cover certain mandatory populations and benefits but allows states to cover other optional populations and benefits. In another example, states can require certain enrollees to share in the cost of certain Medicaid services, but there are limits on (1) the amounts that states can impose (subject to a maximum allowable amount), (2) the beneficiary groups that can be required to pay, and (3) the services for which cost sharing can be charged. Due to this flexibility, there is substantial state variation in factors such as Medicaid eligibility, covered benefits, and enrollee cost-sharing requirements. In FY2023, Medicaid provided health care services to an estimated 97 million

---

292 *CHAMPVA Operational Policy Manual*, CHAMPVA, Chapter 2, Section 31.4, "Kidney Transplantation," in *CHAMPVA Operational Policy Manual*.

293 38 C.F.R. 17.38(a)(1)(iii).

294 For more information, see, CRS Report R42747, *Health Care for Veterans: Answers to Frequently Asked Questions*.

295 CHAMPVA, Chapter 2, Section 30.8, "Immunosuppression Therapy," in *CHAMPVA Operational Policy Manual*.

296 CHAMPVA, *CHAMPVA Program Guide*, p. 45, https://www.va.gov/COMMUNITYCARE/ docs/pubfiles/ programguides/CHAMPVA-Guide.pdf.

297 For more information about the Medicaid program, see CRS Report R43357, *Medicaid: An Overview*.

individuals at a total cost of approximately $894 billion (including federal and state expenditures).[298]

Does Medicaid Cover Organ Donation?

States are permitted to tailor their organ transplantation benefit coverage through what are referred to as *written standards* included in the Medicaid state plan as approved by Centers for Medicare & Medicaid Services (CMS).[299] (For more information, see "Does Medicaid Cover Organ Transplants?") This results in variability in the types of coverage available across states. CRS could not identify a consolidated summary of organ donation coverage policies across states. However, the following are examples of state variation in organ donation policies.[300]

- *District of Columbia:* Covers procedures and medical care required to retrieve an organ from a living donor for use by a Medicaid enrollee, regardless of the donor's Medicaid eligibility status.[301]
- *California:* Covers donor *and* recipient organ transplant surgeries, as specified.[302]
- *Kentucky:* Covers donor expenses, including physician services, facility costs, and lodging and transportation incurred in connection to the transplant surgery, as long as Medicaid is payer of last resort before all other possible insurance sources.[303]
- *Michigan:* Allows Medicaid enrollees to be an organ donor for a non-Medicaid enrolled recipient, but the acquisition of the organ must be paid for by the organ recipient's health insurance.[304]
- *Mississippi:* Covers all facility and physician charges related to the procurement of an organ, whether from a living donor or from a cadaver. Examples of other charges

---

[298] This enrollment figure is measured according to average monthly enrollment and represents the number of enrollees with full and partial benefits who are enrolled on an average monthly basis. This enrollment measure differs from *person-year equivalents*, which represent the average program enrollment over the course of a year, and from *ever- enrolled counts*, which measure the number of people covered by Medicaid for any period of time during the year. Congressional Budget Office Baseline Projections, *Medicaid*, June 2024, https://www.cbo.gov/system/files/2024-06/ 51301-2024-06-medicaid.pdf. Centers for Medicare & Medicaid (CMS), Form CMS-64 data as of May 29, 2024, https://www.medi caid.gov/medicaid/financial-management/state-expenditure-reporting-for-medicaid-chip/expenditure- reports-mbescbes/index.html.

[299] The Medicaid state plan is an agreement between the state and the federal government that details how the state will administer its program (e.g., eligibility requirements, benefit coverage, provider reimbursement, delivery systems) and certifies that the state has met program requirements set forth in federal statute and regulations. If a state wants to change how its program operates (e.g., by adjusting eligibility levels or benefit coverage) or if Congress modifies a requirement (e.g., adds a new state plan option), the state must submit a state plan amendment describing the change to CMS for approval.

[300] The state organ donation policies listed here are not comprehensive or complete. They are intended to provide an illustration of the range of policies that states have adopted through CMS-approved written standards. For more complete information on a given state's coverage, see the source materials associated with each state.

[301] For example, see CMS, Letter to State, "District of Columbia State Plan Amendment (SPA) 20-0008," June 2, 2021, available at DC SPA 20-0008 APPROVAL.pdf (medicaid.gov). Also see CMS, Letter to State, "South Dakota's State Plan Amendment (SPA) Transmittal #22-0005," July 12, 2022, https://www.medicaid. gov/medicaid/spa/downloads/SD-22-0005.pdf.

[302] California State Statues of 2022, Chapter 47, §126, https://heinonline.org/HOL/P?h= hein.ssl/ssca0412&i=222.

[303] Kentucky Law, Title 907, Chapter 010, Regulation 830, https://apps.legislature.ky.gov /law/kar/titles/907/ 010/830/.

[304] Michigan Department of Health and Human Services, Behavioral and Physical Health and Aging Services Administration, "Organ and Tissue Transplant Services," Bulletin Number MMP 22-44, December 1, 2022, p. 7, https://www.michigan.gov/mdhhs/-/media/Project/Websites/mdhhs/Assistance-Programs/Medicaid-BPHA SA/2022-Bulletins/Final-Bulletin-MMP-22-44-Hospital.pdf?rev=f09538bf929b44bc873b6177d2bdc81f&hash= 6C2BA9EF7AC66E621E5E472A283FD972.

allowable in this state include fees related to searching for matching tissue, bone marrow, or organ; the donor's transportation and hospitalization costs; and fees associated with the removal, withdrawal, and preservation/storage of the organ or tissue. The state also covers medically necessary follow-up care beyond the transplant hospital admission for the living donor, but only in the case that the donor is a Medicaid enrollee.[305]

- *North Dakota*: Covers medically necessary transplants and related services, including "cadaveric or living donor expenses; organ procurement costs, tissue typing, and searches and matches."[306]

Does Medicaid Cover Organ Transplants?

Federal Medicaid funds may be used to pay for "services furnished in connection with organ transplant procedures." States that offer this coverage are required to include written standards defining such coverage in the Medicaid state plan. The Medicaid statute requires that these written standards provide that similar individuals are treated alike and that any restrictions on facilities or practitioners that provide organ transplant procedures are consistent with the accessibility of high-quality care under Medicaid.[307]

The federal Medicaid statute explicitly excludes coverage of organ transplantation services for unauthorized aliens (i.e., noncitizens in Medicaid statute) who are entitled to limited benefit coverage under emergency Medicaid.[308] In general, benefit coverage under emergency Medicaid comprises "medical assistance under Title XIX of the Social Security Act ... for care and emergency services that are necessary for the treatment of an emergency medical condition (as defined in Section 1903(v)(3) of such Act) of the alien involved and are not related to an organ transplant procedure."[309]

States are permitted to tailor their organ transplantation benefit coverage through the written standards included in the Medicaid state plan, as approved by CMS. This flexibility results in variability across state Medicaid programs in terms of state coverage of organ transplantation services. For example, states may limit coverage to specified Medicaid enrolled subgroups (e.g., children under the age of 21, adults with an absence of specified comorbidities), specify the coverage that will be available (e.g., types of organs that can be transplanted, full coverage for some groups and limited coverage for others, limited coverage of experimental or investigative services or multi-organ transplants), specify utilization controls (e.g., prior authorization requirements, requirements that the procedure must be performed at a Medicare-approved transplantation center), among other criteria. The type of coverage available and the level of detail included in the written standards vary across states.

---

[305] Mississippi Division of Medicaid, "Title 23: Medicaid Part 202 Hospital Services," in *Administrative Code*, p. 33, https://medicaid.ms.gov/wp-content/uploads/2021/07/Title-23-Part-202-Hospital-Services-07.01.21.pdf#page=37.

[306] CMS, Letter to State, "RE: North Dakota State Plan Amendment (SPA) 20-0022," August 26, 2020, https://www.medicaid.gov/medicaid/spa/downloads/ND-20-0022.pdf.

[307] Social Security Act (SSA) §1903(i)1 [42 U.S.C. 1396b(i)]; 42 C.F.R. §441.35.

[308] Under emergency Medicaid, states are required to cover limited Medicaid services for the treatment of an emergency medical condition to otherwise eligible aliens (i.e., those who meet Medicaid's other eligibility requirements such as financial, categorical, and state residency requirements), regardless of immigration status or lack of immigration status. See SSA §1903(v)(3) [42 U.S.C. §1396b(v)(3) and 8 U.S.C. §1611(b)(1)(A)].

[309] P.L. 104-193; Personal Responsibility and Work Opportunity Act, §401(a)(1)(A).

Does Medicaid Cover Posttransplant Care?

States are permitted to tailor their organ transplantation benefit coverage through the written standards included in the Medicaid state plan, as approved by CMS, resulting in variability across state Medicaid programs in terms of state coverage of posttransplant care. Examples of state coverage for posttransplant care include the following:[310] all postoperative surgical follow-up care services for liver transplants, including treatment for acute rejection; re-harvesting and/or re- transplantation for up to 120 days following the surgical procedure;[311] transplant services (including evaluations and assessments) after a transplant and follow-up services, as well as medically necessary inpatient services following the discharge for the transplant stay to manage complications from the transplant;[312] and follow-up care for the Medicaid enrollee and live donor.[313]

CMS guidance explicitly addresses requirements regarding federal Medicaid payment for follow- up services (e.g., immunosuppressive drugs, medically necessary care that may be required as a result of the transplant) for a Medicaid-enrolled adult who received an organ transplant that was *not* paid for by the Medicaid program.[314] The guidance specifies that states are permitted (but not required) to cover such services, as long as the services are coverable under Medicaid, meet applicable Medicaid coverage requirements (e.g., are sufficient in amount, duration, and scope to reasonably achieve its purpose),[315] and are included in that state's Medicaid state plan.

Does Medicaid Cover Immunosuppressive Drugs Posttransplant?

States are permitted to tailor their organ transplantation benefit coverage through the written standards included in the Medicaid state plan as approved by CMS, resulting in variability across state Medicaid programs in terms of state coverage of posttransplant immunosuppressive drugs. (For more information, see "Does Medicaid Cover Organ Transplants?") With regard to coverage for immunosuppressive drugs administered after the transplant procedure, CRS found evidence that at least some states offer this coverage.[316] As with the other coverage categories

---

[310] The posttransplant care policies listed here are not comprehensive or complete. They are intended to provide a range of the types of policies that states have adopted through CMS-approved written standards. For more complete information on the specific coverage included in these examples, see the source materials.

[311] Medi-Cal, *Provider Manual*, June 2021, https://mcweb.apps.prd.cammis.medi-cal.ca.gov/assets/8B313A4A-3B84-49DB-B98B-6A51BECCF01C/transplant.pdf?access_ token=6UyVkRRfByXTZEWIh8j8QaYylPyP5ULO.

[312] MoHealth Net, *State of Missouri Transplant Manual*, p. 28, https://mydss.mo.gov/media/pdf/ transplant-provider-manual.

[313] Minnesota, "Transplant Services," in *Provider Manual*, https://www.dhs.state.mn.us/main/ idcplg?IdcService= GET_DYNAMIC_CONVERSION&RevisionSelectionMethod=Latest Released&dDocName=ID_008926#transplant.

[314] HHS, Region V Health Care Financing Administration, Chicago Regional State Letter #52-93, "Coverage of Follow-Up Services for Organ Transplants Not Provided Under Medicaid—Information," December 1993, https://www.hhs.gov/guidance/sites/default/files/hhs-guidance-documents/1993%2520-%2520organ%2 520transplants%2520 not%2520provided%2520under%2520medicaid_221.pdf.

[315] For more information on Medicaid benefit coverage requirements, see CRS Report R43357, *Medicaid: An Overview*.

[316] For example, see Nevada, Medicaid Services Manual Transmittal Letter, "Medicaid Services Manual Changes Chapter 3600—Managed Care Organization," January 28, 2022, https://dhcfp.nv.gov/uploadedFiles/ dhcfpnvgov/content/Resources/AdminSupport/Manuals/MSM/C3600/MSM_3600_01_29_22_ADA.pdf#page =28. See also Michigan Department of Health and Human Services, Behavioral and Physical Health and Aging Services Administration, "Michigan Medicaid Policy Bulletin Number MMP 22-44," December 1, 2022, https://www.michigan.gov/mdhhs/-/media/Project/Websites/mdhhs/Assistance-Programs/Medicaid-

discussed above, coverage of immunosuppressive drugs posttransplant varies by criteria including enrollee group or transplantation procedure type within and across states.

Medicare

Medicare is a federal program that pays for covered health care services of qualified beneficiaries. It was established in 1965 under Title XVIII of SSA to provide selected health care items and services to individuals aged 65 and older, permanently disabled individuals under the age of 65, and persons with end-stage renal disease (ESRD; permanent kidney failure requiring dialysis or an organ transplant), or amyotrophic lateral sclerosis (also known as Lou Gehrig's disease).[317] In 2023, Medicare covered 66.7 million beneficiaries and spent $1.037 trillion.[318] The program is administered by CMS, within HHS.

Medicare consists of four distinct parts:

- Part A (Hospital Insurance) covers inpatient hospital services, skilled nursing care, hospice care, and some home health services.
- Part B (Supplementary Medical Insurance) covers various items and services including physician services, outpatient hospital services, some home health and preventive services, and certain durable medical equipment for home use.
- Part C (Medicare Advantage, or MA) is a private plan option that covers all Medicare Parts A and B services, except hospice.[319] Private insurers (organizations) may offer one or more MA plans, where a plan is a set of benefits and cost-sharing obligations offered for a specific premium in a specific geographic area. Most MA plans provide care through a contracted network of providers. In 2023, approximately 48% (over 32 million) of beneficiaries received their Medicare services through MA.[320]
- Part D is optional and covers outpatient prescription drug benefits. Part D benefits are offered only through private organizations, which offer prescription drugs only or offer drugs through an MA plan.

Services provided under Parts A and B (also referred to as *original* or *traditional* Medicare) generally are paid directly by the government on a *fee-for-service* basis, using different prospective payment systems or fee schedules.[321] Under Parts C and D, Medicare pays private

BPHASA/2022-Bulletins/Final-Bulletin-MMP-22-44-Hospital.pdf?rev=f09538bf929b44bc873b6177d2bdc81f&hash=6C2BA9EF7AC66E621E5 E472A283FD972.

317 HHS, "Who's Eligible for Medicare?," https://www.hhs.gov/answers/medicare-and-medi caid/who-is-eligible-for-medicare/index.html.

318 The Board of Trustees, Federal Hospital Insurance and Federal Supplementary Medical Insurance Trust Funds, Table II.B1: "Medicare Data for Calendar Year 2023," in *2024 Annual Report*, March 2024, p. 11, https://www.cms.gov/oact/tr/2024. Some Medicare beneficiaries are also eligible for and receive Medicaid coverage— dual-eligible individuals. Medicare is the primary payer for these individuals, and Medicaid coverage for dual-eligible individuals can include Medicare cost sharing and/or coverage of services not covered by Medicare.

319 Medicare Advantage (MA) enrollees may choose hospice, but the hospice benefit is paid for through Medicare Part A and not through the MA plan's capitated monthly payment.

320 The Board of Trustees, Federal Hospital Insurance and Federal Supplementary Medical Insurance Trust Funds, *2024 Annual Report*, March 2024, p. 7.

321 A *prospective payment system* is a method of payment in which amounts or rates of payment are established in advance for a defined period and generally are based on an episode of care, regardless of the actual amount of

insurers a monthly *capitated* amount to provide enrollees with required benefits; the insurers then contract with and pay providers to furnish covered health care services and pharmacies to pay for outpatient prescription drugs for enrollees. Payments to contracted providers may vary across providers and may differ from rates paid under traditional Medicare.

Does Medicare Cover Organ Donation?

Medicare, traditional and MA, typically does not pay for health care services furnished to non-Medicare beneficiaries. However, traditional Medicare pays transplant hospitals or OPOs for the costs of acquiring organs, such as excising an organ(s) from a non-Medicare beneficiary who is a living or deceased donor when the organ recipient is a Medicare beneficiary. In addition, traditional Medicare pays for organ acquisition costs related to kidney transplants regardless of whether the recipient is enrolled in traditional Medicare or MA.[322]

The aforementioned Medicare payments are made to health care providers—hospitals, physicians, laboratories, and so on—not to organ donors or recipients. For example, Medicare pays for a hospital's or OPO's organ acquisition costs but does not pay the costs incurred by a donor or donor's family.

Does Medicare Cover Organ Transplants?

In general, Medicare covers reasonable and necessary health care services associated with certain organ transplants, including heart, lung, kidney, pancreas, intestine, and liver organ transplants.[323]

Medicare pays transplant hospitals for the implantation surgery and related preoperative services furnished to an organ recipient who is a Medicare beneficiary, similar to the way Medicare pays for other inpatient hospital services.[324] Specifically, traditional Medicare pays the transplant hospital the Medicare inpatient prospective payment system (IPPS) rate for the inpatient stay and related preoperative outpatient services.[325] Except in limited circumstances, each MA organization pays its network hospitals the rate that was negotiated between each organization and each hospital.[326] Under MA, in-network and out-of-network rules regarding coverage, cost sharing, and payment rates to hospitals may apply.[327]

---

care used. A *fee schedule* is a comprehensive list of maximum payment amounts that Medicare uses to reimburse physicians and other entities; fee schedule payment amounts are based on statutory and regulatory requirements.

322 The costs of organ acquisition for kidney transplants, including the Medicare-covered costs related to the care of a living kidney donor, are covered by original Medicare, even for beneficiaries enrolled in MA. SSA §1852(a)(1)(B)(i).

323 Medicare.gov, "Organ Transplants," https://www.medicare.gov/coverage/organ-transplants. See also CMS, Internet- Only Manuals, *Medicare National Coverage Determinations (NCD) Manual*, publication no. 100-03, https://www.cms.gov/regulations-and-guidance/guidance/manuals/internet-only-manuals-ioms-items/cms014961. MA plans are required to cover all Medicare required services, except hospice and the organ acquisition costs for kidney transplants, consistent with Medicare statutory and regulatory requirements, as well as national and local coverage determinations.

324 For more detail about traditional Medicare and MA, see CRS Report R40425, *Medicare Primer*.

325 For further information about the Medicare inpatient prospective payment system, see Medicare Payment Advisory Commission (MedPAC), "Hospital Acute Inpatient Services Payment System," https://www.medpac.gov/document- type/payment-basic/.

326 In general, MA organizations are required to provide all items and services for which benefits are available under Parts A and B to beneficiaries who are eligible for Part A and enrolled in Part B. SSA §1852(a)(1)(B).

327 An MA organization and a hospital or hospital system decide whether the hospital is in-network or out-of-network, which may determine the payment rates/amounts an MA organization pays a hospital for inpatient and outpatient services.

In addition to the IPPS or MA plan payment for the inpatient hospital services, Medicare pays for other health care services associated with an organ transplant. For example, traditional Medicare pays for physician (e.g., anesthesiologist, surgeon) and laboratory tests separately under two Medicare payment systems—the physician fee schedule and the clinical lab fee schedule, respectively. MA plans pay the negotiated rates to network providers.

All services furnished to the Medicare beneficiary organ recipient are subject to applicable Medicare cost sharing—deductible, co-payment, or coinsurance.[328] Beneficiaries enrolled in MA may be subject to different cost sharing based on the MA plan's requirements.

Does Medicare Cover Posttransplant Care?

Medicare pays for postoperative surgical care for 60 days for organ transplant recipients.[329] Postoperative services furnished to a Medicare beneficiary recipient are subject to Medicare deductible and coinsurance requirements.

For living donors, Medicare pays for postoperative services directly related to the organ donation. Medicare also covers routine follow-up care for organ donors until the donor "no longer exhibits symptoms related to the organ donation." However, Medicare may review claims for services rendered more than three months after the organ donation surgery; follow-up examinations may continue to be covered up to six months after the donation surgery to monitor for complications. Donors do not pay Medicare coinsurance or deductible for the aforementioned services.[330]

Does Medicare Cover Immunosuppressive Drugs Posttransplant?

Medicare coverage for immunosuppressive drugs depends on the type of organ transplant and how the recipient initially qualified for Medicare. This is specifically relevant for kidney recipients who are under the age of 65 and become eligible for Medicare because they have ESRD.[331]

ESRD Medicare beneficiaries who receive a successful kidney transplant no longer have ESRD, and thus their Medicare coverage ends after the 36th month post-hospital discharge.[332] However, beginning January 1, 2023, these individuals may enroll in a new Medicare Part B benefit that covers immunosuppressive drugs (PBID), as long as they do not have other health insurance coverage such as group health plans, Medicaid, or VA coverage.[333] The PBID benefit covers only immunosuppressive drugs and only when an ESRD Medicare beneficiary loses Medicare coverage due to no longer having ESRD and does not otherwise qualify for Medicare. Individuals enrolled in the PBID benefit pay a monthly premium, and the covered drugs are subject to an annual deductible and 20% coinsurance.[334]

---

[328] For further information about Medicare coverage of, payment for, services and applicable beneficiary cost sharing, see CRS Report R40425, *Medicare Primer*.

[329] CMS, Part I, Chapter 31, §3103 in Medicare Provider Reimbursement Manual.

[330] Ibid, §3105.

[331] End-stage renal disease is one of the Medicare eligibility categories,140 as well as persons aged 65 and older, permanently disabled individuals under the age of 65, and individuals who have amyotrophic lateral sclerosis (also known as Lou Gehrig's disease).

[332] Medicare General Information, Chapter 2, §10.4.4, in Eligibility and Entitlement Manual.

[333] Consolidated Appropriations Act, 2021 (P.L. 116-260), §402. See also Medicare General Information, Chapter 2, §40.9.3, in Eligibility and Entitlement Manual; and Chapter 15, §50.5.1, in Medicare Benefit Policy Manual.

[334] GAO, Kidney Transplants: Medicare Coverage of Immunosuppressive Drugs, GAO-24-107230, August 8, 2024, p. 4.

Medicare Part B covers immunosuppressive drugs for non-kidney organ transplant recipients as long as the recipient was entitled to Medicare Part A and is enrolled in Part B and the organ transplant was covered by Medicare (i.e., not by another health insurance plan or program).[335] This coverage is subject to the Part B deductible and coinsurance.[336]

Private Health Insurance

Private health insurance is the predominant source of health insurance coverage in the United States.[337] Nearly 190 million individuals in the United States had private health insurance as of the first quarter of 2022.

Covered benefits (e.g., office visits, surgical procedures, prescription drugs) may differ by plan, subject to applicable federal and state requirements. Common variations include what cost- sharing requirements apply to a given benefit and whether a benefit is covered both *in network* and *out of network*. In addition, a plan's coverage of a benefit generally depends on the benefit being deemed *medically necessary* for an enrollee.

Private health insurance plans are subject to federal and/or state requirements, including certain benefit coverage requirements. Federal requirements on private health coverage may apply to *large-group*, *small-group*, *self-insured group*, and/or *nongroup* plans.[338] Requirements for nongroup and small-group plans apply to plans sold on and off the health insurance exchanges.[339] State-level private health insurance requirements also may apply to large-group, small-group, and nongroup plans but generally do not apply to self-insured group plans.[340] Federal and state private health insurance requirements may vary by type of plan. For example, as discussed below, the federal requirement on coverage of *essential health benefits* is applicable only to small-group and nongroup plans.

Plans may voluntarily cover benefits, including providing coverage that exceeds any applicable federal or state requirements or providing coverage where there is no requirement to do so, as long as there is no applicable prohibition on such coverage.[341]

---

[335] 42 U.S.C. §1395x(s)(2)(J).

[336] CMS, Chapter 17, §80.3, in *Medicare Claims Processing Manual*.

[337] See CRS Report R47507, *Private Health Insurance: A Primer*, for more information on private health insurance, including data on private health insurance enrollment. As further explained (and broken down) in that primer, the enrollment estimate cited above in this report includes large-group, small-group, and self-insured group plans offered by private sector employers, as well as nongroup plans. The primer also explains plan features such as covered benefits (including medical necessity and other considerations, such as medical management requirements), cost sharing, and provider networks.

[338] Broadly, private health insurance includes group plans (largely made up of employer-sponsored insurance) and nongroup plans (i.e., plans a consumer purchases directly from an insurer). See CRS Report R45146, *Federal Requirements on Private Health Insurance Plans*, for more information on large-group, small-group, self-insured group, and nongroup plans; background on federal and state regulation of private health insurance; and summaries of current federal requirements on different types of plans.

[339] The individual exchanges and small business health options program (SHOP) exchanges are virtual marketplaces in which consumers and small businesses, respectively, can shop for and purchase private health insurance coverage. Plans sold in the individual and SHOP exchanges have to meet all the requirements applicable to the nongroup and small-group markets, respectively. Additional requirements apply only to exchange plans. For more information, see CRS Report R44065, *Overview of Health Insurance Exchanges*.

[340] State-level private health insurance requirements are beyond the scope of this report.

[341] This report section focuses on federal requirements relevant to private health insurance coverage of organ transplants. CRS is not aware of data on frequency or scope of such private health insurance coverage (including where it may otherwise be required by states or where plans may voluntarily provide it).

Does Federal Law Require Private Health Insurance to Cover Organ Donation?

There is no federal law that specifically requires private health insurance coverage of benefits related to organ donation—for organ donors or recipients.

However, certain federal private health insurance requirements are, or may be, relevant to such coverage, depending on state implementation, plan variation, and/or individual circumstances. This primarily includes the requirement that certain plans cover a set of essential health benefits (EHB), as discussed in the next section regarding organ transplants for recipients.

To the extent that a plan covers benefits for an enrollee's receipt of an organ donation, the plan also may cover the costs of the enrollee's organ donor. This would likely depend on the terms and conditions of the enrollee's (organ recipient's) plan, any applicable requirements on that plan (EHB or state requirements), and whether the organ donor has another source of coverage.

If a private health insurance enrollee decides to donate an organ to someone, similar considerations may determine whether the enrollee's plan will cover the costs of his or her donation. In general, private health insurance plans cover benefits that are medically necessary for their enrollees' health, so this may be another consideration regarding coverage of the donor's costs, especially if the recipient is not also an enrollee of that plan. See, for example, the coverage exclusion discussed in the next section.

Does Federal Law Require Private Health Insurance to Cover Organ Transplants?

There is no federal law that specifically requires private health insurance coverage of benefits related to organ donation. However, certain federal private health insurance requirements (particularly as related to coverage of the EHB) are, or may be, relevant to coverage of an enrollee's receipt of an organ transplant, depending on state implementation, plan variation, and/or individual circumstances.

Coverage of the Essential Health Benefits

Small-group and nongroup plans are required cover a core package of 10 categories of essential health benefits.[342] The categories of EHB are ambulatory patient services; emergency services; hospitalization; maternity and newborn care; mental health and substance use disorder services, including behavioral health treatment; prescription drugs; rehabilitative and habilitative services and devices; laboratory services; preventive and wellness services and chronic disease management; and pediatric services, including oral and vision care.

The benefits to be covered within each EHB category generally are not defined in federal law; rather, the law requires the HHS Secretary to further define the EHB to include items and services in at least those 10 categories and to be "equal in scope to the benefits provided under a typical employer plan." To date, the HHS Secretary has directed each state to select an EHB benchmark plan, within certain parameters, to serve as the basis for the state's EHB.[343]

[342] 42 U.S.C. §300gg-6; 42 U.S.C. §18022.

[343] For more information on the process for defining the essential health benefits (EHB) in each state, see CMS, Center for Consumer Information and Insurance Oversight (CCIIO), "Information on Essential Health Benefits (EHB) Benchmark Plans," https://www.cms. gov/cciio/resources/data-resources/ehb.

Applicable plans in each state must provide EHB coverage that is "substantially equal" to such coverage in their state's benchmark plan, as specified in regulations.[344] For example, if a state selects a benchmarkplan that includes organ transplant benefits in one or more EHB categories, the applicable plans in that state would have to provide substantially equal coverage, including in terms of any coverage limitations.

Because states select their own EHB benchmark plans, EHB coverage requirements may vary considerably from state to state. Per CRS review of publicly available EHB summary documents, "transplant" is listed as a covered essential health benefit in all 51 EHB benchmark plans.[345] Some of the benchmark plan summaries provide additional detail about transplant coverage and/or exclusions.

For example, Arizona's EHB benchmark plan summary includes explanations on its transplant coverage such as, "organ transplant services include the recipient's medical, surgical and hospital services; inpatient immunosuppressive medications; and costs for organ procurement." It also details certain exclusions such as, "these benefits are available when the Member is the recipient of an organ transplant. No coverage if Member is an organ donor for a recipient other than a Member enrolled under this plan."[346]

Iowa's EHB benchmark plan summary indicates that transplant coverage exclusions do apply and that transplant coverage is subject to case management but does not provide further detail. Some of the EHB benchmark plan summaries do not detail any transplant coverage or exclusions (e.g., Florida, Massachusetts, Washington).[347] In all cases, the full EHB benchmark plan documents may provide more detail than the summary documents discussed here.

In short, as currently implemented, the requirement to cover the EHB effectively includes transplant coverage in all states and the District of Columbia, although the details of this coverage requirement vary across the states. Plans required to cover the EHB—those in the small-group and nongroup markets—must provide transplant coverage according to their state's EHB benchmark plan.

Cost sharing (including deductibles, coinsurance, and co-payments) is possible for most categories of EHB, although certain federal requirements limit enrollees' total cost sharing on the EHB.[348] For example, plans must have annual limits on enrollee out-of-pocket costs that are no higher than federally set amounts ($9,450 for self-only coverage and $18,900 for

---

[344] 45 C.F.R. §156.115(a)(1).

[345] See current benchmark plan documents for each state and the District of Columbia at CMS, CCIIO, "Information on Essential Health Benefits (EHB) Benchmark Plans," https: //www.cms.gov/marketplace/resources/ data/essential-health- benefits#ehb. For each state and DC, see the "EHB Benchmark Plan Information" ZIP file, which generally includes the full benchmark plan and a benchmark plan summary document and also may include other documents. For the analysis and examples in this report, CRS extracted and reviewed the benchmark plan summaries, which list certain benefits (i.e., "transplant") and indicate whether they are covered as EHB, otherwise covered, or not covered. As indicated in the discussion above, additional coverage details may or may not be provided for the listed benefits.

[346] Ibid. See Arizona's 2017-2025 EHB Benchmark Plan Information ZIP file, which includes its summary document, "AZ-BMP-Summary-PY2025-2027.pdf," https://www.cms.gov/marketplace/resources/data/e ssential-health-benefits#Arizona.

[347] Ibid. See the EHB Benchmark Plan Information ZIP files for Iowa, Florida, Massachusetts, and Washington at https://www.cms.gov/marketplace/resources/data/essential-health-benefits#ehb. For these and most other states, the current EHB benchmark plans are dated 2017-2025. Prior-year files are listed separately. For states that have made changes to their EHB benchmark plans in certain years, current and prior files are dated accordingly. See the top of the web page cited here for further discussion.

[348] See the "Enrollee Cost Sharing and Plan Payment for Benefits" section in CRS Report R45146, *Federal Requirements on Private Health Insurance Plans*.

coverage other than self-only, in plan year 2024).[349] This generally applies to most private health insurance plans and only to in-network coverage of the EHB.[350]

Other Potentially Relevant Federal Requirements

Other federal requirements on private health insurance also could be relevant for enrollees seeking coverage of organ transplants. This may depend on the circumstances and/or other factors.

For example, most plans are prohibited from excluding coverage based on an enrollee's preexisting health conditions. This does not mandate a plan to cover particular benefits (such as organ transplants), but with respect to the benefits a plan does cover, a plan may not deny coverage of those benefits based on an enrollee's health condition. In other words, if a plan covers organ transplant benefits, the plan cannot exclude that coverage for an enrollee because the enrollee had a related health condition before enrolling in the plan.[351] Large-group, small-group, self-insured, and nongroup plans are subject to this requirement.

Does Federal Law Require Private Health Insurance to Cover Posttransplant Care?

There is no federal law that specifically requires private health insurance coverage of benefits related to organ donation, but the EHB and other requirements may be applicable. This includes benefits related to posttransplant care.

For example, to the extent that benefits for posttransplant care are included as EHB in a state's EHB benchmark plan, applicable plans in the state would be required to provide substantially equal coverage. See next question regarding coverage of immunosuppressant drugs in particular.

Does Federal Law Require Private Health Insurance to Cover Immunosuppressive Drugs Posttransplant?

There is no federal law that specifically requires private health insurance coverage of immunosuppressive drugs posttransplant. However, the EHB requirement described above is effectively applicable.[352] Although states, rather than the federal government, generally specify the benefits to be covered as EHB, federal regulations have provided specific requirements regarding some EHB categories—including the prescription drugs category.[353]

Current regulation provides that an applicable health plan meets the EHB requirements for the prescription drugs category of EHB if it covers at least one drug in every U.S. Pharmacopeia (USP) category and class, or the same number of prescription drugs in each category and class as the state-selected EHB benchmark plan. Under the USP, immune suppressants are a class within the category of immunological agents, which effectively means that all plans subject to EHB requirements must cover at least one immunosuppressant drug.

---

[349] Ibid.

[350] Ibid. Although large-group and self-insured plans are not required to cover the EHB, they are subject to certain cost- sharing and plan-payment requirements that are related to the EHB.

[351] For more information on this requirement and others related to private health insurance premiums, benefits, cost sharing, provider networks, and other topics, see CRS Report R45146, *Federal Requirements on Private Health Insurance Plans*.

[352] See "Coverage of the Essential Health Benefits" in this report.

[353] See, for example, 45 C.F.R. §156.115 and 45 C.F.R. §156.122.

Federal rulemaking finalized in April 2024 also codified the existing agency stance that "to the extent that a health plan covers prescription drugs in excess of the benchmark, these drugs will be considered EHB and are subject to requirements including the annual limitation on cost sharing and the restriction on annual and lifetime dollar limits."[354] In general, this means that if a plan covers immunosuppressant drugs beyond what is required as EHB, these drugs also are subject to certain cost-sharing protections applicable to the EHB, such as an annual out-of-pocket maximum.[355]

Appendix. Policy Experts and Acronyms

Table A-1. Congressional Research Service policy experts

Issue Area	CRS Contact
Organ Transplantation (General); Organ Procurement and Transplantation Network	Jared Sussman
Organ Transplantation, Legal Issues	Wen Shen
Medicare Oversight of Organ Procurement Organization (OPO) and Transplant Hospitals/Programs	Marco Villagrana
Bureau of Prisons	Nathan James
Department of Defense	Bryce Mendez
Immigration and Customs Enforcement	Abigail Kolker
Indian Health Service	Elayne Heisler
Department of Veterans Affairs	Jared Sussman
Medicaid	Evelyne Baumrucker
Medicare Part A Coverage of and Payments to Hospitals and OPOs for Organ Implantation Surgeries and the Costs of Organ Acquisition	Marco Villagrana
Medicare Part B Coverage of Immunosuppressive Drugs	Cliff Binder
Medicare Advantage	Paulette Morgan
Private Health Insurance	Vanessa Forsberg

Table A-2. Acronyms used in this report

Acronym	Definition
BOP	Bureau of Prisons
CCIIO	Center for Consumer Information and Insurance Oversight
CD	Clinical Director
CHAMPVA	Civilian Health and Medical Program of the Department of Veterans Affairs
CMS	Centers for Medicare & Medicaid Services
DHS	Department of Homeland Security
DOD	Department of Defense
EHB	Essential Health Benefits

354 Departments of the Treasury and HHS, "Patient Protection and Affordable Care Act, HHS Notice of Benefit and Payment Parameters for 2025; Updating Section 1332 Waiver Public Notice Procedures; Medicaid; Consumer Operated and Oriented Plan (CO-OP) Program; and Basic Health Program," Final Rule, April 15, 2024, 89 *Federal Register* 26218. See this preamble discussion for additional information, including on the interaction of state benefit mandates: https://www.federalregister.gov/d/2024-07274/p-1998.

355 See "Coverage of the Essential Health Benefits" in this report. Though large-group and self-insured group plans are not subject to EHB coverage requirements, they generally are subject to the cost-sharing requirements that are based on the EHB. However, in guidance released concurrent to the above-mentioned rulemaking, the agencies indicated that future rulemaking will "address the applicability of this policy to those plans." See Departments of Labor, HHS, and the Treasury, "FAQ About Affordable Care Act Implementation Part 66," April 2, 2024, https://www.dol.gov/agencies/ebsa/about-ebsa/our-activities/resource-center/faqs/aca-part-66.

Table A-2. Acronyms used in this report

Acronym	Definition
ESRD	End-Stage Renal Disease
FDA	Food and Drug Administration
FMC	Federal Medical Center
GAO	Government Accountability Office
HHS	Health and Human Services
ICE	Immigration and Customs Enforcement
IHS	Indian Health Service
IPPS	Inpatient Prospective Payment System
MA	Medicare Advantage
MHS	Military Health System
MTF	Military Treatment Facility
NDS	National Detention Standards
NOTA	National Organ Transplant Act
OIG	Office of Inspector General
OPO	Organ Procurement Organization
OPTN	Organ Procurement and Transplantation Network
PBNDS	Performance-Based National Detention Standards
PRC	Purchased/Referred Care Program
SHOP	Small business health options program
SSA	Social Security Act
UAGA	Uniform Anatomical Gift Act
UNOS	United Network for Organ Sharing
VA	Department of Veterans Affairs
VCCP	Veterans Community Care Program
VHA	Veterans Health Administration

Source: Compiled by the Congressional Research Service.

Index

S

T

U

V

W

X

Y